The Illustrated Book of

Child Health

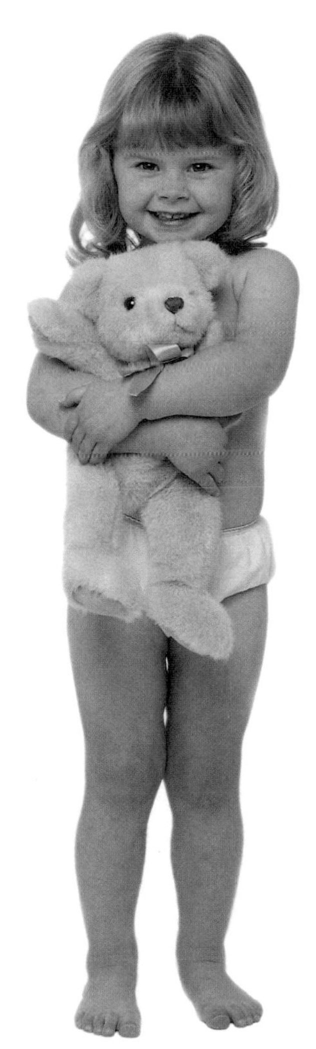

The Illustrated Book of
Child Health

Published in 2004 by Silverdale Books
An imprint of Bookmart Ltd

Registered Number 2372865

Trading as Bookmart Limited
Blaby Road
Wigston
Leicester
LE18 4SE

Produced by Eaglemoss Publications Ltd
Based on *Having Babies*

Consultant for chapters 1 and 2:
Dr Ilona Bendefy MBBS MRCP (Paeds)

Consultant for chapter 3:
Samantha Pearce RGN Cert Ed of Peak Skills,
a first-aid training company.

Cover photography by Belinda Banks/Brightstar

Please note: every effort has been made to ensure that the information contained in this book is accurate. However, the reader is advised to take medical advice as a matter of course. Mention of particular products, or illustrations of them, does not imply endorsement. The publishers can accept no legal responsibility or liability for any accident, injury or other adverse effect arising from the use of information and advice in this book.

Printed in Singapore

ISBN 1 84509 099 3

10 9 8 7 6 5 4 3 2 1

CONTENTS

Chapter One
General Health Care

ENCOURAGING A HEALTHY LIFESTYLE

By encouraging your children to eat well and be active from an early age, you will be helping them to establish lifelong good habits and giving them the best start in life.

Simple ways to keep your child healthy

- **Set an example:** children learn by example so follow a healthy lifestyle yourself as much as possible – for example, walk instead of going by car or bus whenever possible.
- **Educate him:** teach your child respect for his own body, and explain why it's important to stay healthy.
- **Don't set unrealistic goals:** if you enjoy eating pizza, don't deny yourself or your children all the time.
- **Keep him active:** ensure that your child has one daily outdoor physical activity, whether this is going to the park, swimming or playing with friends. Set a daily time limit for watching television or videos.

As a parent, whether you're running after a crawling baby or toddler or lugging nappies and extra shopping home from the supermarket, you may find that you are more active than ever before. However, in turn, it is all too easy to let your children fall into a sedentary lifestyle, which will have a negative effect on their health and energy levels in both the long and short term.

In your eagerness to encourage your children to eat, it is easy to settle for a less than healthy diet. In the best interests of the whole family, it's important to make healthy living a top priority. It is advisable to introduce new measures gradually, to avoid the lifestyle change becoming a passing fad. It may take a few months for it to become an established habit, so don't be too hard on yourself if you and your family lapse from time to time.

Eat your greens

We are continually bombarded with information about a daily intake of fruit and vegetables being good for our health, including evidence that it lessens the risks of various forms of cancer and cardiovascular disease. We are aware of the benefits, but the reality of encouraging children to choose broccoli and apples over chips and crisps is not easy. Children learn by example, so the best way of instilling a love of good food in your children is if you eat healthily yourself.

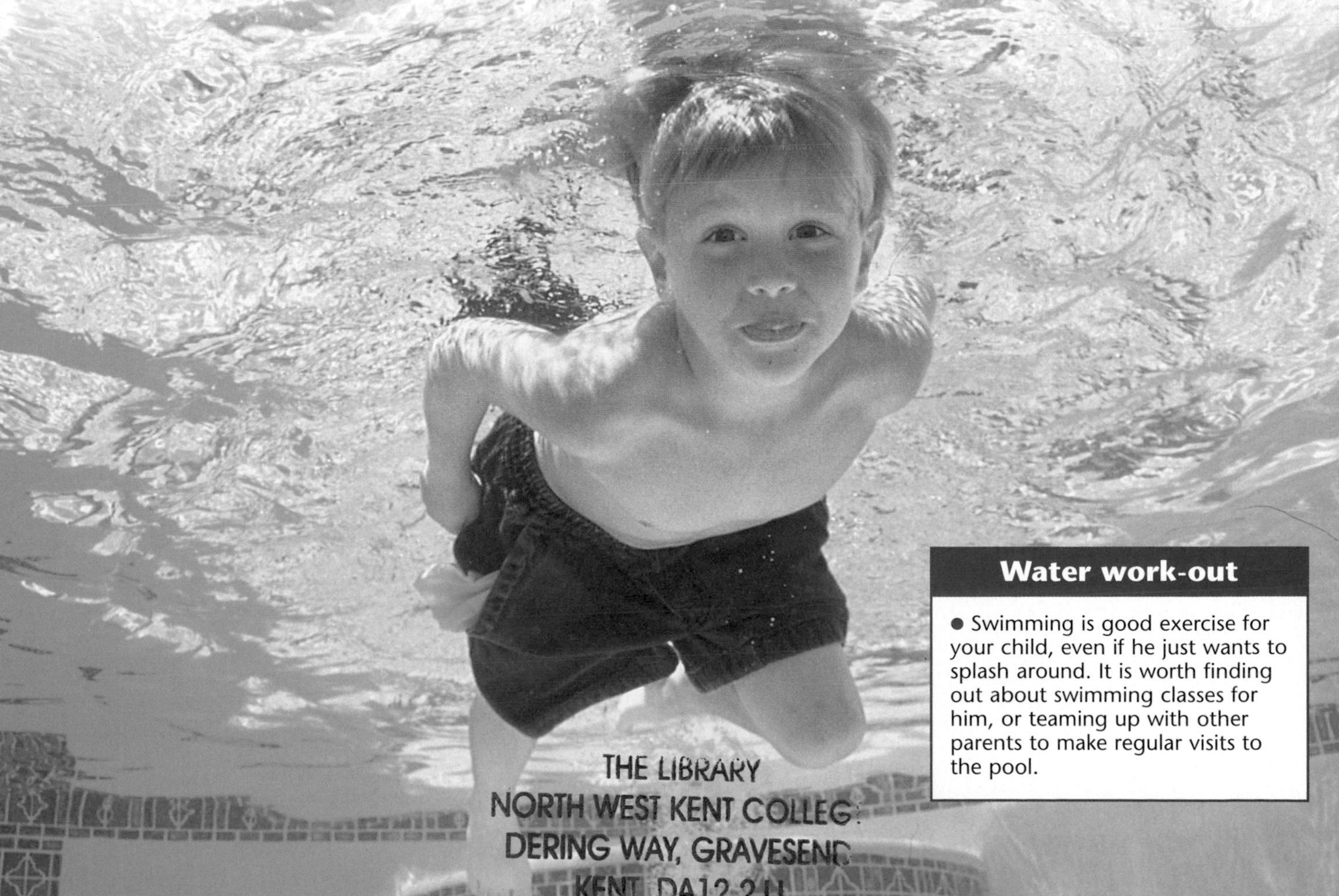

Water work-out

- Swimming is good exercise for your child, even if he just wants to splash around. It is worth finding out about swimming classes for him, or teaming up with other parents to make regular visits to the pool.

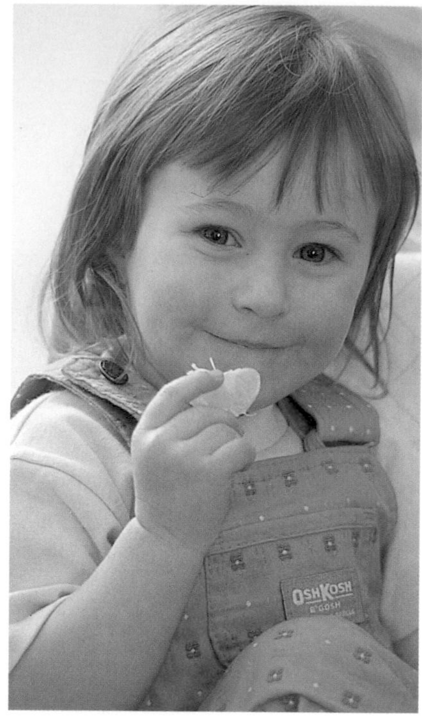

Healthy eating tips

Try to monitor your child's diet carefully to prevent her from falling into bad eating habits. Follow these healthy eating guidelines:

Do:

✔ Make raw vegetables and fruit readily available as snacks.
✔ Always grill rather than fry food.
✔ Limit sweets and cakes.
✔ Provide home-made, wholesome food.
✔ Buy organic whenever you can.
✔ Make sure your child has an adequate intake of iron-rich foods.

Don't:

✘ Add sugar automatically, for example to cereals.
✘ Force food on a child who doesn't want to eat.
✘ Offer comfort food.
✘ Praise your child for finishing a meal.
✘ Use sweets or fizzy drinks as rewards for good behaviour.

Try giving your child small pieces of fruit and vegetables as snacks, rather than sweets. If you and your family persevere with a healthy eating plan, it will soon become a natural part of your lifestyle.

If you want your child to eat fruit and vegetables, make sure you eat them yourself. Encourage your children to take an active part in choosing fruit and vegetables at the supermarket. Put them on display at home, in a bowl or a rack, so that your child will get used to them and regard them as an integral part of everyday life.

Enjoying food

While you don't want your child to be overweight, it's important not to make an issue out of how much he eats. You should try to ensure that your child has a healthy attitude to food and enjoys eating from an early age. Unless under medical guidance, children should not be put on a diet because this can have very adverse effects on health.

Fit for life

All sorts of activities can help to keep your child fit and he is likely to enjoy being active and interacting with others. Why not visit your local playground where your child can run around, and go on the swings, slides and balancing equipment. Go for walks as often as you can and take a ball along too, so your child can play in an open area in the fresh air.

You can make fruit fun by taking your children to a pick-your-own fruit farm. They will enjoy the experience and you will find it economical.

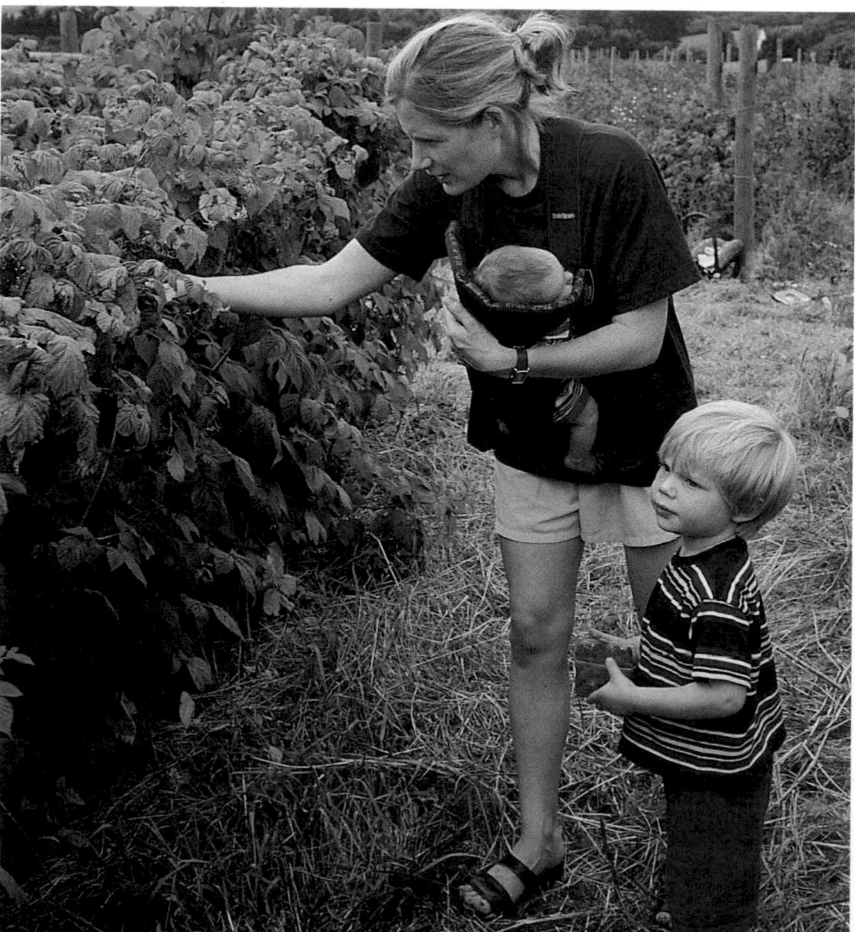

Questions & Answers

Q ***My son always wants to travel in the buggy. How can I make him walk some of the time?***

A Start by encouraging him to walk some of the way to your destination. Distraction often works well so try pointing out interesting things. In shops, encourage your child to get out of the buggy to look at something, but make sure that you are extremely careful and know where he is at all times.

Q ***My son will eat chicken nuggets and chips only for his tea. What can I do?***

A Many children go through a stage of faddy eating so don't worry too much. Try making your own healthy version: use good quality chicken, minced and dipped in breadcrumbs, cut chunky potato chips and fry in olive oil. Tomato ketchup, although sugary, contains nutrients, too. Eat as a family as much as possible. If your child sees you eating different foods, in time he may want to try them.

TEACHING YOUR CHILD ABOUT HYGIENE

Keeping clean and being a toddler don't always go hand in hand, but teaching your child a basic hygiene routine is vital to prevent him picking up too many germs.

When you first introduce your child to the rules of hygiene, it's important to strike a balance between letting him get messy – a valuable part of growing up – and keeping him healthy. Concentrate on the 'must-dos', such as washing his hands before eating and after using the toilet, and don't fuss about his muddy knees. Remember, you can't create a completely sterile environment and some contact with germs is beneficial because it helps to build up his immune system.

Basic cleanliness

By around the age of three, your child will respond to reasoning. Explain that he should, for example, wash his hands after playing in the garden as dirt carries germs that could give him tummyache. You will have to tell him this many times before hand-washing becomes a habit, but persistence and consistency will pay off.

After breakfast, encourage your child to brush his teeth at the same time as you do – you may need to follow up his efforts by brushing them again yourself. Let him choose his own brush and toothpaste, but don't buy toothpaste that contains sugar or artificial sweeteners. It's important that your child brushes his teeth at the end of the day because food particles left in the mouth overnight will cause decay.

In the evening, if your child isn't having a bath, wash his face, hands and knees with a sponge or flannel. Check the state of your child's nails and make using a nailbrush fun. Clip his nails regularly, too, as short nails collect less dirt.

It is vital to teach your child toilet hygiene to reduce the risk of him picking up germs. At first, you'll empty the potty and wipe his bottom (from the front to the back) but help him to do it himself as soon as he shows an interest. Leave a step by the basin to encourage him to wash his own hands, and show him how to turn on the cold tap, rub the soap into a lather, rinse and dry with a towel.

Making bathtime fun

Most young children love splashing around in the bath, and for them getting clean just happens in the

Don't have daily battles over keeping clean. As long as he hasn't cut or grazed himself, a bit of dirt on your child's knees will do no harm.

Know your enemies

There are three basic types of germ. Whether germs are harmless or potentially dangerous is dependent on the specific organism.

- **Bacteria:** these tiny, single-celled organisms are everywhere, including inside the body and on the skin. Many types of bacteria are harmless, and some are even helpful, but they can also cause illness. Our skin acts as a barrier but, if it is broken, harmful bacteria can enter the body. Antibodies produced by the immune system will try to overcome the bacteria but, if they fail, antibiotics can be prescribed.
- **Viruses:** these organisms are smaller than bacteria, and they cause illness by getting inside the body's cells and changing the way the cells work. Viruses are beaten when the body's immune system produces antibodies to attack them (in immunisation, a weakened form of the virus is injected into the body to stimulate the production of antibodies and help protect the body). Viruses do not respond to antibiotics.
- **Fungi:** types of fungi can cause infection, such as thrush, and are treated with antifungal creams and medicines.

If you have more than one child, let them have a bath together. If your children learn that bathtime is also playtime, they'll be much more willing to keep clean.

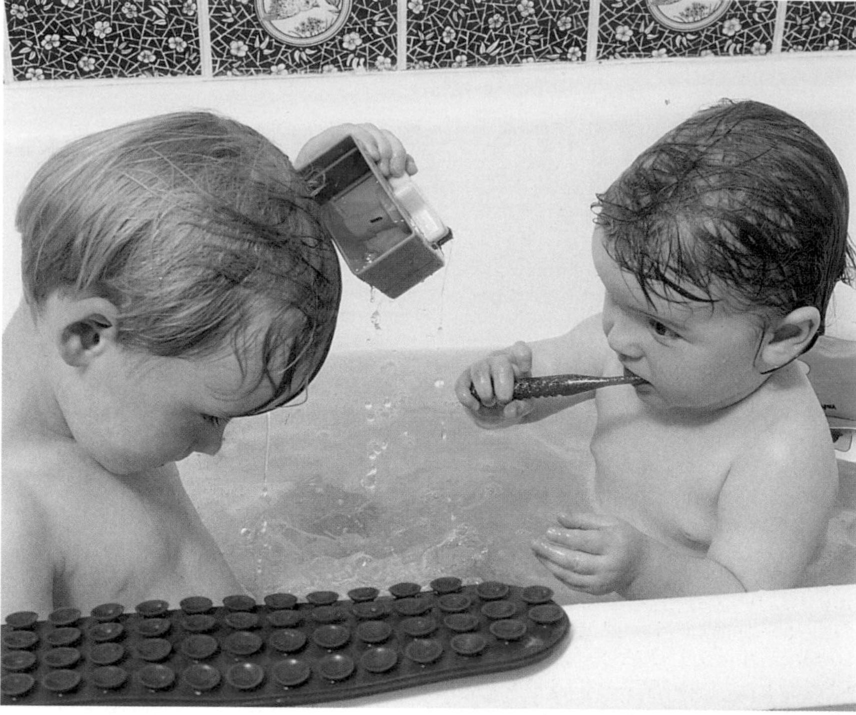

process. Show your child how to wash his body, remembering to rinse off the soap. Let him practise on toys in the bath. It can be difficult to persuade an older child to have a bath because he may be absorbed in a game or a book that he doesn't want to interrupt. Use bath toys, such as floating ducks, and bubble baths to lure him into the water.

If your child still hates having a bath, try the shower, or just give him a stand-up wash, which will be over quickly.

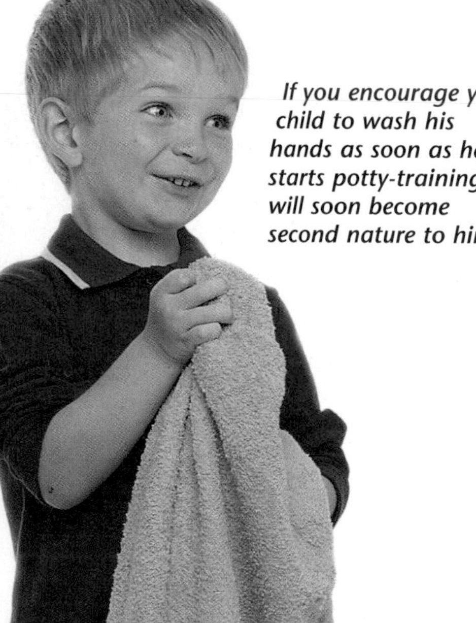

If you encourage your child to wash his hands as soon as he starts potty-training, it will soon become second nature to him.

Bad hair days

Little girls are usually more amenable to haircare than boys. However, hairwashing can be a battleground for both sexes. Conflict is eased once your child is old enough to participate.

Washing your child's hair once a week is quite often enough. Use a baby shampoo and if your child hates the suds in his eyes, buy a hair shield or swimming goggles. Some children like to get the ordeal over as quickly as possible, in which case you can use a shower for rinsing. Others prefer a more gentle approach. Singing songs together can help.

Clean clothes

Some children are very visually aware, so use this to encourage an interest in keeping clothes clean. Keep old clothes handy for extra messy play.

- Dress your child in clothes that are appropriate for what he's doing – there's no point putting him in a smart outfit for playgroup if he comes back covered in paint.
- For hygiene purposes, make sure your child wears clean socks and underwear every day, and show him that dirty clothes belong in the linen basket.
- Ask your child to help you put clothes into the washing machine, and add soap powder and conditioner, so he knows how dirty clothes are cleaned. You could also let him handwash his teddy's clothes in the sink and peg them on the line, just like a grown-up.

Questions & Answers

Q *I get furious when my child gets dirty. Am I overreacting?*

A Perhaps a little. Getting dirty is just a natural part of growing up. An over-anxious girl who cries because she has spilt something on her dress, or the boy who rushes in for his hands to be washed every five minutes, is not going to enjoy his or her early years. Remind yourself that the human body is incredibly efficient at keeping out infection, and that raising a happy child is infinitely more important than raising a clean one.

Q *Should I be teaching my son how to clean his penis?*

A Special care isn't needed to clean a penis, circumcised or not. Don't be tempted to pull back the foreskin or clean under it with cotton buds or antiseptics.

Q *We have a pet cat and dog. Are my children at risk of infection?*

A Yes. Children can pick up a number of infections from pets, including ringworm. If your children have been playing with your pet, make sure they wash their hands before they eat anything. They should also wash their hands after playing in the garden, where there may be faeces (a source of toxoplasmosis). Finally, teach your children never to touch a pet's mouth or bottom.

AVOIDING SUNBURN

WHAT IS SUNBURN?

Sunburn occurs when people spend too much time in the sun or under sun lamps. Sunburn makes the skin red, sore and blistered and can often cause sickness and fever. Continued over-exposure to the sun not only ages the skin prematurely, but can also cause skin cancer.

The sunlight that reaches the Earth's surface includes two kinds of invisible ultraviolet light, called A and B. UVA rays are deeply penetrating and remain relatively constant all year round. UVB rays penetrate less deeply, but are the ones that cause sunburn. They are at their highest levels in the summer and, like UVA, cause skin cancer. It is important to protect the skin and eyes from both UVA and UVB rays.

Symptoms of sunburn

Initially, there may be no sign that your child's skin is burning except for a slight pinkness to the skin. Several hours after the exposure he may start to complain that his skin feels hot and painful. The skin may feel itchy and tight, and look red and burnt.

How to protect your child from the sun

Some children are more sensitive than others to the sunlight, especially those with fair skin. Following these guidelines will help you to ensure your child is protected in the sunshine.

1 The sun is at its hottest between 11 a.m. and 3 p.m., so seek shade or keep your child covered up during this time.

2 Apply a sunscreen with a sun protection factor (SPF) of more than 25, half an hour before going out in the sun.

3 Use sunblock on your baby's skin and on parts of your child's skin that are likely to burn, e.g. the nose, ears and shoulders.

4 Cover your child in clothing made of tightly woven fabrics that will both absorb and reflect the sun's harmful rays.

5 Make sure that your child is wearing a hat with a wide brim to shade his ears, neck, face and head.

6 Encourage your child to wear sunglasses, which filter out both UVA and UVB light.

7 Do not assume that because it is cloudy your child is safe from the sunlight – 80 per cent of ultraviolet light will get through the clouds.

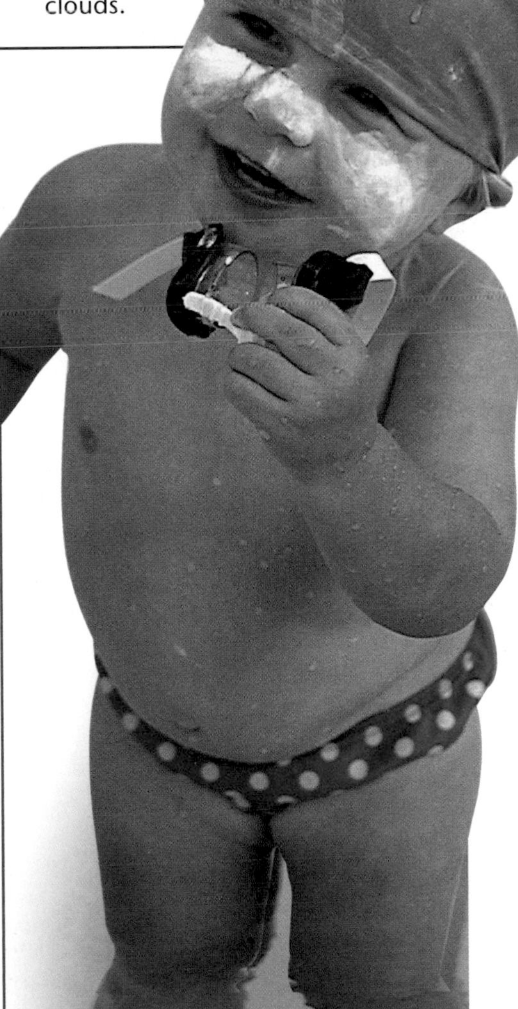

Sunblock completely cuts out the sun's harmful rays. Apply to babies who are exposed to the sun, and children's noses, cheeks and shoulders, in addition to suncream applied to the whole body.

Factors that make the sun more dangerous

- **Skin moles:** children with moles, or whose parents have moles, are more at risk of getting skin cancer, especially malignant melanoma. You should, therefore, be particularly careful with these children in the sun.

- **Sweat or water on the skin:** any kind of liquid on the skin will not only reduce the effectiveness of a sunscreen lotion, it will attract more sunlight, which will make the skin more vulnerable.

- **Water, sand, wind, snow and pavements:** these all increase the sun's strength by reflecting the rays, therefore doubling its strength.

- **CFCs** (chlorofluorocarbons): these are chemicals emitted by machines such as refrigerators, and used in various aerosols and solvents. They increase the destruction of the ozone layer, allowing more UV rays on to the Earth's surface.

- **The angle of the sun:** this applies only if you are at the equator where the sun's rays are a lot stronger.

- **Altitude:** the higher you are, the thinner the atmosphere, therefore the greater the exposure to both UVA and UVB rays.

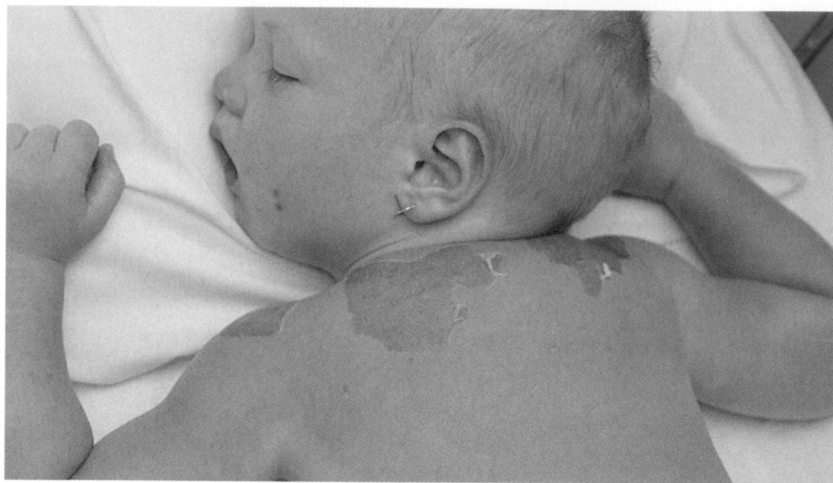

LEFT: If your child is sunburnt, give her plenty of fluids and treat the skin with flamazine cream. See your doctor if the area of skin blistered is more than the area of the palm of her hand.

BELOW: Your child's head, neck and eyes are very sensitive to the sun, so use a sunblock, high-factor suncream, sunglasses and cap to protect against the rays.

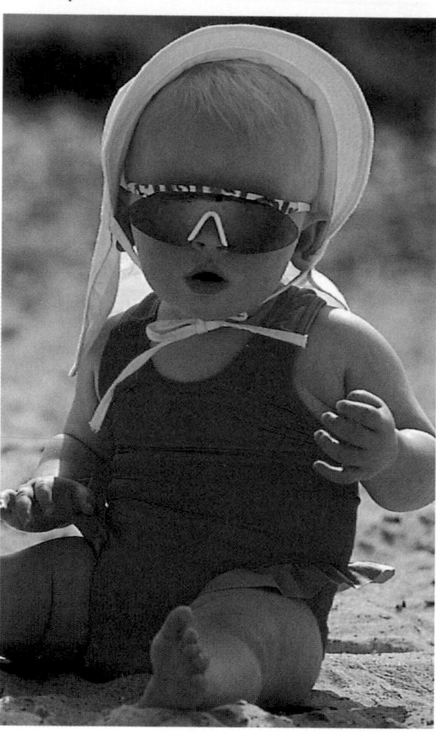

Hazards of sun exposure

Sunburnt skin might seem to be a mild effect of sun exposure, but there are more serious long-term effects of spending too much time in the sun.

- **Reduced immunity:** over-exposure to ultraviolet rays may affect the body's immune system in the long term.

- **Premature ageing:** the sun can have a ravaging effect on skin. It causes premalignant skin changes called solar keratoses.

- **Skin cancers:** three types of skin cancer are directly linked with sun exposure. These occur mainly in the 50–60 age group, but, particularly with malignant melanoma, young people are affected. Malignant melanoma may be linked to one or two episodes of blistering sunburn in our youth, which sensitise the skin, leading to melanoma.

Effects of sunburn on the skin

The skin protects the body against injury and infection, as well as regulating body temperature. Over-exposure to the sun is a major cause of skin damage to the top layer, the epidermis, and a deeper layer, known as the dermis.

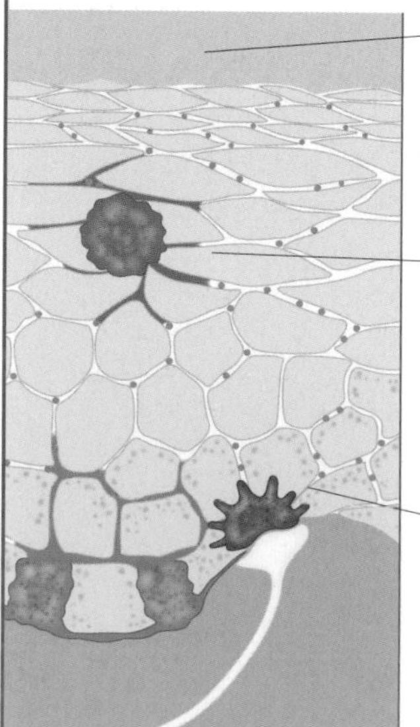

Upper layer of skin
UVB rays permeate the upper layers of the skin, damaging cells and causing burning and blistering.

Langerhans cells
These cells are part of the immune system and fight off infection. Exposure to the sun can cause damage to the cells contributing to the risk of skin cancer.

Dermis
UVA rays can penetrate deep into the layers of the skin and damage the dermis, which can cause the skin to lose its elasticity.

What does SPF mean?

Most sunscreen lotions display an SPF (sun protection factor) rating. SPF is measured by timing how long skin covered with a sunscreen takes to burn compared with unprotected skin. If your skin normally burns after 10 minutes, then a sunscreen with an SPF of 15 would provide your skin with protection from the sun for 150 minutes (i.e. 10 x 15). Even if waterproof or water-resistant, these products will lose their effectiveness once in the water.

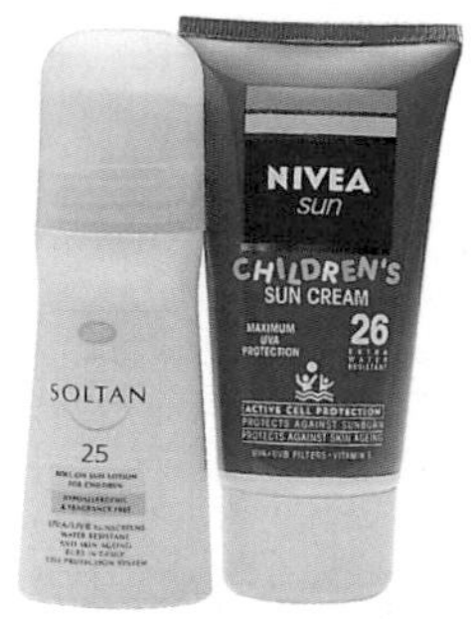

CAR SAFETY

MINIMISING THE RISK OF ACCIDENTS

By observing safety measures you can often avoid accidents in cars and prevent serious injury to passengers.

- Ensure that safety features built into your car (e.g. seat belts) are checked regularly and used according to the manufacturer's guidelines.

- Ensure that child locks fitted to the rear doors of your car are in operation. These prevent the doors from being opened from the inside, but allow someone to open the door from the outside. Child locks should be used until children are at least eight years old.

- For safety, install a separate wide-angle mirror in your car so that you can observe children in the back of the car without having to turn round.

- Check the car regularly for mechanical safety. In particular, check that the tyres are properly inflated and are not showing signs of wear.

- Never leave a child of any age unattended in a car.

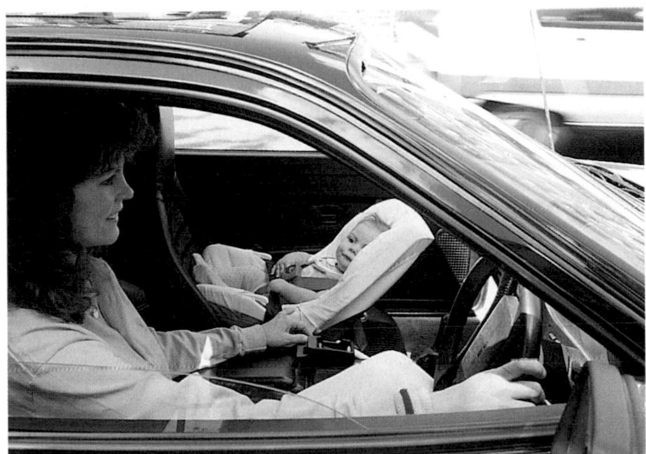

- Carry a torch, a warning triangle, a first-aid kit and an empty fuel can in the car, in case of emergencies.

It is vital that your child is secured safely when in a car. Use a baby seat in the front only if there is no air bag, or if the air bag has been disabled.

Securing your child

An unrestrained child can be killed by being thrown forwards in a car at a speed of just 8kph (5mph). Even on a short trip, secure your child in an appropriate seat or restraint.

- For babies less than a year old and weighing less than 10kg (21lb 5oz) you must use a rear-facing seat, secured with the car seat belt. In a forward-facing seat, sudden deceleration can cause the head of a small baby to be thrown forward violently, stretching the spinal cord by up to 5cm (2in). A baby should be kept rear-facing for as long as possible.

- An infant-only seat has a harness that can be adjusted to fit your baby snugly. A convertible seat can be used later when your baby is bigger, but the slots for the shoulder and crotch straps are generally not as close to the child's body.

- A baby should never in any circumstances be placed on the front seat of a car that has an airbag; an inflating airbag can crush a baby's skull. The baby should be placed in the back of the car in a rear-facing seat.

- A baby that is at least a year old and weighs 9–18kg (20lb 8oz–41lb) can be placed in a forward-facing seat on the rear seat of the car and secured to the anchor points provided.

- A child weighing 15–25kg (34lb 8oz–58lb 4oz) who is able to stay properly seated in a car can be secured on the rear seat using the car seat belt. Until about the age of eight, a booster seat is needed to raise the child so the seat belt fits across the lap and chest.

Choosing a car seat

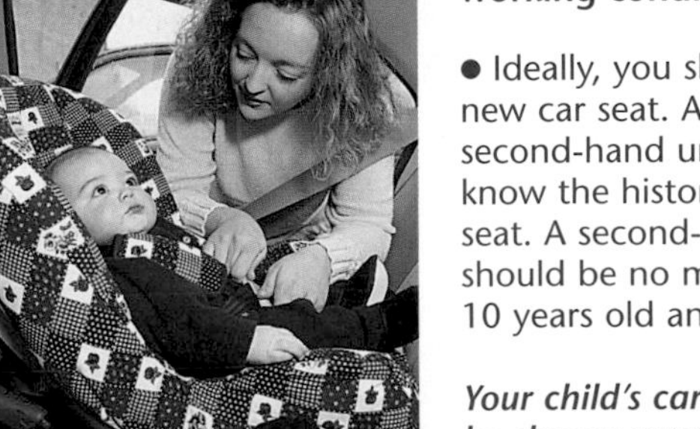

The 'best' seat is one that is suited to your child's age and weight, is in good working condition and fits the seat of your car and your child comfortably.

- Ideally, you should buy a new car seat. Avoid buying second-hand unless you know the history of the seat. A second-hand seat should be no more than 10 years old and should never have been involved in a crash. Check the seat has all its parts and look for possible damage. Buckles and harness adjusters should work easily.

- Most experts recommend a convertible seat equipped with a five-point harness. When buying a convertible seat, choose one with a maximum rear-facing weight that will allow your baby to face to the rear for as long as possible.

- Make sure that the seat is fitted correctly. You can either fit it yourself by carefully following the instructions, or get a reputable garage to fit it.

Your child's car seat should be chosen carefully, and fitted according to the manufacturer's instructions.

Garage safety

Children are often attracted to playing in a garage. But even when stationary, a car is a potential hazard and the garage often contains items that are dangerous in the hands of a child.

1 Keep the garage locked and discourage your child from going in there.

2 Keep the car locked when it is in the garage or standing in the drive.

3 Fuel is a potential fire hazard – always avoid keeping fuel stored in containers. If this is necessary for any reason, use only clearly marked metal containers designed for the purpose.

4 Place any fuel, chemicals and tools out of the reach of a child.

5 When driving the car into or out of the garage, make sure that you know where your child is before starting the car.

6 Children have been known to climb into freezers when playing. If you keep a freezer in the garage, make sure that it is kept locked at all times, even if it is switched off. The same advice applies to the boot of a car.

Safe driving

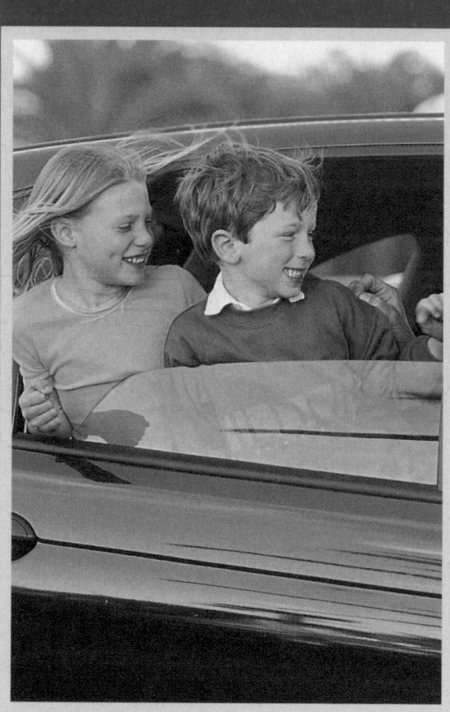

Taking precautions when driving reduces the chances of having an accident. It also reduces the possibility of injuries to children and other passengers if an accident does happen.

- Ensure that all passengers wear the seat belts provided. Children must be restrained in a manner appropriate to their age and size. Headrests for the driver and passengers must be properly positioned to reduce the possibility of neck injuries.
- Position rear-view mirrors and wing mirrors so that you have a clear view of the road behind you when driving.
- Ensure that children under the age of 12 do not travel in seats that have either front airbags or side airbags.
- Do not allow children to lie down in the car – they cannot be secured by seat belts in this position.
- Never store loose items, such as books and stereo equipment, on the shelf at the back of the car. If you have to brake suddenly, these items could be thrown forward and cause injuries to your children.
- On a long journey give children small toys and books to keep them occupied. You could also play games and listen to story tapes.

By law, children must wear the seat belts provided. Never allow them to travel unrestrained.

What to do in the event of an accident or breakdown

If you are involved in an accident or your car breaks down, you must continue to think of the safety of your passengers and yourself.

1 Switch off the engine and check to see what danger there is from other vehicles travelling on the road.

2 If you have been involved in an accident, check to see if anyone in your car has any injuries and consider giving appropriate first aid.

3 If it is necessary and safe to do so, get your passengers out of the vehicle. Remember though that there are certain situations where it is safer to remain in the car. The hard shoulder of a motorway, for example, is potentially a very dangerous place and passengers should not be allowed to leave the car unless they can move to a safe place away from any traffic.

4 If possible, place a warning triangle 50–100m (164–328ft) behind your car, where it is clearly visible.

5 Carry a mobile phone to call for help, or ask someone else to call.

Carry a warning triangle in case you break down or have an accident in a place where it is dangerous to stop.

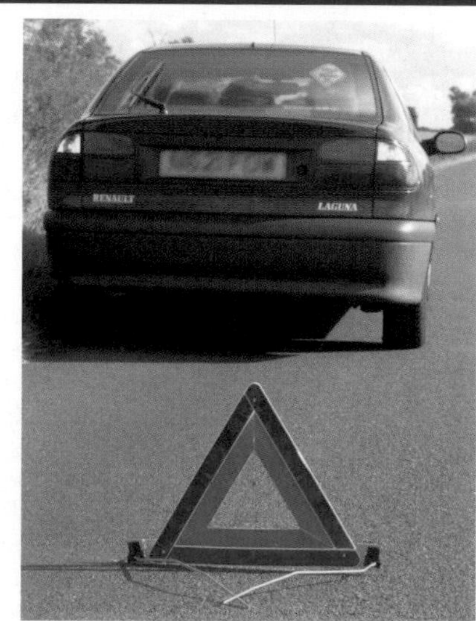

HOME SAFETY

ACCIDENTS CAN HAPPEN

According to the Child Accident Prevention Trust, over two million children aged under 14 go to casualty each year after suffering an accidental injury. There are many reasons why children are at risk.

- They lack experience and have no conception of risk. For example, they may see water as fun and flames as pretty.
- Small children are very curious about anything new. This leads them to stick their fingers into holes, put objects in their mouths and explore cupboards.
- They lack stability and co-ordination. As a result, bumps, falls and tumbles tend to be a regular occurrence.
- They are unaware of dangers. For example, if they see a toy across the room, they'll head for it, not necessarily seeing the table with hot cups of tea in their path.

Young children, particularly toddlers, are often oblivious to danger. Child-proof your home to prevent accidents occurring.

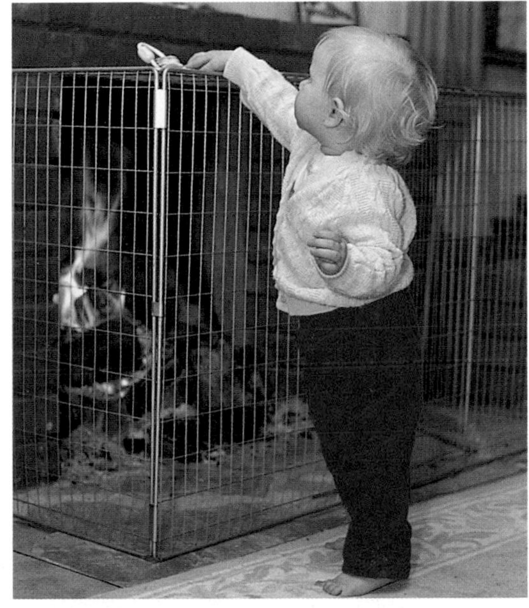

Prevention

Accidents are not always random events over which we have no control. In most cases they can be predicted and prevented. Take a tour around your home from your child's level.

- **The living room:** the fire and fireplace can present a danger to your child, as can electrical items, such as the television, stereo and sockets. Be aware of sharp edges too, for example on ornaments and on furniture.
- **The kitchen:** be extra careful when your child is around any electrical appliances, such as the cooker, kettle, microwave, freezer, washing machine and drier. Other danger areas are cleaning materials and drawers with sharp utensils.
- **The toilet and bathroom:** potential dangers include bleach, shampoos, razors, hot taps, the medicine cabinet, the radiator and the slippery floor.
- **The bedroom:** potential dangers here include an open window, a plugged-in hairdryer, bedside lamps and toiletries.
- **The garden:** make sure the gate is kept closed. Be aware of the hazards posed by garden chemicals, the lawn-mower and garden tools.

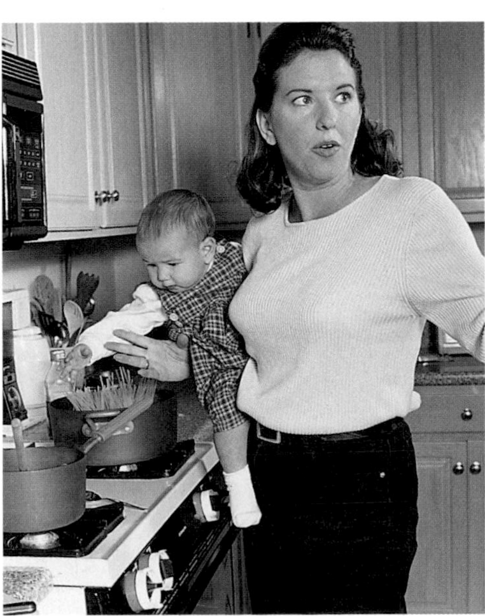

As a rule, it is wise to keep your baby out of the kitchen. Accidents can very easily occur, especially when you are cooking.

Your mobile child

Be aware that once your child becomes more mobile, the dangers change. You need to stay one step ahead.

- **Young babies:** although they may seem to be most vulnerable in the early months, their limited mobility helps to keep them safe. But don't be complacent, as even very young children surprise their parents by rolling over or grabbing objects. Never leave babies unattended on any raised surface. Always use the harnesses in car seats, high-chairs, prams and buggies.
- **Crawlers:** once babies become more mobile, sharp objects on the floor are a problem, as are doors and stairs. Fires and sockets are major dangers and the video may be a source of fascination.
- **Toddlers:** in addition to the hazards already stated, you can now add in the dangers when children pull themselves up on the furniture. Tablecloths are a no-go, as are trailing wires, cords and curtains. Once toddlers can reach higher levels, all ornaments need to move up a level. Watch out for slippery floors, too.
- **Older children:** you can explain about dangers to older children and they will understand more, but don't rely on this. A youngster can easily forget all he knows about crossing a road when he's chasing a ball or rushing to the ice-cream van.

Fire hazards

House fires are the biggest single cause of accidental death at home. Many could be prevented, or reduced in severity, by early detection. Make sure you take all the necessary precautions.

- **Fit smoke detectors:** install at least one per level in your house. The best places are at the foot of the stairs and outside bedrooms. Check the batteries regularly.
- **Fit socket guards:** these inexpensive plastic guards fit into unused electrical sockets and prevent children sticking anything into them.
- **Fit a fireguard:** this should be fixed to the wall. One with a horizontal guard on top helps to prevent youngsters dropping things too near the fire.
- **Keep matches and lighters out of reach:** preferably store them high in a cupboard.
- **Take care with candles:** they are very appealing to children, so it's probably wise to avoid them altogether or use them only in the evenings after your child is asleep. Make sure candles are extinguished properly before going to bed.
- **Empty ashtrays:** if someone is smoking, make sure all ashtrays are kept out of a child's reach and that they are emptied regularly, especially at bedtime.
- **Buy a household fire extinguisher:** store it out of reach and make sure you know how to use it – reading the instructions in an emergency will waste time.

NOTE: take care with bonfires and barbecues. Never leave a child unattended near a bonfire or a barbecue.

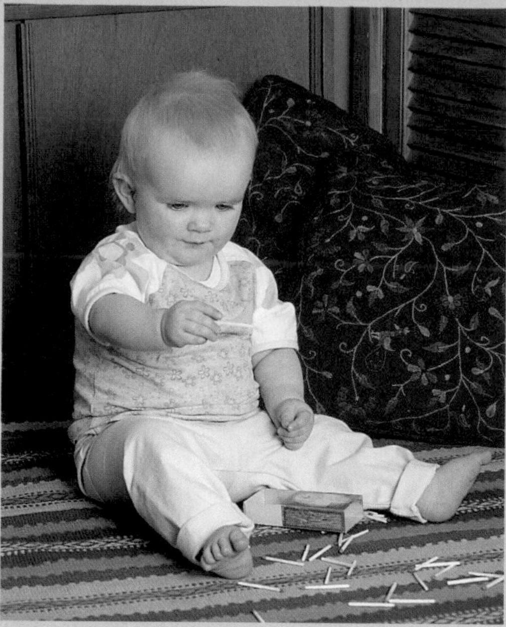

Matches, lighters and candles will all have an irresistible appeal to a young child, and she will have no qualms about making them her playthings. Keep them out of reach, for example in a drawer fitted with a child lock.

Garden safety

Backyards and gardens can be a source of potential danger for young children.

- Every year a small number of children under the age of five drown in garden ponds, according to figures from the Royal Society for the Prevention of Accidents (RoSPA).

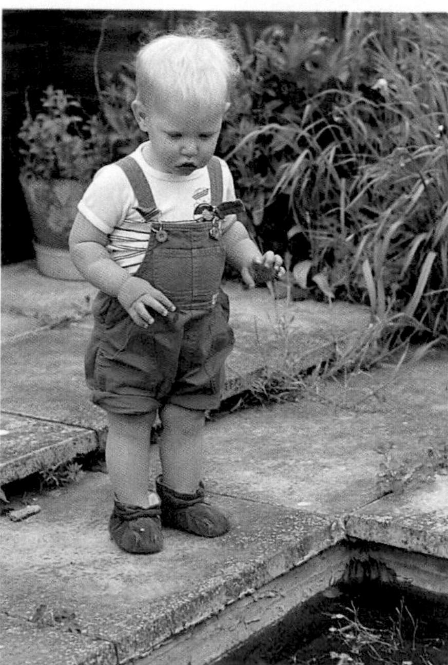

- In the under-fives, drowning is the third largest cause of accidental death in the home in the UK.
- Young children can drown in just 2.5cm (1in) of water – watch for containers that may have collected rainwater and ensure that paddling pools are emptied at the end of the day.

Young children are fascinated by water. Make sure that your child is never left unattended around water and that your garden is as safe as it can be.

- Government figures show that 80 per cent of pond drownings happen in the garden of a friend, relative or neighbour.
- Check that all garden tools are stored away in a locked shed.
- Make sure all garden chemicals – weedkillers and slug pellets, for instance – are well out of reach of your child. Never store these substances in old soft-drink bottles or other household containers in case your child mistakes them for the real thing.

Useful addresses

For more information on how to keep your child safe, contact the following organisations:

Child Accident Prevention Trust
4th Floor
18–20 Farringdon Lane
London EC1R 3HA
Tel: 020 7608 3828
www.capt.org.uk

or in Northern Ireland:
Child Safety Centre
23a/b Mullacreevie Park
Killylea Road
Armagh BT60 4BA
Tel: 028 3752 6521

Royal Society for the Prevention of Accidents (RoSPA)
Edgbaston Park
353 Bristol Road
Edgbaston
Birmingham B5 7ST
Tel: 0121 248 2000
www.rospa.com

WATER SAFETY

DROWNING

In the UK, drowning is the third largest cause of accidental death in the home in the under-fives.

- About eight children a year drown in garden ponds, usually those of a friend or neighbour.
- It is possible for a young child to drown in just 2.5cm (1in) of water.
- Drowning can occur undetected as it is usually silent; a child can slip under the water and become unconscious without making a noise.
- Under water a child will lose consciousness after two minutes and suffer irreversible brain damage after four to six minutes.
- A child may survive longer in cold water due to the 'diving reflex', which diverts blood to essential organs. A child has been known to survive after 66 minutes of submersion in ice-cold water.

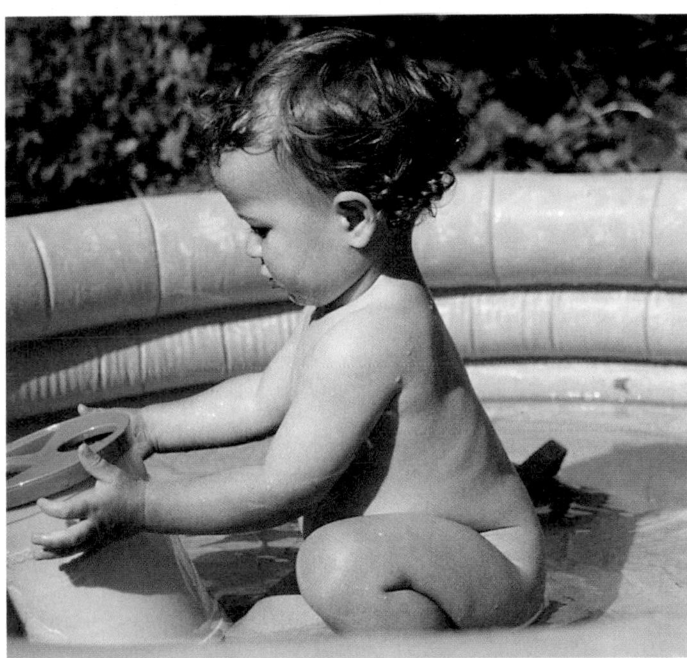

Your child may love splashing in his paddling pool, but it's important that he is supervised at all times because a child can drown without making a noise.

Bathtime safety

Bathtime is usually one of the high points of a young child's day. Most children enjoy the sensation of being in water and the close attention they receive. However, it is also a time of potential danger so take some simple precautions to avoid any accidents.

1 NEVER leave your baby or pre-school child unsupervised, even for a minute. In the time it takes you to answer the phone or doorbell your child could slip under the water and stop breathing. If you have to leave the room, wrap him in a towel and take him with you.

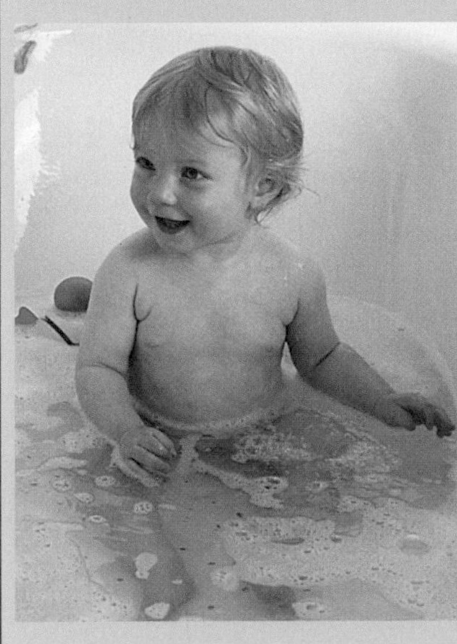

2 Get everything you need ready first, such as bath products and towels, so your attention is not distracted once he is in the water.

3 Use only 7.5cm (2–3ins) of water in the bath for babies and toddlers; older children should not sit more than waist deep.

4 Use supporting rings as an 'extra hand' only. Do not rely on them to keep your baby safe because he may lose his grip, or he could slip and become trapped underneath them. A non-slip bathmat may also be useful, but again, don't rely on it to support your child.

5 Teach your child never to touch taps and always to stay seated while in the bath.

A baby's skin is five times more sensitive than an adult's. Always test the temperature of the bath water with your elbow to check that it is comfortably warm.

In the home and garden

Toddlers and young children are fascinated by water, whether it is in your mop bucket, the toilet, a garden pond or a large puddle. It is up to you to make your home and garden safe.

- Fit a lid lock to your toilet.
- Fit a strong cover to a garden pond. Fence it in well or, better still, drain it until your child is older.
- Make sure containers of water (or other liquids) are never left unattended and empty them immediately after use. Pull out the plug as soon as you get out of the bath.
- Supervise your child at all times in a paddling pool; then empty it after use and store in an upright position so it can't collect rainwater.
- Check your garden for large puddles or collections of water after it has been raining.
- Be extra careful when visiting friends and neighbours as they may not have made their homes and gardens safe for young children.

Swimming pools

A visit to the swimming pool can be a great treat for you and your child. Having fun in the pool is also an important first step in learning to be safe in water. Enjoy your time in the water together, but remember some common-sense steps to keep your child safe.

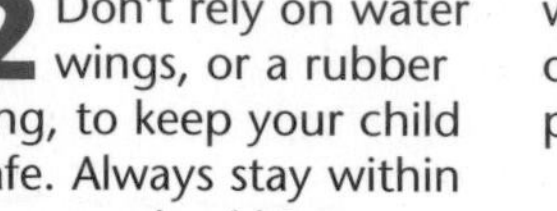
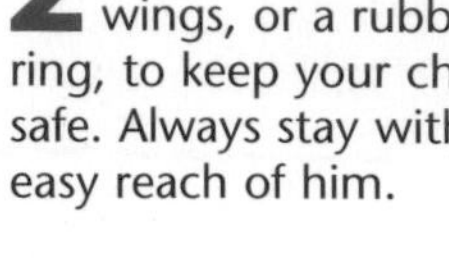

1 NEVER leave your baby or pre-school child unsupervised in the pool. The area of the pool can be very noisy and distracting, but you must watch him closely at all times.

2 Don't rely on water wings, or a rubber ring, to keep your child safe. Always stay within easy reach of him.

3 Try to make sure there is one adult per child. It's difficult to watch over more than one small child in a pool at a time.

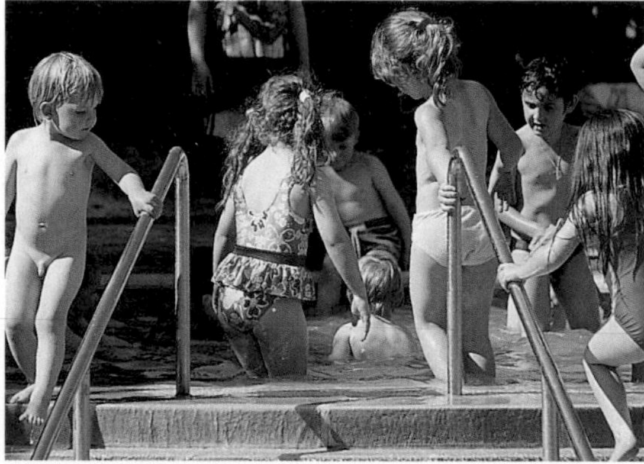

4 Enrol your child in swimming lessons when he is three to four years old, but don't assume he will then be safe in the water alone. You will still need to supervise him closely.

5 Learn to swim, if you can't already.

Keep a close eye on your child and remember that swimming pools can be hectic and crowded, and attention can be diverted easily.

The great outdoors

From time to time you will probably go on outings to the seaside, or to ponds, rivers or lakes. Such outings are fun, but be aware of possible dangers.

1 NEVER leave your child unsupervised near water, for any reason.

2 Never let your child approach the edge of the water unless you are holding him tightly.

3 If your child wants to go into the water, go with him and hold his hand. Waves can easily sweep a small child away.

4 Use recognised bathing spots only, where you can see the surface you are walking on.

5 Babies and children can get very cold quite quickly. Stay in the water for a short time only and then dry your child well and wrap him in warm clothes.

Emergency action

If you supervise your child carefully it is very unlikely that he will come to any harm during bathing and water play. However, anyone who cares for children should know what to do in an emergency.

- If you see your child slip under the water, pull him up immediately. He will probably react by coughing and spluttering and will need no more than a reassuring cuddle.
- If he has been under water for longer, you will need to act quickly and calmly; pull him out and check to see if he is conscious.
- If he is conscious and breathing, take off any wet clothes and wrap him warmly. Even if he appears to be fully recovered, you should take him to see a doctor straightaway just in case he has inhaled water.
- If he is unconscious, check to see if he is breathing and if he has a pulse. Shout for someone to call for an ambulance, but don't leave him alone.
- If your child is not breathing, give mouth-to-mouth resuscitation, or 'mouth-to-nose and mouth' in the case of a baby under one year. Start as soon as possible – while your child is still in the water, if necessary.
- If there is no pulse, begin CPR (cardio-pulmonary resuscitation).
- Continue resuscitation until the ambulance comes or until your child begins to breathe on his own.

A first-aid class will teach you how to administer CPR, as well as other resuscitation techniques.

- If your child begins to gasp and breathe again, it is likely that he will vomit. Hold him with his head lowered, or place him in the recovery position to stop him inhaling vomit.
- When the ambulance arrives, try to remember exactly how long your child was submerged. This is important information for the medical staff. He will then be taken to hospital to receive expert care and the doctors there will do everything they can to help him.

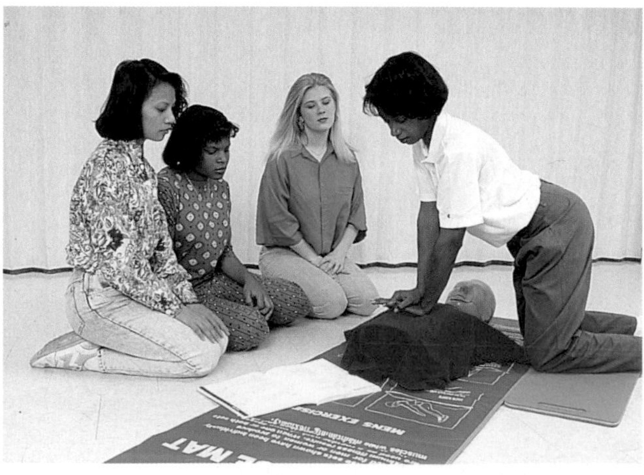

YOUR MEDICINE CABINET

BE PREPARED

Illness in childhood often strikes suddenly. Giving immediate attention at home may mean that there is no need to seek medical help.

As well as relieving a child's distress, prompt action may stop a relatively minor worry – such as a high temperature – from spiralling into a much worse one, for example, febrile convulsions. In the case of an accident, it may save a frantic, and often dangerous, dash to the local accident and emergency centre.

Your medicine cabinet should be placed out of reach of children and preferably locked. Ideally, all contents should be listed on the door, and dated if they have a short life. That way, missing items can be replaced and you can avoid keeping others beyond their use-by date. Equipment, such as scissors, must to be kept clean and dry and preferably in its own container.

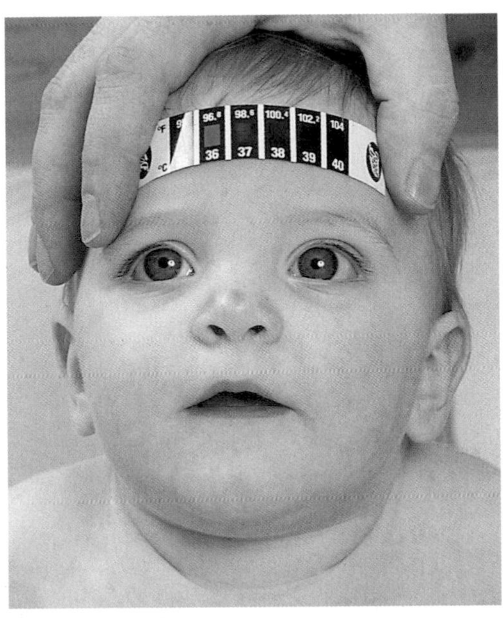

A forehead temperature strip is easy to read and simple to use, especially with a wriggling child. If your child's temperature is higher than 37.5°C (100°F) for 24 hours, you should contact your doctor.

Keeping a well-stocked medicine cabinet

- **Pain relief mixture (paracetamol):** helps to relieve aches and pains, such as teething, stomach ache, fever and cold.
- **Gripe mixture:** can be given to babies to relieve wind and soothe gripe. Recommended for babies aged 1–12 months.
- **Infant cough mixture:** to be used for infants over the age of three months only.
- **Medicine spoon:** ideal for cough medicines, gripe mixture and liquid paracetamol, it measures 2.5mls and 5mls.
- **Vapour rub:** gently massaged into your child's chest, this helps to clear the airways.
- **Rehydration powder:** for babies or young children suffering from dehydration as a result of vomiting or diarrhoea.
- **Calpol:** a branded paracetamol, which, on doctor's advice, may be given to babies under three months, e.g. after immunisation.
- **Ibuprofen:** lowers fever and relieves pain. Available in syrup form but use for infants on doctor's advice only.
- **Thermometer:** skin adhesive thermometers are the least frightening for a small child.

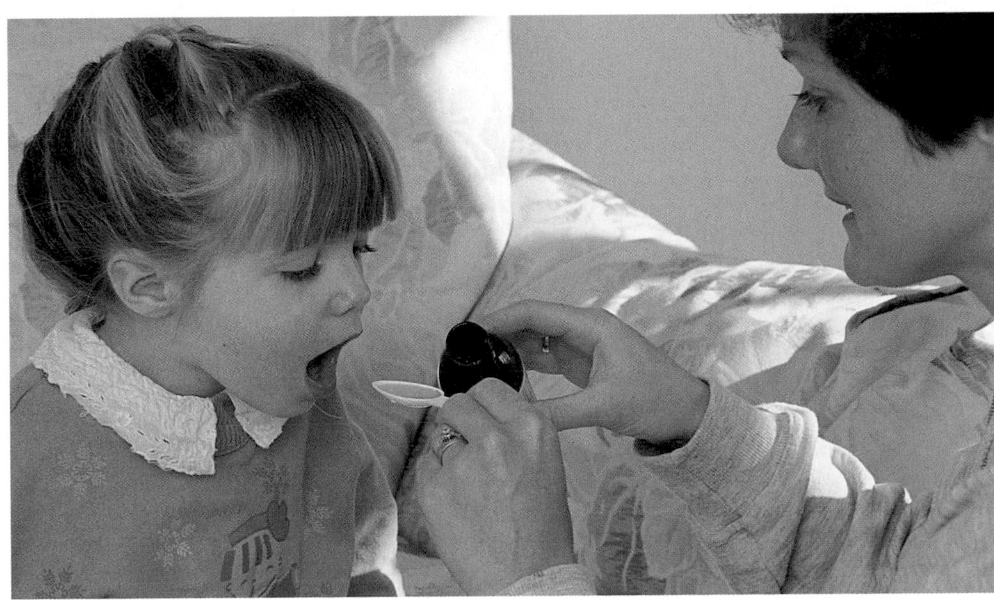

A medicine spoon will enable you to give the correct dosage of cough mixture, or any other liquid medicine your child may need.

First-aid kit

• **Bonjela:** this pain-relieving gel can soothe the teething process and help heal mouth ulcers. Do not give to babies under four months old.

• **Arnica cream:** available from major chemists and health-food shops, this herbal remedy reduces bruising and pain from a bruise.

• **Calendula cream:** another herbal remedy that helps to relieve sore and dry skin.

• **Plasters:** keep a box of different sizes, shapes and types, e.g. waterproof and digit-shaped.

• **Bandages:** preferably in various sizes and types, such as strips of adhesive and non-adhesive bandage, crêpe and elasticated tubular bandage, which is useful for supporting a sprained limb and keeping swelling down.

• **Sharp scissors:** ensure one side is rounded so that dressings – or clothing, for example, if the child is scalded – can be cut off without harming the skin further.

• **Antiseptic cream:** helps to soothe burns and scalds, as well as chapped, dry skin and nappy rash.

• **Sterile gauze:** for placing over a non-adhesive dressing on an open wound.

• **Adhesive tape:** waterproof tape is useful on areas, such as the hands, that will invariably get wet over time. Never totally encircle a digit with tape because this could cut off the blood supply.

• **Antiseptic wipes:** useful for cleaning cuts and grazes.

• **Nappy rash cream:** nearly all babies suffer from nappy rash and this cream can help to clear it up at the first signs of redness.

MOBILE FIRST AID

As well as keeping a good stock of medicines and first-aid equipment at home, it is important to have a basic first-aid kit in the car for outings because accidents can happen at any time. The kit should be a pared-down version of your medicine cabinet.

You can buy ready-assembled first-aid kits in containers of various sizes at all major chemists. However, if you decide to put together your own kit, a large lunchbox makes an ideal container. The contents of the kit should be listed on the box and checked regularly. Store the kit out of the reach of children.

It's a good idea to keep a first-aid manual close at hand, too. Try to read up on common injuries, such as those to the head, scalds and ankle sprains, so that you can remain calm in the event of an accident. Knowing what to do in advance could mean the difference between life and death. Make sure that you have an updated list of emergency numbers – your local GP, nearest casualty department – to hand both in the car and at home.

Keeping a first-aid kit means you are prepared should your child have an accident. Store the items in an air-tight container and check the kit regularly.

TAKING YOUR CHILD'S TEMPERATURE

TEMPERATURE CHANGES

Most children have a raised temperature at some point in their first few years. It is a normal response to the infections that children face.

- Being able to check your child's temperature can help you to identify whether he is ill.

- The normal body temperature of a child is 36–37.2°C (97–99°F). This may vary slightly with the time of day or the amount of exercise your child has had.

- Any temperature over 37.2°C (99°F) indicates that your child is unwell; consider giving him some paracetamol syrup.

- Seek medical advice if your child's temperature is higher than normal for over 24 hours. If his temperature rises above 40°C (104°F), sponge him down with tepid water and seek urgent medical help.

- Bear in mind that even with a normal temperature, a child may still be unwell. Be guided by your own feelings and knowledge of your child and seek medical advice if you are at all concerned.

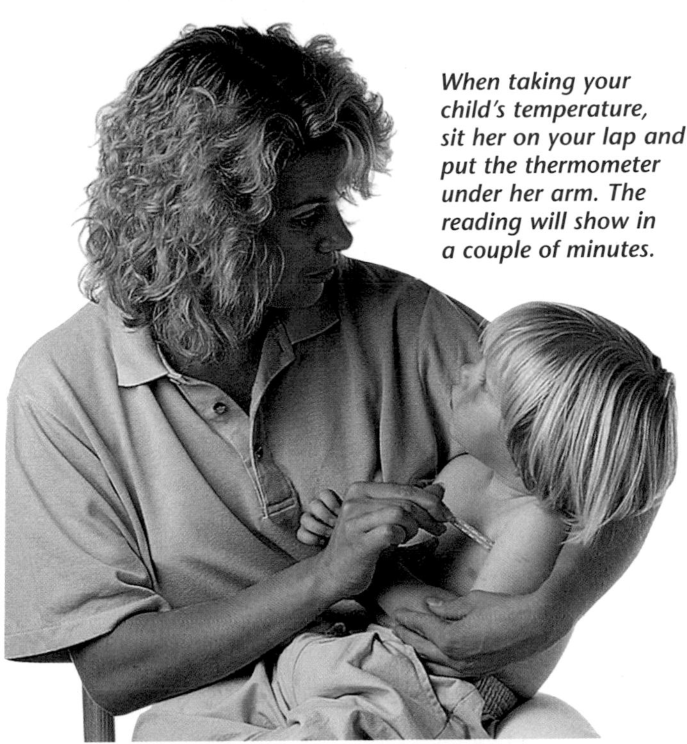

When taking your child's temperature, sit her on your lap and put the thermometer under her arm. The reading will show in a couple of minutes.

When should I take my child's temperature?

There is no harm in taking your child's temperature if you are concerned.

- **Symptoms:** if your child has the following symptoms, he may have an infection: sore throat, rash, vomiting, diarrhoea, runny nose, earache, achiness, shivering, headache, flushed appearance or tummy pain. He may, of course, have none of these symptoms, but still be ill.

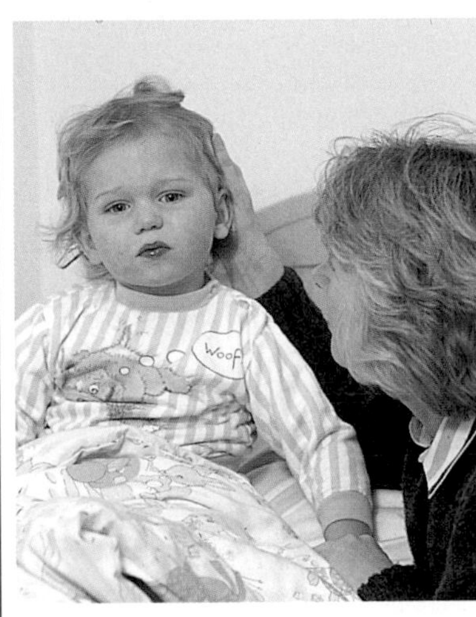

- **Method:** take your child's temperature using whichever method suits you and your child best (see overleaf).
  Make a note of the reading and take the temperature again half an hour later.

If your child feels hot when you touch her, take her temperature to judge whether she has a fever. Do not overwrap your child; allow air to cool her skin.

Where should I take my child's temperature?

You can buy thermometers to use in the mouth, under the armpit, on the forehead or in the ear.

- **Mouth:** putting a thermometer under the tongue gives a good indication of a child's temperature but is not suitable for young children, especially if a mercury thermometer is used.

- **Armpit:** using a thermometer under the armpit is a safe and easy method if your child can sit still for long enough.

- **Forehead:** this is the easiest way to take your child's temperature but the reading is not very accurate and should be used as a rough guide only.

- **Ear:** this is a quick and accurate method but the thermometers are expensive.

NOTE: thermometers should be cleaned after each use and stored in a cool place out of the reach of children. Always read the instructions. Different types of thermometer may require special care and may need to be cleaned in different ways.

Digital thermometer

This works with batteries and displays the temperature in a window. It does not contain mercury, so is safe to put into your child's mouth, but it is often easier to take the temperature under the armpit. An underarm temperature may be slightly lower than the true internal temperature.

1 Remove your baby's upper clothing and sit her comfortably on your lap.

2 Place the thermometer under your baby's armpit and hold it there until you hear a beeping sound. This usually happens within one or two minutes. A digital thermometer can be put under the tongue, but it may be difficult to persuade a baby or young child to keep it there for long enough.

3 Once you hear the bleeping noise, remove the thermometer and your child's temperature will be shown on the digital display. Once you have noted the temperature, turn the thermometer off to conserve the batteries.

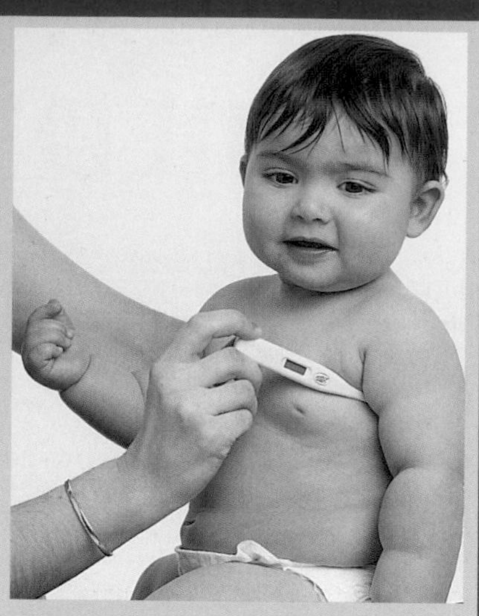

Digital thermometers are easy and safe to use under the arm. They give a more accurate reading than a forehead strip thermometer.

Forehead strip thermometer

This is a flexible plastic strip with heat-sensitive panels. It is quick and easy to use, especially for very young children, but it may not give as accurate a reading as other types of thermometer.

1 Place your child in a comfortable position, hold the heat sensitive strip at both ends and press closely against his forehead. Make sure that the whole strip is in contact with the skin.

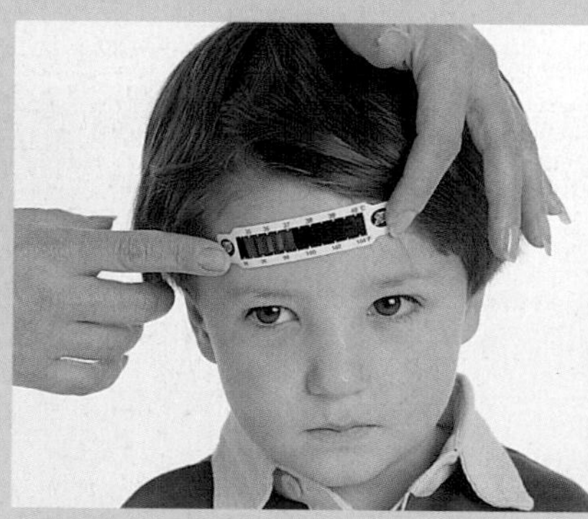

2 Hold the strip in place until there is a complete colour change in one of the panels; this usually takes about 30 seconds. Note which panels light up while the strip is still in place, because the reading will be lost as soon as you remove the strip.

3 The highest panel that lights up indicates the temperature.

This thermometer is a small heat sensitive plastic strip, but it may not give a very accurate reading.

Ear thermometer

An ear thermometer is a quick way of taking a child's temperature. These are available from chemists.

- This type of thermometer measures the temperature near the eardrum, inside the ear canal. It works by measuring the infra-red radiation in the ear canal and is a very quick and accurate device.
- Always follow the manufacturer's instructions carefully and precisely.

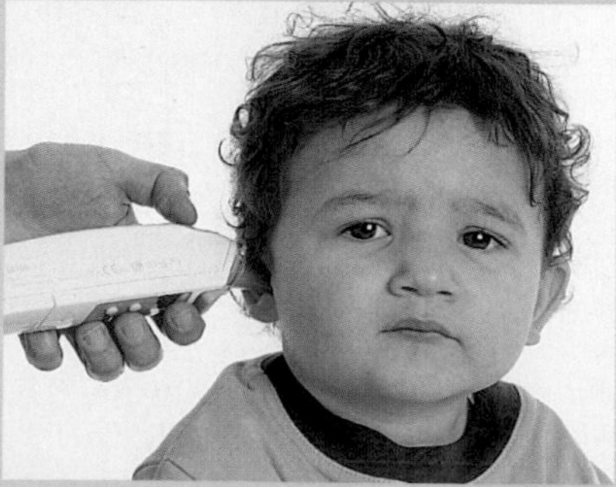

Ear thermometers will give a quick and accurate reading, but they are expensive to buy.

Mercury thermometer

This thermometer is made of glass and contains mercury, which expands when warmed. This type of thermometer should not be used in the mouths of babies or young children, because they might bite down and break it, releasing the mercury, which is poisonous.

1 First shake the thermometer down to return the mercury to the bulb after its last use.

2 To take an underarm temperature, seat your child in a comfortable position. If possible sit him on your lap – this way you will be able to cuddle him and keep his arm still.

3 Gently lift your child's arm, tuck the end of the thermometer with the silver bulb into his armpit then bring his arm down and fold it across his chest. The thermometer should stay in position for at least three minutes so you may need to hold his arm gently in place.

4 Remove the thermometer and read off the temperature against the scale. You may need to slowly rotate the thermometer until the mercury becomes visible.

TAKING YOUR CHILD TO THE DOCTOR

Going to the doctor may not be an enjoyable experience for your child, but it shouldn't be something that he dreads. The key is to prepare him well in advance for what will happen.

At some point, it is highly probable that you will have to take your child to see a doctor, whether that means going to the local GP practice or a hospital outpatients department. You may find that you feel particularly anxious when your child is the patient, but it's important that you don't transfer your own fears to him.

Finding the right doctor

Some GPs are excellent at helping children to feel relaxed, but others relate better to adults. Often this is simply because they are busy and don't have time for the kind of small talk that helps to put children at ease. However, if your doctor seems insensitive to the needs of your child, you may want to consider using a different doctor. You could ask friends and neighbours to recommend a GP who is good with children. Alternatively, your health visitor should be able to advise you.

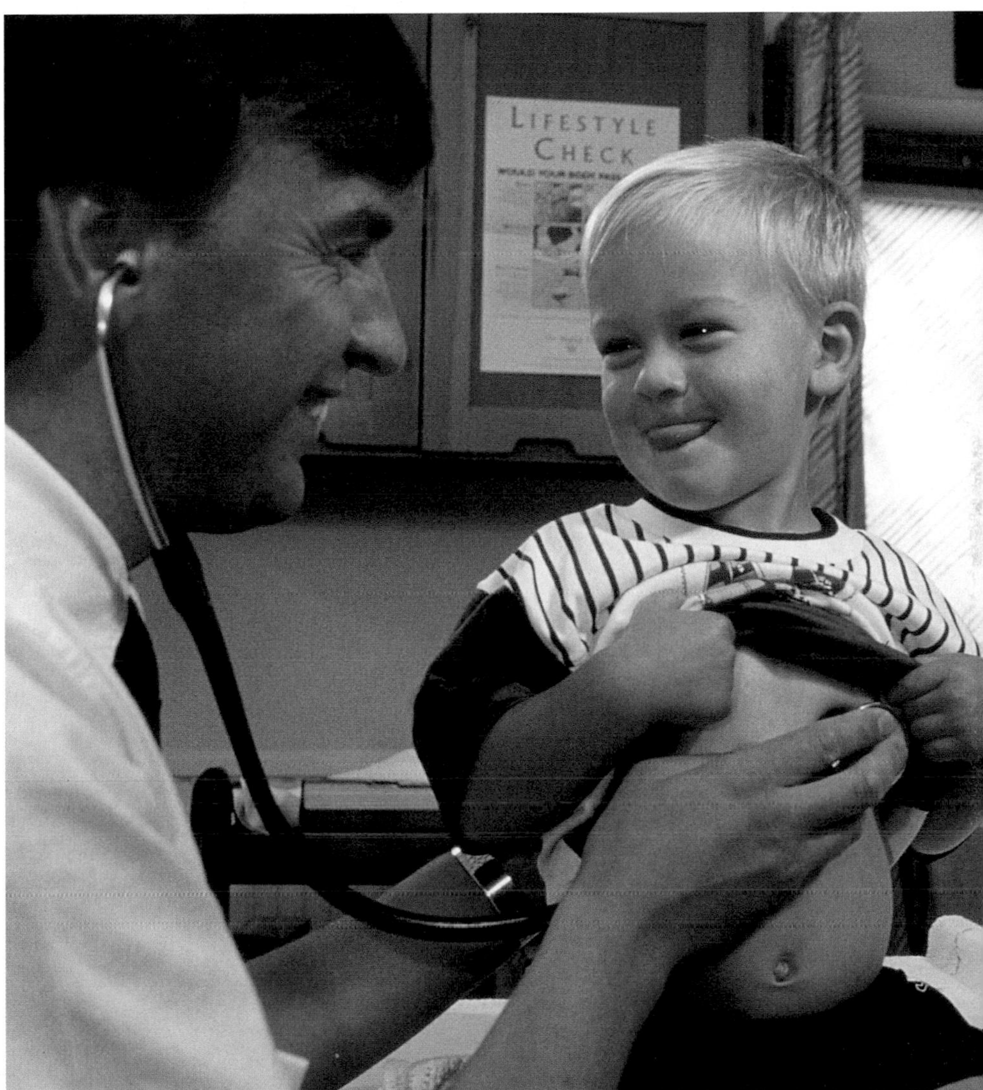

It's quite natural for a child to feel nervous about going to the doctor, who will probably be a stranger to him. Try to find someone with whom your child feels at ease.

Dos and don'ts

You can prepare your child for a visit to the doctor in the following ways:

✔ Do be honest about where you are going.

✔ Do give him a simple explanation of what is likely to happen at the surgery.

✔ Do encourage him to talk about any fears he may have.

✔ Do take along favourite toys to keep him occupied and distracted.

✘ Don't emphasise the fun – he could be very disappointed.

✘ Don't promise him it won't hurt.

The waiting game

One of the worst aspects of taking a child to the doctor is the long wait you may have to face. To avoid this, try to arrange an appointment either at the beginning or end of surgery. Receptionists are usually sympathetic to the fact that the patient is a small child and do their best to be helpful.

However, if that isn't possible, you will have the chore of keeping your child quiet in a roomful of people who don't want a noisy child disturbing the peace. Some surgeries and medical centres make a real effort to cater for children by providing a play area with books and construction toys, but others may have just a selection of very old magazines. If yours is the latter, make sure you take some favourite toys and books and any comforter along with you.

It's a good idea to dress your child in clothes that are easy to take off, not just because it will make the doctor's examination easier, but to stop him from becoming too hot in an over-warm waiting room. If you have older children, try to arrange for them to be looked after by a friend or relative rather than taking them, too, as this may make the visit even more stressful.

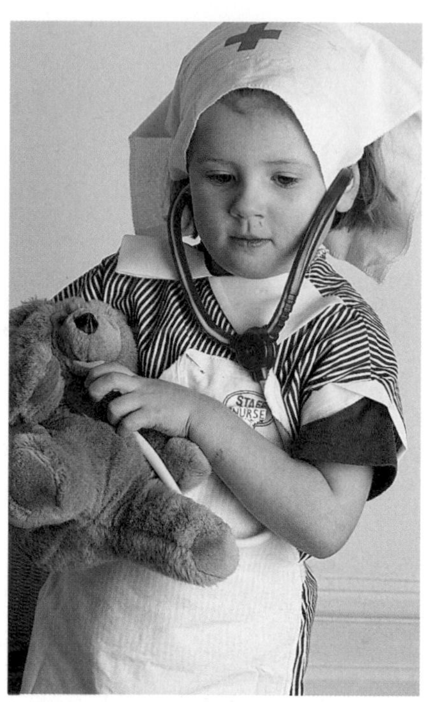

Meeting the doctor

A young child may feel anxious about going to see the doctor, but you can offer reassurance in the following ways:

- Make it clear that you will be with your child throughout the doctor's consultation and will not leave him even for a moment.
- While you explain the problem, sit your child on your knee facing the doctor so that he feels involved in the conversation.
- If the doctor asks your child questions, give him time to give his own answers rather than responding for him.
- If your child has to lie on the bed to be examined by the doctor, stand close by, holding his hand or stroking his head to soothe him.

To help your child overcome fears about the doctor, buy her a nurse's kit with pretend stethoscope and thermometer, and play simple games, such as listening to teddy's heart.

Being honest

While you do not wish to say anything that may frighten your child, it's equally important that you don't mislead him about the purpose of a visit to the doctor. If he is going to have an injection and asks if the needle will hurt him, it pays to be honest and agree that he will feel the prick but only momentarily. Follow this up quickly by promising him that he can have a treat immediately afterwards. This treat should not be conditional on his being a brave boy; let him know that it is all right for him to cry when he is hurt.

Playing doctor

It's important that your child understands that the doctor is a kind, caring person who is there to help him feel better or prevent him from becoming sick. Role-play with dolls or teddies is invaluable in helping children come to terms with their fears of doctors and hospitals.

For an older child, you might also invest in a special doll that, when taken apart, reveals the organs of the body. As well as being fascinating and educational, it will help to familiarise your child with his anatomy and make it easier for him to tell you and the doctor where he feels pain.

Fighting the fear

Some children may need the help of a psychologist to overcome fear of the doctor. Seek advice if:

- He becomes distressed at the mention of the doctor's name.
- He denies that he is feeling unwell even when it's clear to you that he's poorly.
- He becomes panic stricken if you are just passing by the surgery on your way to somewhere else.
- He is also fearful of nurses, dentists, even hairdressers.

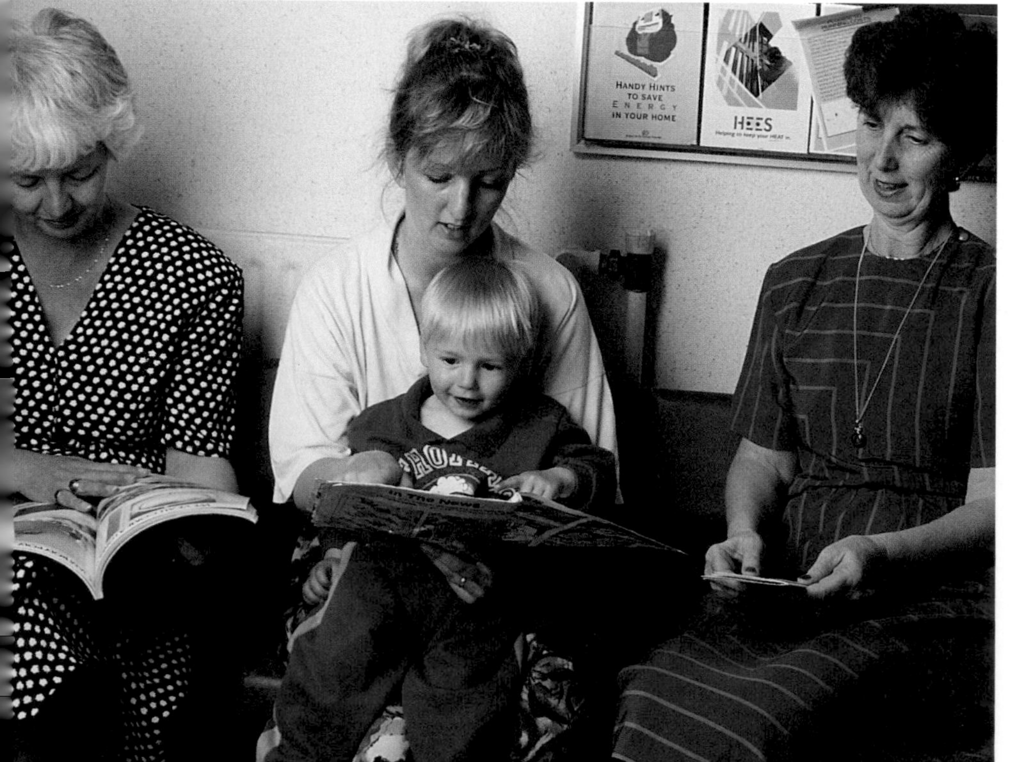

Even if you have an appointment, you may be kept waiting at the GP's surgery. Take along a book or toy to distract your child, as not all practices have a play area.

NHS Direct

If you need urgent or additional help regarding your child's health, call NHS Direct. This 24 hour telephone line gives you access to experienced nurses who can give you medical advice over the telephone.

NHS Direct: 0845 4647

TAKING YOUR CHILD TO THE DENTIST

Regular dental check-ups are an essential part of your child's overall health care. It is important to ensure that going to the dentist is a positive experience for your child from an early age.

Most dentists suggest that children start their visits from the age of about two-and-a-half years. This is because toddlers usually have a full set of baby teeth by then. However, if you have any concerns about your child's teeth or gums before this age, don't hesitate to consult a dentist.

Fear of the dentist

Thankfully, being frightened to go to the dentist is becoming less common. This is mainly due to falling levels of tooth decay in recent years, which has meant fewer children requiring treatment at an early age. Consequently, visits to the dentist are much less traumatic than in the past. Indeed, many young children positively enjoy the experience.

If you don't mind dental checks, taking your child to the dentist with you – even before she needs check-ups – can be a very positive move.

Parents are not always so relaxed about visiting the dentist, perhaps because they had bad experiences as children themselves. Children are very sensitive to a parent's anxieties, so if you do have any fears, try to avoid showing them. Alternatively, find someone else to take your child.

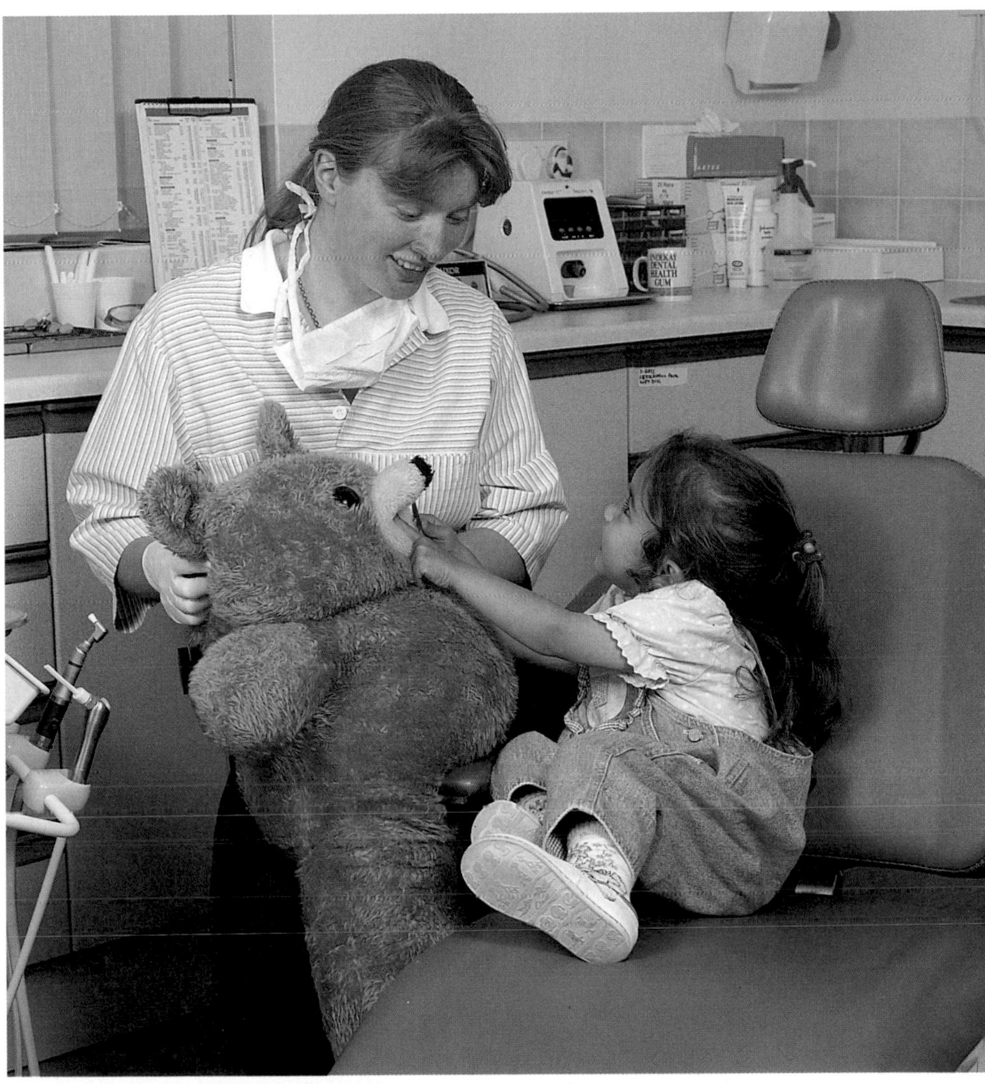

Some dentists will try to make your child's visit less of an ordeal by showing her toys or playing games. This is especially comforting if it is your child's first visit or if she needs some dental work.

Dental milestones

All children develop at different rates. Below is a general guide:

AGE	TOOTH DEVELOPMENT
6 months	First baby teeth usually come in – often the front upper or lower teeth.
2½ years	There is a full set of baby teeth (also referred to as 'milk' or deciduous teeth), consisting of 20 teeth, five in each half of each jaw at the top and bottom. This includes eight front incisors, eight back molars and four canines.
4–12 years	Baby teeth begin to fall out to make way for a full set of 32 adult teeth.

Making it fun

One of the other factors making children's visits to the dentist more acceptable is the way in which some dentists approach the check-ups. Rather than beginning with an intimidating examination, they try to create a relaxed environment with some fun activities, such as a 'ride' in the chair.

The dentist may also give 'prizes', such as balloons or colouring sheets, to reward good behaviour.

Accidents to baby teeth

Most children will have their baby teeth until they are around six years old. Injuries to these teeth usually happen to toddlers, or children who are generally unsteady on their feet. A child falling and hitting his mouth on the corner of furniture is a common accident.

1 If a baby tooth is loosened in a fall, the dentist is unlikely to recommend treatment, but he will advise specific care of the affected area. The tooth may take a week or two to tighten again, and during this period your child may find a softer diet easier to eat. The dentist will show you how to keep the area around the tooth clean with cotton buds. If the tooth is knocked out of position, the chances are that it will go back into position by itself, but do go back to the dentist again if it doesn't.

2 If a baby tooth is knocked back into the gum, the dentist may X-ray your child's mouth to assess exactly what has happened. Remarkably, the tooth will usually grow back into place over a number of weeks or possibly months. Until this time, the dentist will probably recommend that your child has a diet of soft food and that the affected area is carefully cleaned. He may ask to see your child again sooner than usual to check the tooth's development.

3 If the tooth is completely knocked out, attempt to find it and take the tooth and your child to the dentist. Carry the tooth in a container with some milk, which will give it a better chance of survival. (If your child has swallowed the tooth, you must take your child to the dentist or a hospital casualty unit.) Don't attempt to put the baby tooth back into the socket as it might harm the developing adult tooth.

As your child becomes mobile, he'll be more likely to knock his teeth. However, baby teeth are extremely resilient.

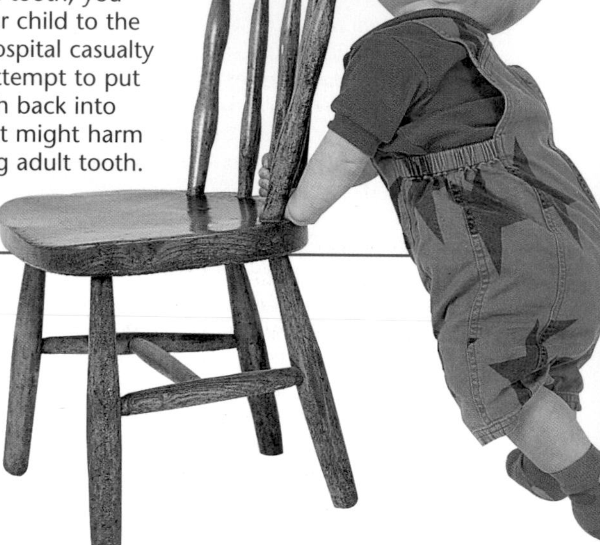

If your child is particularly nervous, find a sympathetic dentist. One of the best ways of finding a child-friendly dentist is by word of mouth.

It may also help your child if you talk to her about what she might expect to happen at the dentist's. In addition, taking a cuddly toy can be useful as it provides comfort for your child.

Your dentist may give your child a reward for being brave, such as a sticker or a badge. This should help to make him more willing to return.

Dentists skilled in dealing with children will use gradual techniques to persuade a child to allow an examination and treatment, each visit building on the previous one. The first check-up might even start in a completely non-clinical environment, such as a play area or waiting room.

The dentist will advise on the most appropriate interval between check-ups. Usually this will be at least six months but it will depend on the needs of your child and the rate at which her teeth are developing.

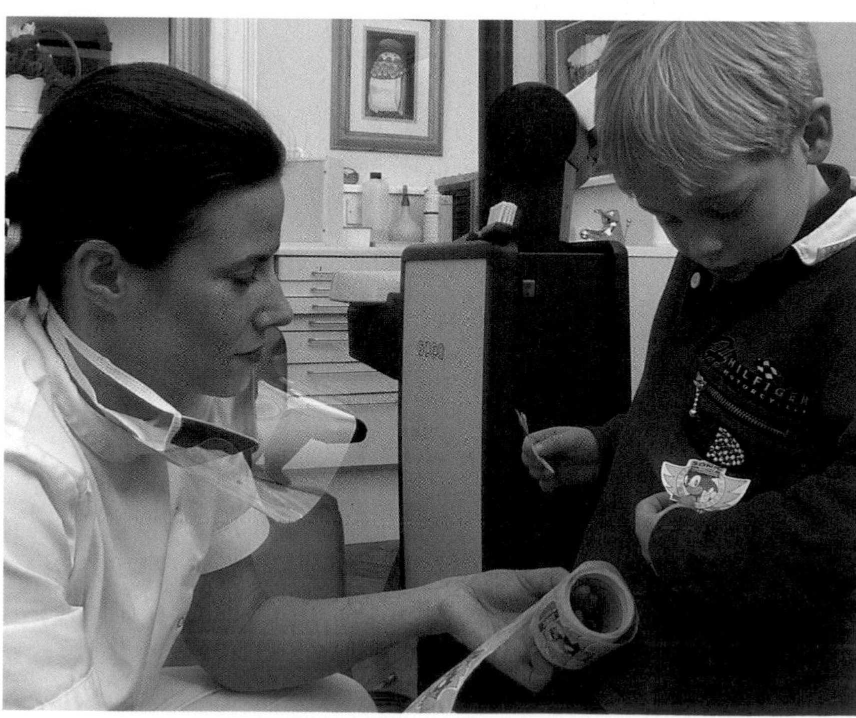

Questions & Answers

Q ***Can thumb sucking cause teeth to stick out?***

A Not necessarily. Although really prolonged thumb sucking into the early teen years can cause difficulties, the 'problem' generally solves itself without the need for any intervention. If teeth have been moved forward slightly due to thumb or dummy pressure, as soon as the habit ceases the teeth tend to drift back to their original position. Corrective treatment is almost never required.

Q ***Why can't my child use the same toothpaste as me?***

A The main reason is that young children require different levels of some of the ingredients, especially fluoride. Young children need a much smaller intake of fluoride than adults. Flavouring is a further reason. The flavour of some 'adult' toothpastes is too strong for the delicate lining of a young child's mouth.

TAKING YOUR CHILD TO THE OPTICIAN

All children should have a sight test before they start school. The first visit may be intimidating for your child, so it is advisable to prepare her in advance.

Most preschool children undergo eye tests carried out by the local health authority. These are usually arranged by the health visitor or baby clinic and may take place before your child's first birthday, and again between the ages of 1½ and 2½ years. These tests are often inconclusive, so your child will need a sight test before she starts school, but it's unlikely that she will need glasses.

If there is a family history of squint, amblyopia or other visual problems, it is important to have your child's eyes tested regularly. Under the NHS, all children are entitled to free yearly eye tests, increasing to six monthly if they need spectacles.

It's not necessary for your child to be able to read, or even to be co-operative, for an eye examination to be carried out. The optometrist will vary the tests according to your child's age and abilities.

Choosing an optician

Ideally, take your child to the same optician as you go to yourself; otherwise, ask for a recommendation from your GP, health visitor or friends. Opticians who specialise in treating children often create a child-friendly environment, and should stock a good selection of children's frames.

To prepare your child for a visit to the optician, take her with you when you go for an eye test. Ask the optometrist if your child can watch the test to see what happens.

There are also storybooks about visiting an optician and these can help

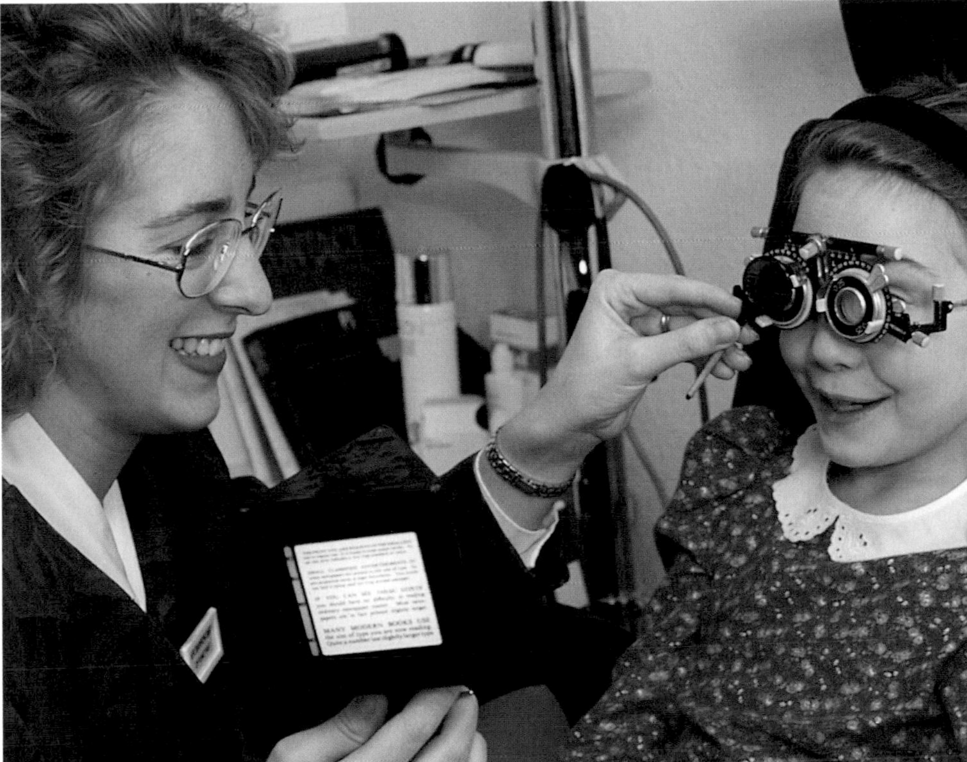

ABOVE: An optometrist will check your child's vision and the health of her eyes.

BELOW: Your child will eventually get used to wearing glasses, even though he may be reluctant to do so in the beginning.

Preparing your child for an eye test

Some of the tasks that the optometrist (an optician who examines eyes) will ask your child to do as part of the sight test may seem a little strange to her. So, before you go to the appointment, it might help to recreate similar activities at home:

- Write down big letters on pieces of card, and give your child a piece of paper with the same letters on. Go to the end of the room, hold up each card and ask your child to point to the matching one on her piece of paper.
- Hold a small toy in front of your child's face, and slowly move it. Ask her to follow the movement with her eyes, without moving her head.
- Get your child used to having a hand placed over one eye while she focuses with the other – make it part of a game.
- Place a pair of glasses on your child's face for a second or two so that she gets used to the feeling of wearing them.

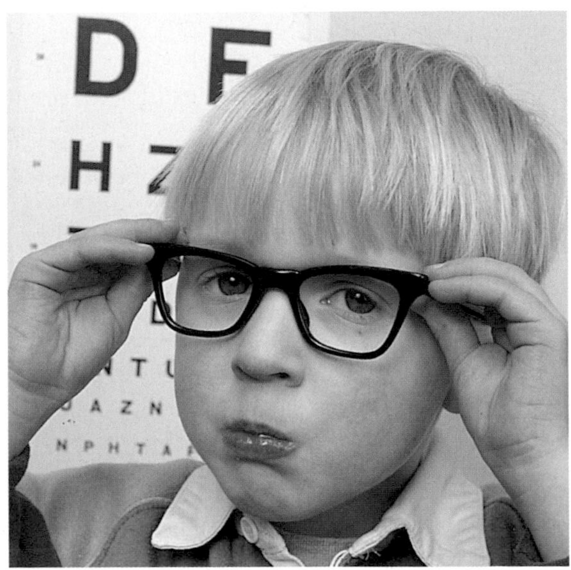

Looking after glasses

- Your child's glasses should be cleaned at least once each day with warm soapy water, and dried using a soft cloth. Special cleaning solutions and cloths are available from the optician, but warm water is usually just as effective.
- When not in use, the glasses should be kept in a hard case to protect them.
- Glasses do need to be looked after carefully, but breakages are inevitable and, if they happen, your child shouldn't be scolded. This will only result in your child being too nervous to wear her glasses at all.

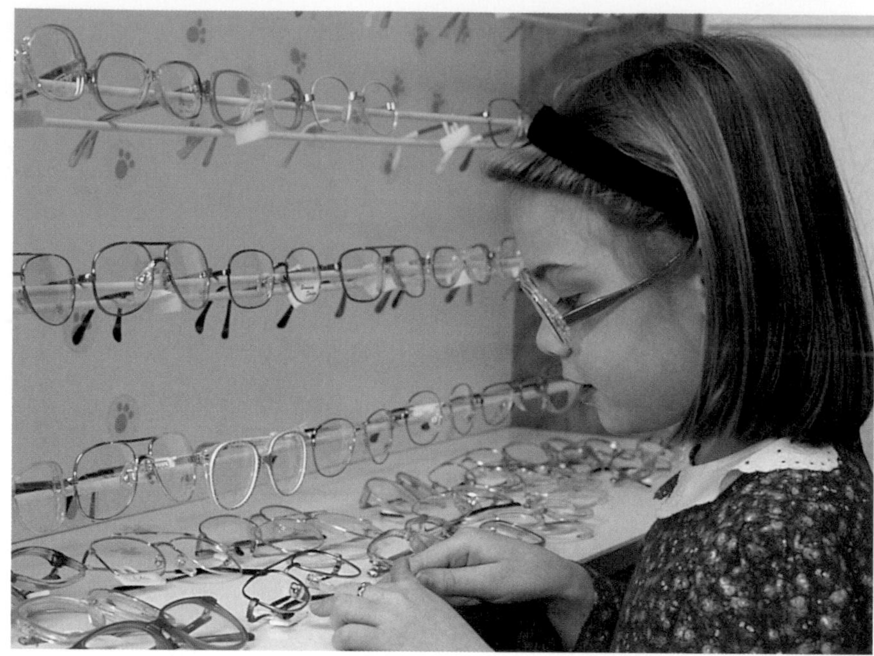

Most opticians stock a wide range of children's glasses so you should be able to find a design that suits your child. Always involve her in the selection.

to familiarise your child with the test procedures. Another way to prepare your child is to draw her attention to people who wear glasses and explain why they are needed.

The visit
The equipment in the room can be intimidating, so it may be better if your child sits on your lap for the examination. Most of the tests will be carried out in a darkened room so, if your child is afraid of the dark, prepare her for this beforehand.

The optician may insert eye drops as part of the test. Very few children have an allergic reaction to the drops, but if your child has any allergies, inform the optometrist. Eye drops do sting for a few minutes and you need to prepare your child for this because she may find it upsetting.

Like most children, your child is unlikely to need glasses and the optometrist may just recommend a further test in a few months' time. If glasses are necessary, the optometrist will advise on when they should be worn. The NHS provides a voucher towards the cost of children's glasses. This usually covers the cost of the lenses and a basic frame.

Ordering the glasses
You can buy the glasses from the optician who carried out the test or take the voucher to another outlet. If you choose to purchase a more expensive frame, you will have to pay the difference between the value of the voucher and the cost of the glasses.

The lenses in children's spectacles are usually made of plastic to reduce the risk of breakage and potential injury to your child's eyes or face should an accident occur. Contact lenses are not usually recommended for young children and should be fitted on medical advice only.

The optician will ensure that the frames fit properly and are comfortable. Regular visits will probably be necessary as young children often break their glasses, and also the glasses may need to be adjusted as your child grows.

Questions & Answers

Q ***Will wearing glasses make my child's sight weaker?***

A No, but not wearing spectacles when necessary could result in poor sight. The visual pathways of young children are still developing and clear vision is necessary for this to happen.

Q ***Can children grow out of squints?***

A There is one eye condition that looks like a squint but is normal and caused by folds of skin near the nose. This will resolve itself. All other squints require early treatment, which often means wearing glasses, or possibly a patch. If an eye appears to 'turn', a test is essential to decide whether treatment is needed.

Q ***If I take my child to the optometrist, will glasses always be prescribed?***

A No, the optometrist will only prescribe glasses to improve your child's vision or to ensure proper development of the eyes. Some children will need to do eye exercises to improve the function of their eyes. In some cases, the optometrist will just give advice on eye care.

Q ***Why is it important to have my child's eyes tested before she starts school?***

A Unless a child can see properly, she is unlikely to fulfil her full potential at school. Research has shown that there is a correlation between difficulties with reading and poor co-ordination of the eyes.

NURSING A SICK CHILD

All children are ill at some stage in their lives, some more often than others. Fortunately, most illnesses are not serious and can be treated at home without the help of a doctor.

You will probably know when your child is ill – he is likely to be off-colour, off his food and may be listless, irritable and more demanding than usual. He may have a fever, complain of pain, vomit or have diarrhoea. While he is feeling unwell, his behaviour may become more babyish than usual and he will probably want help with things that he can usually do for himself.

Plenty of rest

Unless your doctor advises otherwise, or your child wants to go to bed, let him rest on the sofa. This way he won't feel too lonely and will be reassured by being near you or your partner. You should dress him in light, loose, comfortable clothes.

When to call the doctor

Contact your doctor if your child has any of these symptoms:

- **Temperature:** if it is above 37.5°C (100°F) or below 35°C (95°F) for more than 24 hours.
- **Vomiting:** if it occurs more than twice in six hours or if it is yellow/green or bloodstained.
- **Diarrhoea:** if this occurs for over 48 hours or contains blood.
- **Pain:** if there is a persistent headache, particularly if it is accompanied by blurred vision, nausea or severe abdominal pain.
- **Difficulty breathing:** if this occurs with sharp drawing in of the ribs and noisy, rapid breathing.
- **Loss of appetite:** particularly if your child refuses food for 24 hours and seems lethargic.
- **Rash:** if a rash appears over a few hours or there are purple spots that don't fade when pressed by a glass.

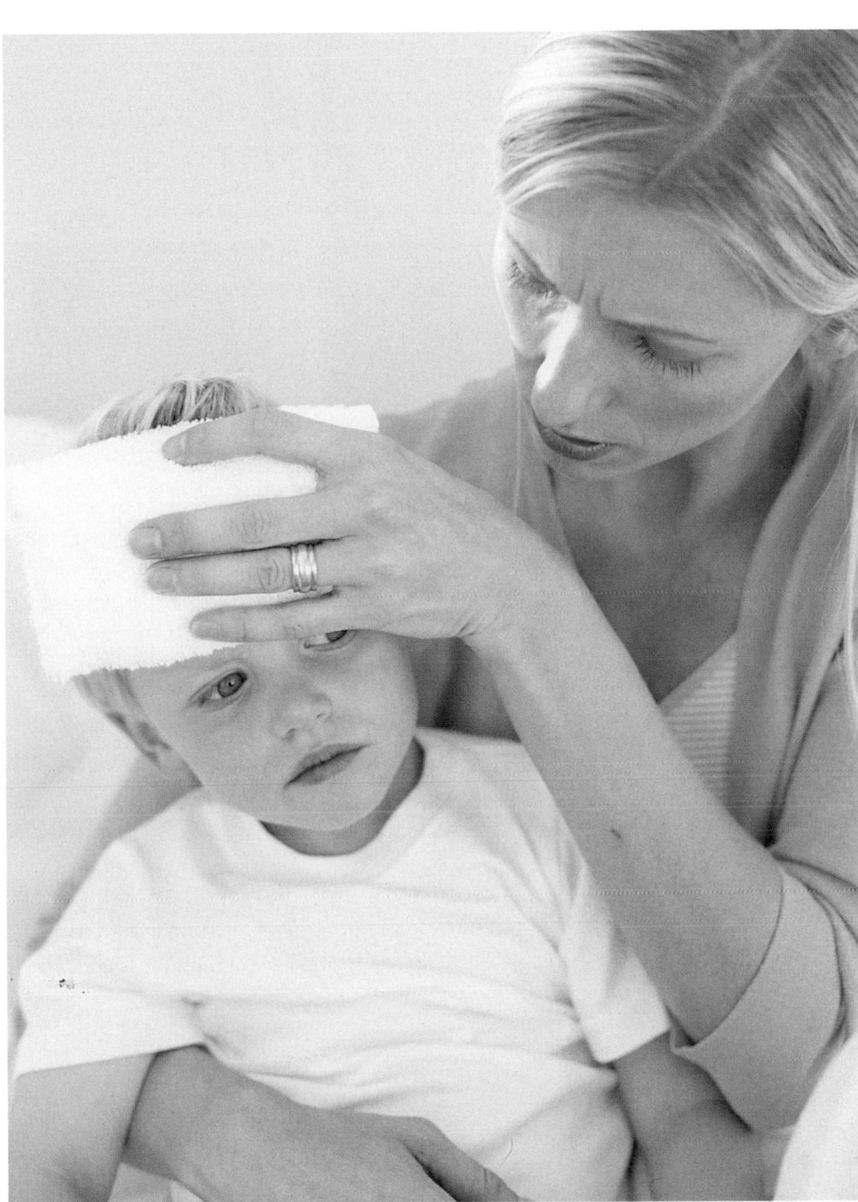

If your child is ill, he is likely to 'regress' and become irritable and demanding. He will need to be kept comfortable, warm and well hydrated and will require lots of love and attention.

Make sure that you keep the room warm, but not too hot, and well ventilated.

Ill children tend to become dehydrated quite quickly, and should be encouraged to drink plenty. You can offer your child something to eat, but if he has lost his appetite just concentrate on maintaining his fluid intake for now.

Once your child is feeling better, you will need to find some gentle activities to occupy his time. Read him stories, or let him listen to tapes of nursery rhymes and stories, or watch a favourite video. Provide materials for quiet play – for example, colouring-in books and crayons, play-dough and jigsaws. Playing doctors and nurses with teddies and dolls may also help your child to understand he is ill and make him less fearful of being nursed.

Raised temperature

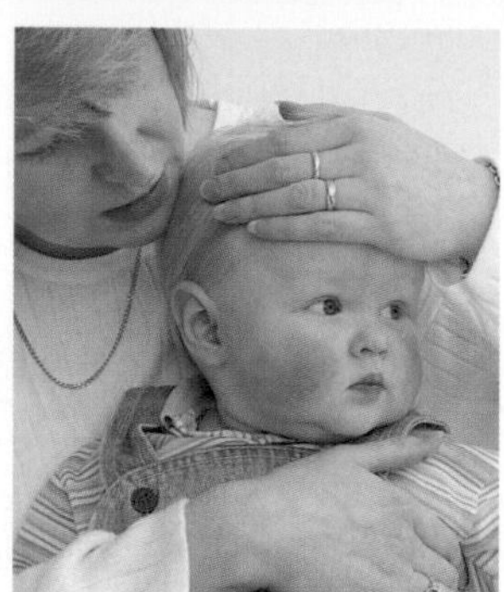

High temperature: a high temperature is a sign that your child's immune system is fighting infection. Check for other signs of illness. If his temperature is above 37.5°C (100°F), he has a fever.

A high temperature can give your child a flushed, 'feverish' look, and he can feel hot to the touch.

Fever: symptoms include feeling hot or cold, headache, dizziness and a rapid pulse. Monitor his temperature and ensure he is drinking. See your GP if his fever exceeds 39.5°C (103°F) or lasts more than 24 hours, or if he is vomiting floppy and unresponsive.

Febrile convulsions: these can occur when your child's temperature rises rapidly. Symptoms include rigidity and twitching.

Pain and temperature control: sponge your child with tepid water. Liquid paracetamol and ibuprofen are safe for children over six months of age. Avoid ibuprofen if your child is vomiting. Never give aspirin.

Sore throat and a cold

Sore throat: most sore throats are caused by viral infections and will disappear within five days. You can nurse your child at home by giving regular liquid paracetamol or ibuprofen and offering frequent sips of cold fluid. Lozenges and ice-cream may be soothing. Seek medical advice if the sore throat lasts for longer than five days, there are spots, discharge or swelling on the tonsils or at the back of the throat, or swallowing or breathing difficulties.

Colds: a cold is a common childhood ailment, spread by tiny droplets of virus in the air passed on by sneezing. Symptoms include a runny nose, sore throat and sneezing. Your child may also have a cough – warm honey and lemon drinks tend to be just as soothing as an over-the-counter remedy. Seek medical advice if the cough persists for over a week or there are breathing difficulties.

It's important to keep an ill child hydrated, giving fluids little and often.

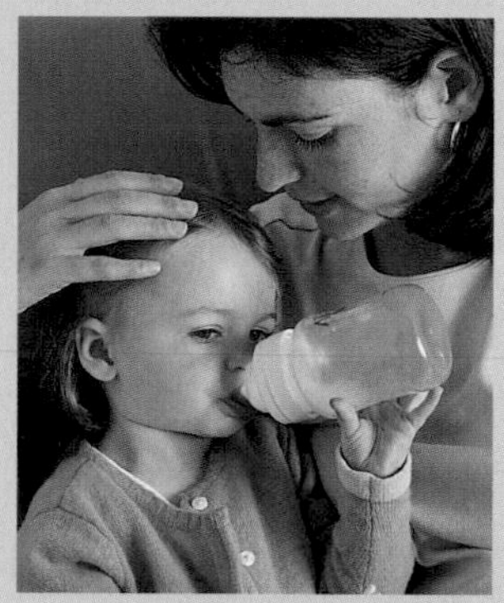

Earache

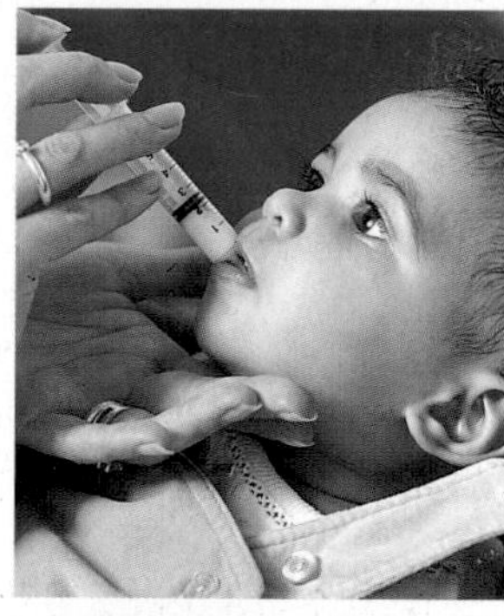

It is common for young children to have earache, but it is not always caused by an ear infection. The nerve supply to the ear is shared with the throat and upper jaw and teeth, so problems there can often be felt in the ear. During a cold, or sometimes with nasal allergies, such as hayfever, the tube that connects the middle ear to the throat becomes congested, causing tension in the eardrum as it is sucked in or pushed out. This in turn can cause an earache. Most of these cases are caused by viruses and do not respond to antibiotics. If you suspect your baby has an ear infection, take him to the doctor on a same-day appointment.

With children, the majority of earaches settle in 24 hours. If the earache carries on for longer, or a discharge flows out of the ear, seek medical advice. Liquid paracetamol or ibuprofen can relieve pain and treat a fever.

Liquid paracetamol can help to soothe some of the symptoms of earache and is easy to swallow.

Chickenpox

Chickenpox is a common, mild viral infection that most children have had by the age of 10. The virus is spread by airborne droplets. It is not usually serious but in very rare cases it can lead to encephalitis (brain inflammation).

If your child has chickenpox, spots will appear, mainly in crops, over three to four days. These change to blisters and crust over. She will have a slight fever, appear unwell and may have a headache. Chickenpox is highly contagious. The incubation period is 12–21 days.

To nurse your child at home, give liquid paracetamol or ibuprofen for a fever and plenty to drink. Never give aspirin as this can cause complications. To soothe the itching, apply calamine lotion, or give a tepid bath with a cup of bicarbonate of soda or oatmeal added. Discourage scratching as it can cause scarring.

Calamine lotion can help to relieve the itching and prevent scratching.

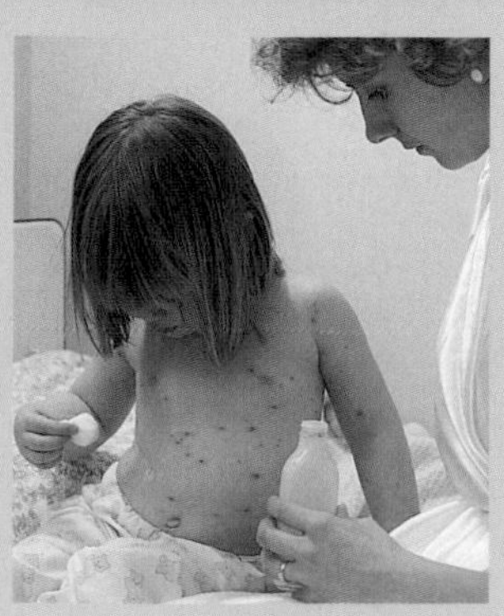

ATTENDING A FIRST-AID COURSE

BECOMING A FIRST AIDER

Children are adventurous by nature, and the younger they are the less idea they have of the risks of being injured.

If your child has an accident, it is vital that you remain calm and take the appropriate steps to ensure his wellbeing until, in more serious cases, the emergency services arrive. A first-aid course will provide you with the knowledge and the confidence to cope should an accident occur.

If you are a parent or carer of a child, a first-aid course designed for the care of babies and children is highly recommended. These courses teach you invaluable skills, which could help you to save a child's life.

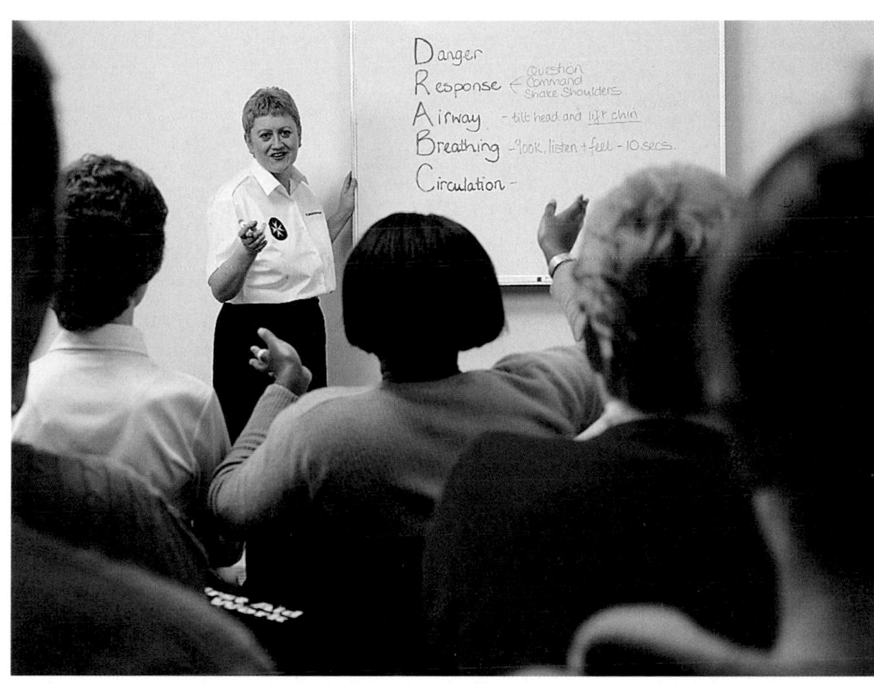

Where to attend a course

The three main organisations that run first-aid courses are the British Red Cross Society, St John Ambulance and, in Scotland only, the St Andrew's Ambulance Association. Some commercial organisations also offer courses.

- You can become a qualified first aider by attending a four-day course, then passing a theoretical and practical exam. You will receive a certificate which is valid for three years, after which time you must attend a two-day refresher course.
- Some organisations run basic courses that concentrate on first aid for children. Although you won't be recognised as a qualified first aider, you will learn many invaluable first-aid skills to help your child in an emergency situation.
- If you decide to attend a course run by a commercial organisation, check that it has either been licensed by the Health and Safety Executive or that its teachers have been professionally trained. Many run courses specifically for parents and childminders.

What you will learn

A first-aid course designed especially for the care of children and infants will teach you how to react in many medical emergencies. It provides hands-on practice, using resuscitation dummies and you will be shown how treatments and techniques vary between babies and children. The first-aid methods you will be taught should include:

- Checking for consciousness.
- Resuscitation techniques.
- The recovery position.
- What to do when a child has an asthma attack.
- Treating burns and scalds.
- How to break an electrical circuit safely.
- Treating a child who has swallowed a poison.
- Dealing with bleeding, from deep wounds to nose-bleeds.
- How to ensure your own safety.

The basic rules

Even if you do not have first-aid training, there may be something you can do to help an accident victim. Always follow these basic rules.

1 Make sure you do not endanger yourself when attending the accident victim.

2 Use your common sense and don't panic.

3 Do not move a child who may have injured her neck or back.

4 Place an unconscious, breathing person in the recovery position unless you suspect a neck injury.

5 When putting a pregnant woman in the recovery position, place her on her left side – this has been shown to be safer for the unborn child.

6 If you are in any doubt about the severity of the problem, get medical help as soon as possible.

7 Do not attempt to do too much yourself. Instead, contact the emergency services.

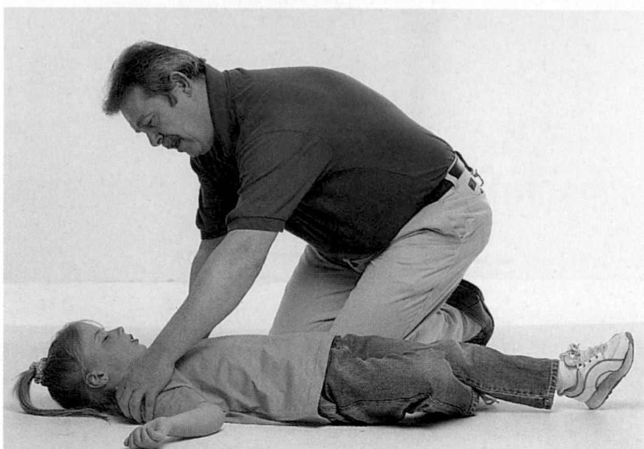

If your child does become unconscious, gently shake her to check for any response. If she is still breathing, place her in the recovery position and contact the emergency services.

Sensible safeguards for your child

As the majority of childhood accidents happen in the home, take steps to make sure your home is as safe as possible:

- Place a fixed guard around any fires, whether open, gas or electric.
- Keep all cleaning fluids locked away.
- Fit safety sockets to all unused power points.
- Never leave an iron that is in use unattended. Always keep a hot iron out of your child's reach.
- Fit a safety gate to the top and bottom of the stairs.
- Place a hob guard around your cooker and fit a safety catch to the oven door.
- Make sure that you have a well stocked first-aid box, both in your home and in your car.
- Keep all medicines out of your child's reach.
- Keep all plastic bags and sharp objects safely out of reach.

To further reduce the risk of accidents:

- Don't allow your baby to pick up small, hard objects, such as beads and nuts, on which he may choke.
- Don't give your baby or child nuts, toffees or chewing gum as they might stick in the throat.
- Don't allow a child to move about with anything hard in his mouth.
- Teach your child the safety drill for crossing the road as early as possible.

First-aid organisations

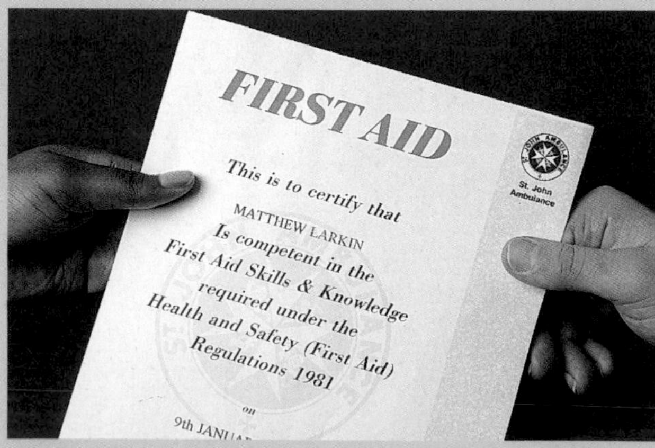

A first-aid certificate is valid for three years. When it expires you will need to attend a refresher first-aid course in order to renew it.

The three main organisations have local branches throughout the country (the St Andrew's Ambulance Association in Scotland only). Contact the organisations, listed below, to find out about your local branch.

St John Ambulance
27 St John's Lane,
London EC1M 4BU
Tel: 0870 010 4950
Fax: 0870 010 4065
www.sja.org.uk

The British Red Cross
9 Grosvenor Crescent,
London SW1X 7EJ
Tel: 020 7235 5454
Fax: 020 7245 6315
www.redcross.org.uk

St Andrew's Ambulance Association
St Andrew's House
48 Milton Street
Glasgow G4 OHR
Tel: 0141 332 4031
Fax: 0141 332 6582
www.firstaid.org.uk

Chapter Two
Common Complaints

ALLERGIES

WHAT ARE ALLERGIES?

An allergy is a disorder in which the body becomes hyper-sensitive to a particular allergen. Allergies include hayfever (allergic rhinitis) and allergy-induced asthma.

- Allergies can develop in the first few months of life, and it is not uncommon for symptoms to start in babies as young as six months. Generally, however, allergies first develop in the second year. After this, attacks become increasingly frequent.

- Allergies have become considerably more common over the last 20 years. It is now estimated that between 20 and 25 per cent of children suffer from an allergy.

- Unfortunately, only around 10 per cent of children with allergies grow out of them. This normally occurs around the age of puberty. In the majority of cases, the allergy persists, but often in a less severe form.

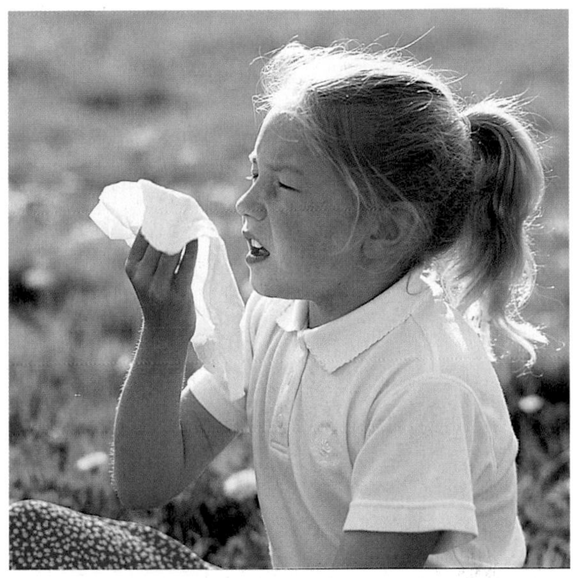

Allergies such as hayfever are becoming more commonplace, with a large percentage of children suffering from them. These allergies occasionally subside around puberty.

Why have allergies increased?

Since humans have not changed in any identifiable way during the last 20 years, it is thought that environmental or lifestyle factors must be responsible for the increase in allergies.

- **East and West:** one theory was developed from observations made after the unification of East and West Germany. After the unification, the rate of allergies among poorer East Germans increased as they moved to the industrialised West. It appears that something in the Western lifestyle may be responsible.

- **The Hygiene Theory:** this theory claims that cleanliness and the use of antibiotics to control minor infections has led to the immune system being less exposed to challenges. This, in turn, has made it unable to develop responses that protect against allergies. The theory is boosted by the fact that three groups of children who are exposed to more infectious agents than others have fewer allergies: children living on farms; children who are the youngest of three or more siblings; and children who regularly attend daycare centres.

- **Urban areas:** the Hygiene Theory does not fully explain the rise in allergies, however, because urban children, who are likely to be exposed to infectious agents frequently, now have more allergies. In such cases it is thought that air pollution, in particular from tobacco smoke and diesel fumes, is likely to be responsible. No link has yet been proved with other environmental pollutants.

Allergy symptoms

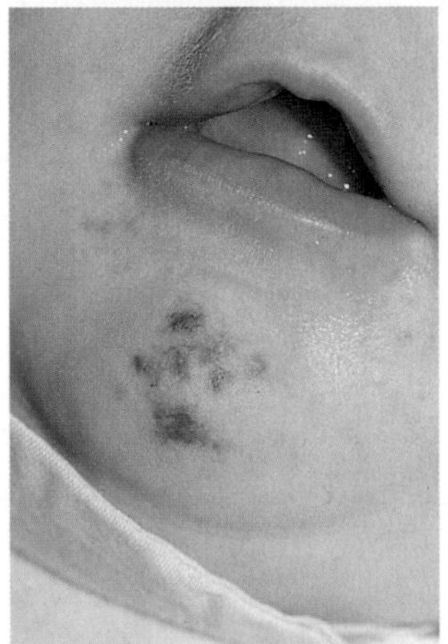

The precise symptoms of an allergy depend on the nature of the allergen and the strength of the allergic response.

- Allergy symptoms are caused, in the first instance, by the release of histamine by the body to combat what the immune system identifies, incorrectly, as a threat.

Allergic eczema causes skin rashes, which can itch. The sufferer is likely to scratch or rub the affected area and exacerbate the condition.

- The range of symptoms is wide. Hayfever, for example, is likely to cause an itchy, stuffy nose, itchy, red eyes and a watery nasal discharge, with bouts of sneezing occurring intermittently.

- These symptoms may also be present in allergic asthma, with the addition of shortness of breath, tightness of the chest and wheezing.

- Other allergies, such as allergic eczema and urticaria, can cause skin rashes, which often itch. These rashes can occur on specific parts of the body or all over it.

What to do if your child has an allergy

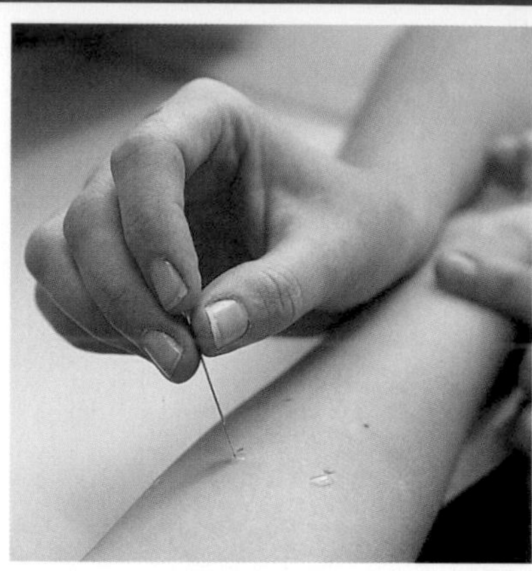

The most important step is to identify what your child is allergic to and take steps to avoid it.

1 The best way to identify an allergy is to keep a diary, noting what your child eats, what possible environmental allergens she is exposed to and when any symptoms appear. A pattern may emerge to reveal the allergen responsible.

A scratch test – when an allergen is scratched on to the skin – can be carried out to discover the cause of an allergy.

2 Ask your GP to refer your child to an allergy clinic. A skin test may be performed to check the cause of her allergy.

3 Thereafter, all possible steps should be taken to keep your child away from the allergen. Medication, e.g. an antihistamine, may be prescribed for use if your child does come into contact with it.

Desensitisation

Desensitisation therapy is a last-resort treatment for long-term allergies, but it is not without its dangers.

- Hyposensitisation involves injecting allergens in increasing doses beneath the skin of an allergy sufferer over a period of about 10 weeks. The therapy is usually successful, but has to be repeated every four or five years. However, there is a slight risk that the patient will go into anaphylactic shock, which is potentially fatal, so the treatment is confined to just a few specialist centres in this country.
- Neutralisation involves either injecting or placing drops of allergen beneath the tongue in decreasing dilutions until there is no allergic reaction – this is known as the 'neutralising dose'. The allergy sufferer takes two or three drops a day of this dose.
- Enzyme-potentiated desensitisation (EPD) is an allergy treatment that has a success rate of about 50 per cent. It is more widely available than other desensitisation treatments, but has to be repeated each year for up to five years. Various different allergens are mixed with an enzyme – which is a substance that helps chemical reactions take place – and injected beneath the skin.

Are allergies preventable?

Allergies cannot realistically be prevented from developing, but they can be delayed if the sufferer effectively avoids the allergens.

- A tendency to allergies (atopy) is inherited. If one parent has an allergy, there is a 30–35 per cent chance that the child will develop an allergy; if both parents have allergies, the chances increase to 50–60 per cent. If a parent is atopic, special precautions can be taken to reduce the risk of the child being exposed to the allergen. This reduces the chances of the child becoming sensitised to the allergen.
- There is no direct evidence that what you eat during pregnancy can induce allergy in your child. However, it is known that the children of mothers who smoke during pregnancy actually have a higher chance of developing allergic asthma.
- Breast-feeding for the first year helps to prevent allergies, but only if the mother avoids eating foods that can cause allergies (allergens), such as dairy products and peanuts.
- If there is a strong family history of allergies, ask your GP to refer your baby to an allergy clinic or dietitian. Certain foods may need to be excluded from his diet for up to two years. Alternative foods, vitamins and minerals may be necessary.
- Keep your child away from animals – cats in particular. Don't use bedding that contains down. If possible, use 'anti-allergy' bedding.
- Do not smoke in the house or near to your child. Smoking sensitises the immune system to allergens.
- Vacuum regularly, using a machine with a fine filter, and dust frequently.
- Keep humidity low, below 35 per cent if possible (humidity meters can be bought cheaply).

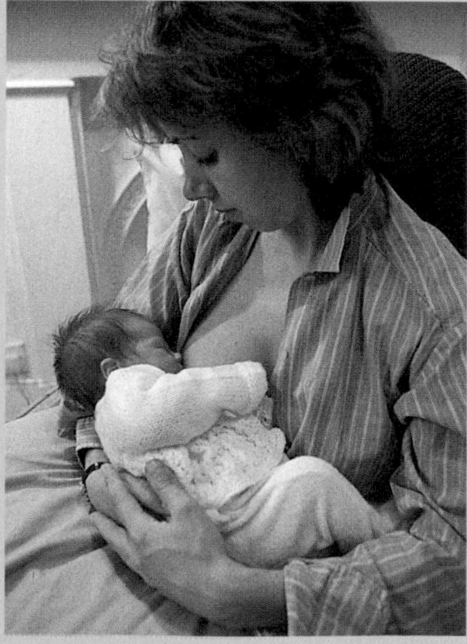

Breast-feeding can help to prevent allergies in babies, but only if the mother takes care to avoid allergy-inducing foods.

APPENDICITIS

WHAT IS APPENDICITIS?

The appendix is a small, thin outpouching of the large intestine, about the size and shape of your child's little finger. It lies in the lower right side of the stomach and it is not thought to have any function. Appendicitis is inflammation of the appendix.

- Normally the liquid contents of the intestine pass into and out of the appendix quite freely. However, sometimes the narrow mouth of the appendix becomes blocked either by a hard piece of faecal matter or swelling of the tiny 'lymph follicles' in the intestinal wall.

- When the appendix is blocked, faecal substances get trapped inside and the appendix becomes inflamed and swollen. This swelling is made worse by the action of the millions of bacteria that are present. Eventually the appendix may burst, allowing bacteria to enter the abdominal cavity, and cause peritonitis, which is a serious infection.

- Most cases of appendicitis occur in children aged between six and 10. Appendicitis is uncommon in the under-fives and rare in infants of less than two years. Appendicitis is more serious in young children because the appendix has often burst by the time a doctor operates to remove it.

- You cannot prevent your child getting appendicitis, although it may be linked with a diet low in fibre.

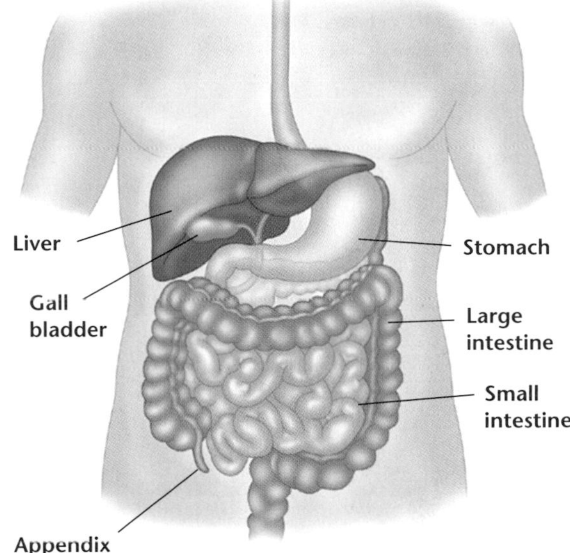

The appendix is a short thin tube attached to the intestine. It has no known function and can become inflamed and swollen.

Signs and symptoms

Appendicitis is difficult to diagnose as the symptoms may be present in other conditions, but look out for the following:

- **Stomach pains:** these may start as a constant, dull ache in the region of the tummy button; later this may worsen and move to the lower right side of the abdomen.

- **Nausea:** with or without vomiting.

- **Loss of appetite:** your child may lose his appetite and refuse food.

- **A fever:** this will be low grade at first, but will increase if the appendix bursts and infection spreads within the abdominal cavity.

- **Constipation or diarrhoea:** the infected appendix can irritate the neighbouring intestine.

- **Tenderness:** pressing gently on the tummy, especially on the lower right, may identify a sore area; the tummy may even feel hard as the muscles contract to protect the painful area.

- **Frequent urination:** irritation of the bladder by an inflamed appendix may make your child want to pass urine more frequently than usual.

Diagnosing appendicitis

When you take your child to your GP, the doctor will try to diagnose whether your child has appendicitis.

- The doctor will ask you about your child's symptoms, particularly about the pain. Encourage your child to tell you how she feels while the doctor listens.

- The doctor will need to feel your child's tummy gently while she is lying down. This may hurt if there is inflammation, so don't tell her that it won't hurt and be ready to comfort her.

- The doctor may want to take a sample of urine from your child to check for a bladder infection.

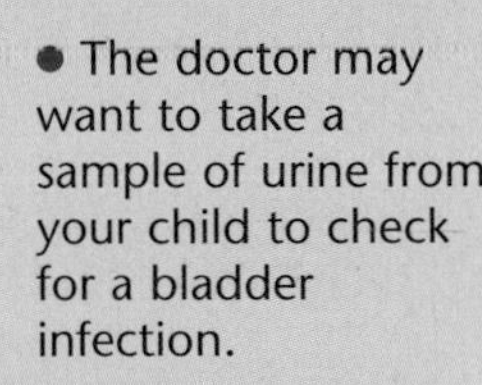

- If appendicitis is suspected, you will be asked to take your child to the hospital. The doctors there will make the final decision and decide whether or not to operate.

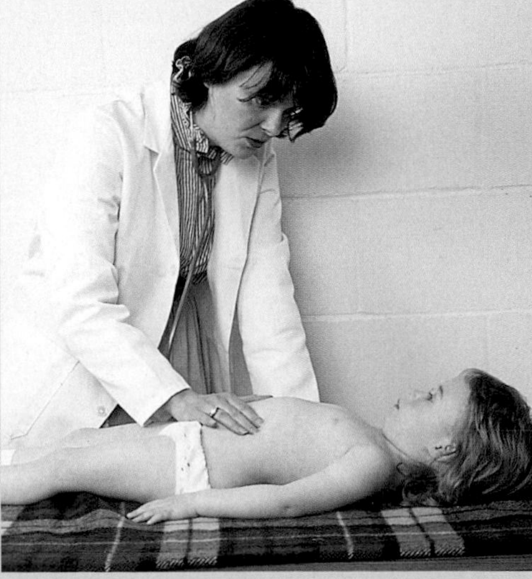

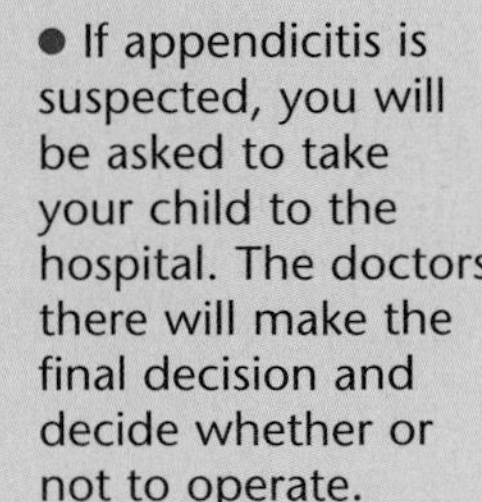

Appendicitis is a condition that can be difficult to diagnose. A doctor will feel your child's tummy gently while asking her questions.

Dos and Don'ts

If you have any reason to suspect that your child has appendicitis, you must seek medical help straightaway.

✔ Do keep your child cool by sponging him with tepid water, if there is a fever.

✔ Do act quickly and seek urgent medical advice, if necessary by going to the accident and emergency department of your hospital.

✘ Don't give anything to ease the pain, as the location and severity of the pain are important clues in the diagnosis of appendicitis.

✘ Don't give your child anything at all to eat or drink in case he needs an operation.

Treatment of appendicitis

The only sure way of treating appendicitis is to remove the appendix, in an operation known as an 'appendicectomy'. This is usually a straightforward operation.

- There are two ways to do an appendicectomy. The first is the 'open' method, which involves an incision, or cut, in the tummy. The second is 'keyhole' surgery, where a telescope is used and only two very small cuts are needed. The doctor will discuss with you which is the most suitable.
- In either case your child will be given a general anaesthetic and so will be asleep during the surgery.
- During the operation the appendix will be removed and then the wounds stitched up again.
- Your child will probably be given some antibiotics to kill any infection, especially if the appendix has burst because this can be dangerous.

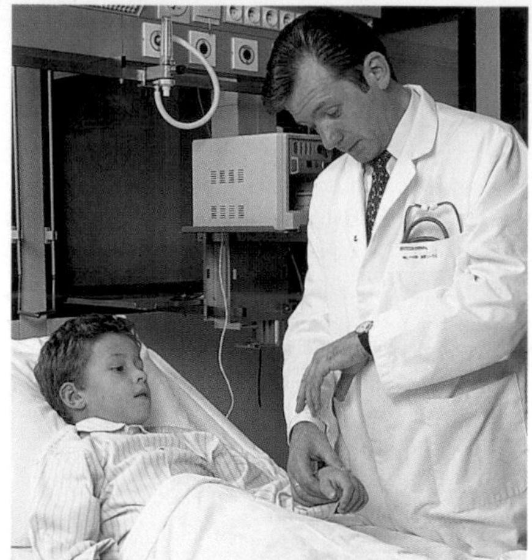

The removal of the appendix is a simple operation, but your child will be monitored closely in hospital.

Recovery in hospital

After surgery your child will probably be in hospital for three to five days, depending on how quickly he recovers. You will be encouraged to stay with him.

- Any general anaesthetic can leave a child feeling a little forgetful, tearful and 'groggy' for around 24 hours.
- Your child may have a 'drip' in his arm to give him fluid.
- A tube may be coming out of the skin near the wound to help drain tissue fluids from under the skin.
- The wound may be held together with clips or stitches and will be covered with a dressing, which the nurses will change regularly.
- Your child may need some mild painkillers to help with discomfort.
- Your child will be up and about fairly soon, probably just climbing gently out of bed on the first day and spending much of the second day up.
- He should pass urine within 12 hours, but may not have a bowel movement for two to three days.

Recovery at home

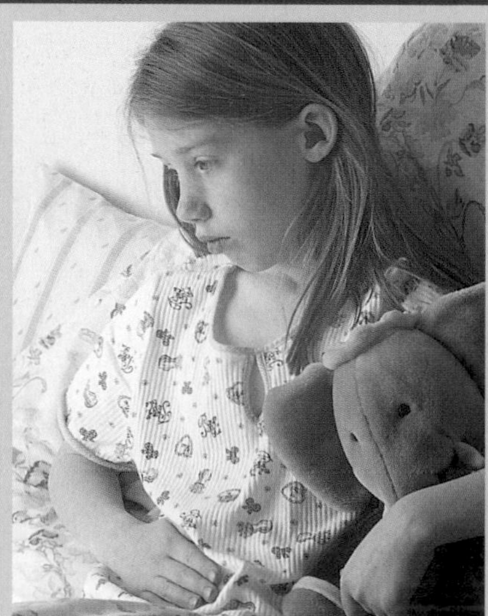

Young children usually get better from an appendicectomy quite quickly, although the recovery time may be longer after a burst appendix. Your child will be back to normal in about six weeks.

1 The wound can be gently cleaned in the shower or bath, using just soap and water.

2 You can expect your child to be tired for a week or two as a result of the surgery. She will perhaps need more daytime naps than she did before.

Your child will take a few weeks to recover from an appendicectomy. Contact your doctor if your child is in any pain or if there is redness or discharge from the wound.

3 In two weeks your child may go back to nursery or school, although she must not be allowed to lift anything heavy or be involved in 'rough and tumble' play for another two weeks.

4 When you leave the hospital you will be told about arrangements for removing the stitches and any follow-up treatment.

5 The wound should heal fairly quickly, although it may look bruised for a time.

ASTHMA IN CHILDREN

WHAT IS ASTHMA?

Asthma is a condition that causes the airways in the lungs to become narrow and inflamed, making breathing difficult. Approximately one in seven children in the UK have symptoms of asthma that require treatment. In the majority of children, asthma causes nothing more serious than mild wheezing as air is squeezed in and out and, as long as they are receiving treatment, they can lead normal lives. However, severe cases must be kept under control or it can be fatal.

What causes it?

The causes are unknown, although scientists have found a possible asthma gene. It is more common in families who suffer from allergies, and if you or your partner have asthma, the likelihood of your child developing it is greater. People with asthma have lungs that are particularly sensitive to certain triggers, which range from common allergens, such as pet hairs, smoke or pollen, to changes in air temperature, exercise or colds.

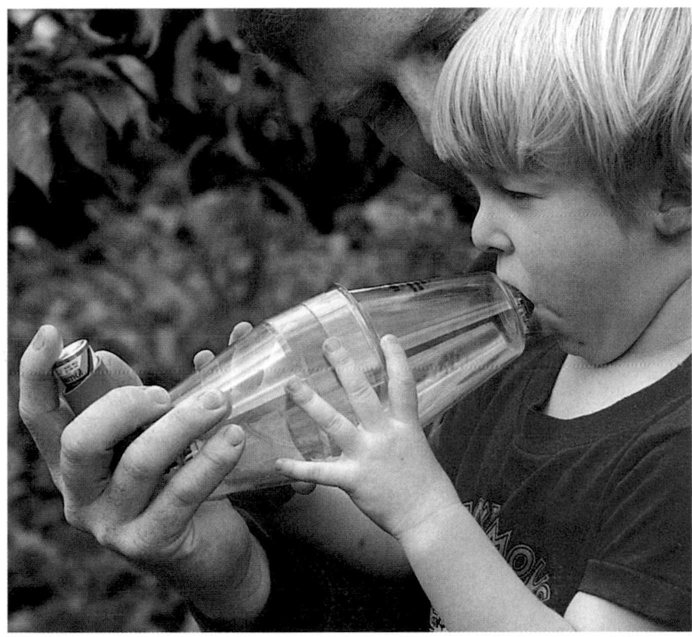

Young children often have difficulty using an inhaler, and may be given a large plastic container called a spacer instead. It has a mouthpiece at one end and a hole at the other end for an inhaler.

How to help your child

To help keep your child's asthma under control, try to take the following measures:

✔ **Do keep rooms well ventilated:** also deal with any damp spots (mould spores can be a trigger).
✔ **Do let your child exercise:** it will help strengthen her body, keep her fit, build confidence and counteract stress.
✔ **Do provide a healthy diet:** also watch out for food allergies and intolerances (main culprits are nuts, wheat and dairy products).
✔ **Do be aware of stress:** starting playschool or school, the death of a pet, or even a new baby in the family can make the symptoms worse.
✘ **Don't smoke:** even a child who doesn't have asthma is more likely to develop it if one or both parents smoke.
✘ **Don't keep furry or feathery pets:** this may make your child's asthma worse.
✘ **Don't let your house be a haven for dust mites:** vacuum and use a damp cloth to wipe away dust frequently, wash your child's bed linen and soft toys often, and replace curtains and carpets, which harbour mites, with blinds and bare boards.

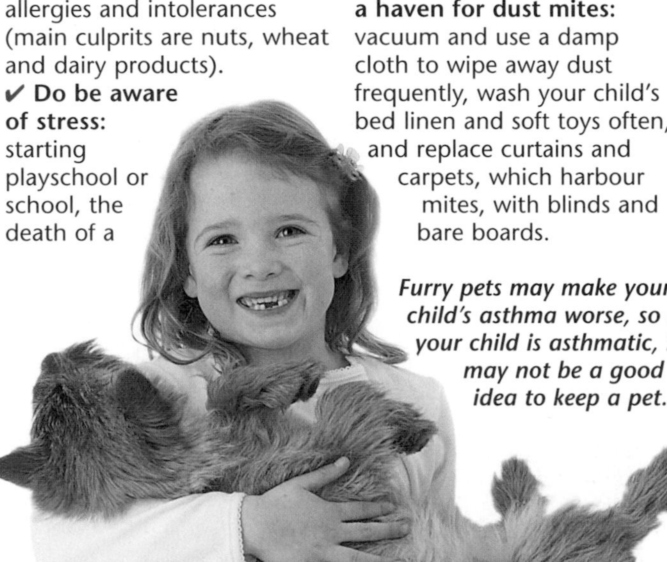

Furry pets may make your child's asthma worse, so if your child is asthmatic, it may not be a good idea to keep a pet.

Symptoms

A child may have asthma if he:

- Coughs, particularly during the night or after exercise.
- Wheezes or produces a whistling or hissing noise from his chest.
- Is frequently short of breath, especially after exercise (he may avoid exertion and frequently ask to be carried).
- Complains of a 'tightness' in his chest.

How is asthma diagnosed?

Around 30 per cent of children up to the age of five experience wheezing and yet the majority of those will not go on to develop asthma. Other illnesses, such as acute bronchitis, can produce similar symptoms, making it difficult to diagnose.

- Measuring a child's lung function is a problem. In adults, a device called a peak flow measure is used, but this is not suitable for children under six years of age.
- Your GP may wish to observe your child's symptoms over a period of time before deciding whether he has asthma. You may be asked to keep a record of your child's symptoms to see whether any pattern is developing.

What treatment is available?

Although there is no cure for asthma, a range of treatments can control it quite effectively. These work in two ways: preventers calm down inflammation in the lungs, which reduces the chance of an attack; relievers act quickly to open the airways in the event of an attack.

When your child is diagnosed as asthmatic, your GP may ask you to keep a record of potential triggers, in order to avoid or reduce contact with them. Your GP may also prescribe one or both types of medicine – a reliever (or bronchodilator) and/or a preventer (corticosteroid or steroid).

Preventers and relievers

- **Preventers:** these work by reducing the swelling and inflammation of the airways, so that they are less likely to react badly when they come in contact with a trigger. Your child will usually be asked to take his preventer twice a day in the morning and the evening to protect the airways and to prevent attacks.

  It may take up to two weeks before he begins to notice an improvement in his symptoms. Although preventers usually contain steroids, the dose is so low that there are no side effects. If your child's asthma is severe, he may be prescribed a short course of steroid tablets.

- **Relievers:** these are taken only when your child has trouble breathing (or when he anticipates having trouble, such as before exercise). They work very quickly to relax the muscles surrounding the airways. This makes breathing instantly easier, but has no affect on inflammation in the airways.

Taking the medicine

Relievers and preventers are usually given via an inhaler or 'puffer', which your child breathes directly into his lungs. This method is very effective as the medicine is delivered to the area affected and very little is absorbed into the bloodstream.

- However, inhalers can be difficult for young children to use, so normally a device called a spacer is used. This is a large plastic container with a mouthpiece at one end and a hole at the other end for the inhaler to fit in (if your child is under three years, he may need to wear a face mask, too).
- The inhaler is pressed once, the medicine is released into the spacer, and your child breathes in and out to the count of 10.

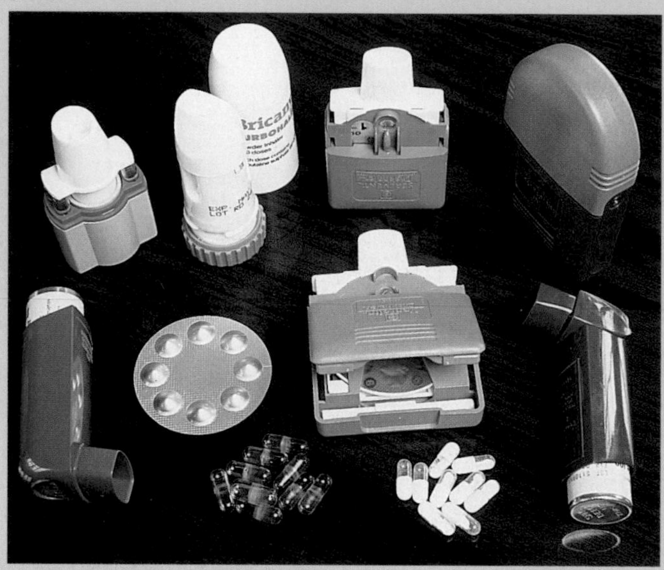

A selection of inhalers for treating asthma; spinhalers or turbohalers; disc inhaler; aerosol inhalers; disc with eight capsules together with capsules containing drugs.

What to do in an attack

An attack may occur when your child's asthma has worsened over time and is no longer easily controlled by inhalers. It can be very frightening, so it's important for you to stay calm and reassure him.

- Give your child his reliever. Sit him in an upright position and encourage him to breathe slowly and calmly.
- The reliever should work within five to 10 minutes but if there is no sign of improvement, or if your child is extremely distressed or exhausted, or has blue lips, call an ambulance. Continue to give the reliever every few minutes until help arrives.

Useful addresses

National Asthma Campaign
Providence House
Providence Place
London N1 0NT
Helpline: 0845 701 0203
www.asthma.org.uk

Action Against Allergy
PO Box 278
Twickenham TW1 4QQ
Tel: 020 8892 2711
E-mail: AAA@actionagainstallergy.freeserve.co.uk

ATTENTION DEFICIT DISORDER

WHAT IS ATTENTION DEFICIT DISORDER?

Attention deficit disorder (ADD) is a behavioural disorder characterised by excessive activity. Most children are easily distracted and often fidgety, but in ADD sufferers these traits are so pronounced that they can make learning and education virtually impossible.

ADD sufferers often have difficulty making friends because they have a tendency to interrupt games and conversations. As children, they will always be easily distracted and forgetful, yet many grow into perfectly 'normal' adults, with good jobs and social lives. Hyperactivity is often associated with ADD. The hyperactive form of ADD is known as Attention Deficit Hyperactivity Disorder, or ADHD.

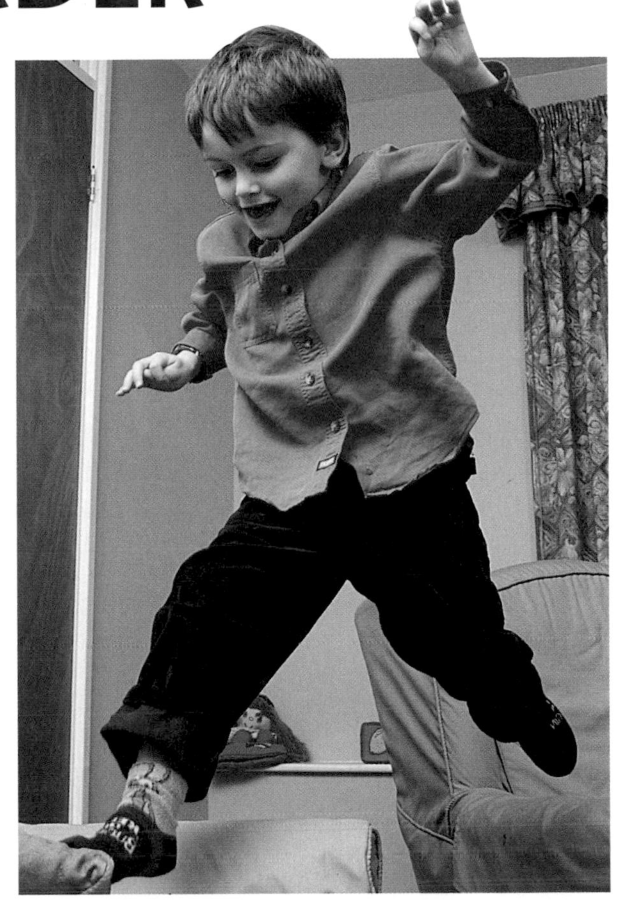

A child who is excessively active and finds it hard to concentrate may have attention deficit disorder. The condition is found in three times as many boys as girls.

What causes ADD?

There are two main reasons why young children can suffer from attention deficit disorder:

1 Scientists have noted that abnormal amounts of certain chemicals (dopamine, serotonin or norepinephrine) can result in ADD-like symptoms. The release of these chemicals is controlled by enzymes, so ADD sufferers probably have an enzyme which is not functioning as it should. There is also some evidence of a genetic link.

2 Food intolerance is sometimes implicated and, although it cannot cause ADD, it may aggravate the symptoms. If you notice that your child's behaviour deteriorates after eating a certain type of food, for example, food containing tartrazine, try excluding it for a week or two to see if there is any improvement.

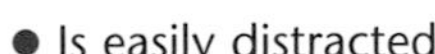

Symptoms

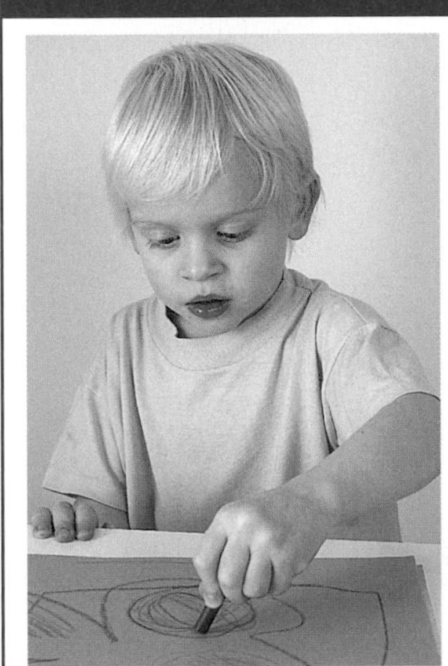

A child with true ADD will display at least eight of the following symptoms consistently for at least six months, before the age of seven:

- Is easily distracted
- Never sits still
- Is always fidgeting
- Has poor concentration
- Rarely waits his turn in games
- Blurts out answers to questions whether right or wrong
- Has difficulty following instructions
- Is chronically inattentive
- Rarely completes a task before starting another
- Has difficulty playing quietly
- Talks incessantly
- Often interrupts
- Doesn't listen properly
- Demonstrates reckless, risk-taking behaviour

A child with ADD may often play alone because he has difficulty making friends with other children. He may frustrate other children by frequently interrupting games and conversations and by not understanding that he has to wait his turn.

NOTE: some children develop ADD-like symptoms following a trauma, such as bereavement, moving home or school, illness or even the arrival of a new baby sister or brother. Such psychological reactions may need professional attention, but they are not caused by ADD.

How is ADD diagnosed?

If your child's behaviour fits the criteria listed overleaf, consult his nursery or school to find out whether he displays similar behaviour patterns there, as well as at home. If so, you will need to consult your GP.

- Your GP can refer your child to a paediatrician, child psychologist or psychiatrist, who will need to confirm that your child is suffering from ADD. Your GP may be involved in prescribing medication.

- Be aware that although acceptance and understanding of ADD is on the increase, a few GPs are still doubtful about its existence. Parents may even find themselves under suspicion for 'causing' their child's symptoms by the way they are bringing him up.

- Questions about your home life may be necessary in order to establish whether your child is simply reacting to a trauma.

- The specialist may test your child for a whole range of conditions with similar symptoms.

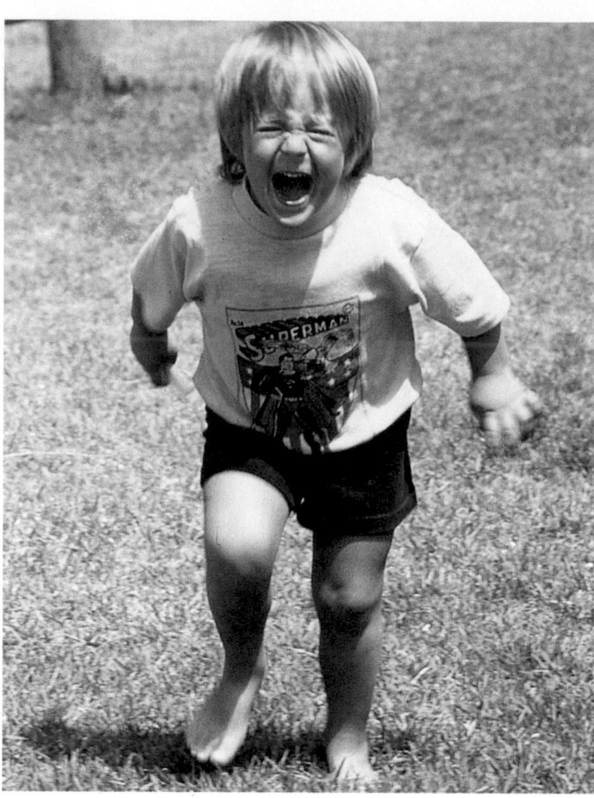

ADD can be very frustrating for a child, leading to frequent temper tantrums. All toddlers have tantrums but a child with ADD will experience them for longer.

How is ADD treated?

Once ADD is diagnosed, your child may be put on medication, which will help to control but not cure the condition.

- At school, your child should have access to teachers who fully understand ADD. Ideally, a network of care should be available, including counselling for parents.

- The availability of treatment and care can vary according to where you live.

- Different drugs and dosages may be tried in order to find out which is most effective for your child's particular condition.

- However, medication should be used only as a supplement to behavioural therapy and parental support.

Useful address

If you require support and advice, contact:

ADD/ADHD Family Support Group
1a High Street, Dirton Marsh,
Westbury, Wilts BA13 4DL
Tel: 01373 826045

Coping with ADD at home

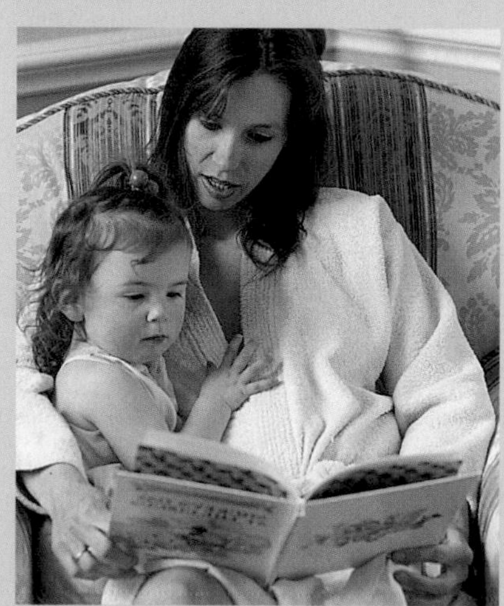

It is important that you try to carry out a normal, everyday routine with an ADD child. This will give her security and help her focus on certain activities.

The following methods can all be used to help a child who has attention deficit disorder:

- **Routine:** develop a simple daily routine that includes activities such as washing and dressing at a regular time each day. This may seem impossible with an ADD child, but persevere. Encourage your child and avoid criticism. Also, try to avoid situations where your child may find it hard to cope, such as long church services.

- **Relaxation:** gentle techniques can help a hyperactive child wind down. Lie on the floor or make yourselves comfortable on the sofa, and try counting backwards, or reciting a story, with your voice getting slower and deeper. See who can speak the slowest.

- **Focusing techniques:** these can help to improve concentration. Encourage your child to examine simple objects closely and describe how they look, how they feel, how they smell and how they sound. Ask him to visualise a scene or an object and describe it.

- **Physical exercise:** this is particularly important if he is hyperactive. Exercise helps him focus his energies and can provide a sense of achievement. Solitary sports are best; team games involve social co-operation, which can be difficult for ADD sufferers and further aggravate their sense of low self-esteem.

AUTISM

WHAT IS AUTISM?

Autism or autistic spectrum disorder is the diagnostic term used to describe a specific type of developmental disorder affecting about one in 300 of the population. Symptoms are far ranging and vary dramatically from case to case.

- Some children with autism have a low IQ, associated learning difficulties, little or no speech and display challenging behaviour. People at the high end of the spectrum have a variety of the condition called Asperger's syndrome.
- Those with Asperger's syndrome usually have fewer language problems than those with autism, often speaking fluently, although their words can sometimes be formal and stilted. They are often of average or above average intelligence but may be solitary and emotionally detached.

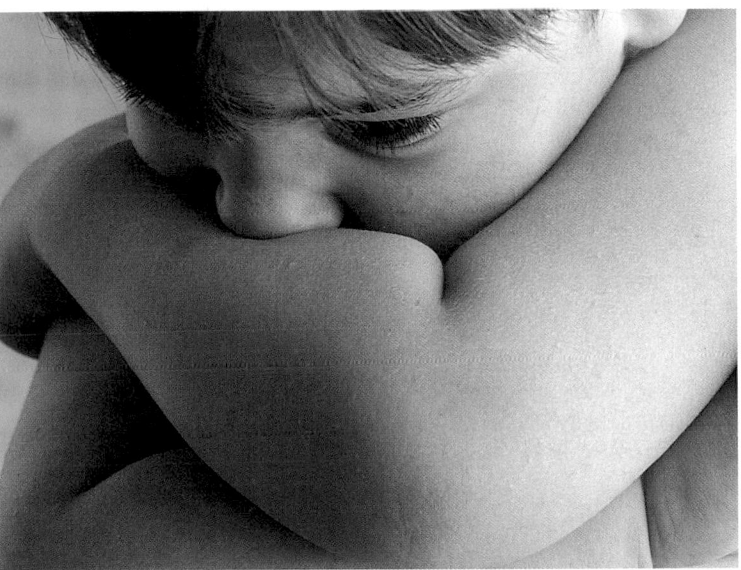

Children with autism have some level of disability in the areas of social interaction, communication and imagination. Onset is before the age of three years.

Possible causes of autism

Autism is thought to be due to developmental problems occurring in the womb or at birth. Although the cause is unknown, the following have been linked to the condition:

- Genetic factors mean that autism occurs more frequently within affected families, and boys are four times more likely to be affected than girls.
- A link between the MMR vaccine and autism has been suggested, as the symptoms of autism typically appear at 12 to 14 months of age, which is when the first dose of vaccine is usually given. However, extensive research, including evaluation of all children vaccinated so far, has not proved any link and has not shown an increased incidence of autism in children receiving MMR vaccination.
- There are possible links with a variety of disorders affecting the central nervous system, such as encephalitis and allergic reactions.
- Some hormonal imbalances in pregnancy may affect the brain's development.
- The pregnant mother may have been exposed to the rubella virus.

Useful address

The National Autistic Society can provide details of your nearest local support group for parents of children with autism.

393 City Road
London EC1V 1NG
Tel: 020 7833 2299
(Mon–Fri 10 a.m.–4 p.m.)
www.nas.org.uk

Signs and symptoms

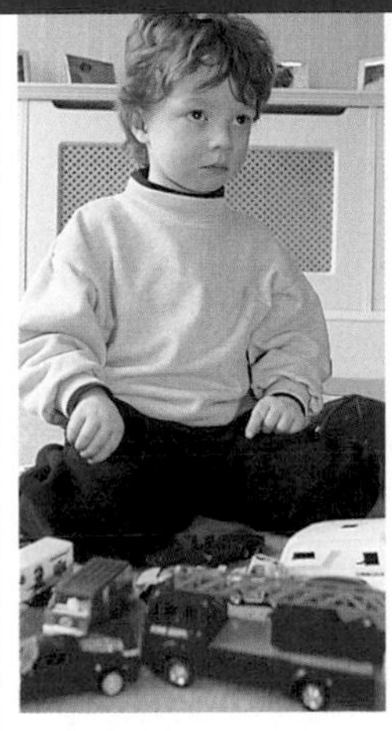

Some areas of disability are more marked than others and change with the child's age and general development. The following, however, will be apparent to some degree in most cases:

- Inability to recognise that other people have thoughts and feelings.
- A lack of, or inappropriate, eye contact.
- Appearing to live in their 'own world'.
- Objections to physical contact and hypersensitivity to taste, noise, lights and smells.
- Lateness in reaching developmental milestones.
- Disturbed behaviour, such as marked aggression, and, in some cases, self-injury.
- Repetitive behaviours or movements.
- A tendency to become anxious and upset when normal routines are changed.
- Obsessive hobbies, such as collecting bottle tops or memorising odd facts.
- Inability to initiate imaginative play – preferring to line up toy cars rather than playing racing cars.
- Absence of speech, especially in toddlers, or inappropriate use of language.
- Poor motor co-ordination.

A child with autism may find it difficult to interact with others.

Diagnosing autism

If your GP suspects that your child may be autistic, he will refer him to a paediatric specialist, who will ask a series of questions which aim to:

1 Provide a detailed history of your child's development.

2 Establish that your child is impaired in the three areas of social interaction, use of imagination and social communication.

3 Identify aspects of repetitive stereotypical behaviour.

4 Gauge the severity of the condition.

What you can do

When you take your child to see the specialist, the diagnostic process can be helped by the following:

- If health professionals or care workers share your concerns, ask that they state this in writing for the specialist to read.
- If your child is assessed in a controlled environment, ask if he can be seen in more natural, less structured, surroundings (or take with you a video recording of him at home). This way, autistic behaviour will appear more marked, which should aid the diagnosis.
- Ask for a written diagnosis. Some specialists claim labelling a child 'autistic' is unhelpful, but it does make it easier for teachers and carers to address your child's needs.
- Be prepared for the diagnostic process to take time. Many parents say it took longer than two years.
- Make use of local support groups or charities even before diagnosis. Sharing your fears and expressing your frustration will help you to cope better with the situation.

Treatments and therapies

An autistic spectrum disorder (ASD) is a lifelong disability. There is no cure but several training programmes have been devised that can aid development:

- The EarlyBird programme, for pre-school children, teaches parents to recognise and deal with the symptoms of autism. Every aspect of development is addressed, from the fear of change in routine, to potty training and speech difficulties.
- The Options Programme involves several carers and parents staying with the child for 24 hours a day. They copy the child's behaviour in order to access his 'world', before encouraging him to engage in their world. Unfortunately, this treatment costs £10,000 per child and involves travelling to the United States.
- Portage is a home-visiting service for pre-school children with special needs. Based on the principle that parents are the key figures in the care and development of their child, Portage builds on the abilities of the child.
- An injection of Secretin, a naturally occurring hormone produced in the digestive system, has been promoted as a 'cure' in the United States. But in the only independent double blind study conducted, children injected with a harmless salt-water solution were shown to be no better or worse off than those given Secretin.

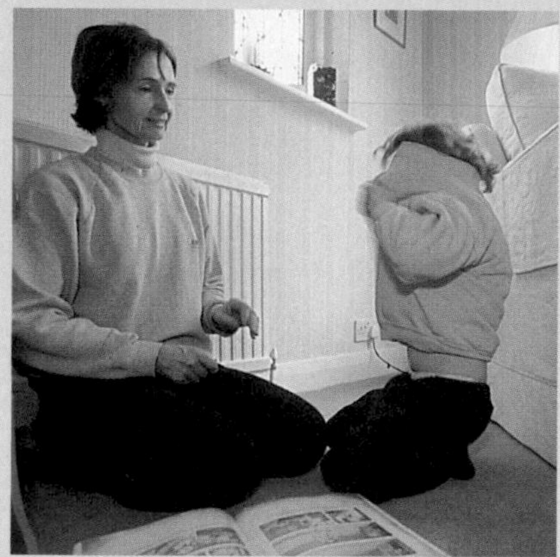

As a parent, you will benefit from the advice, support and guidance provided by specialists in the care of children with autism.

Education and employment

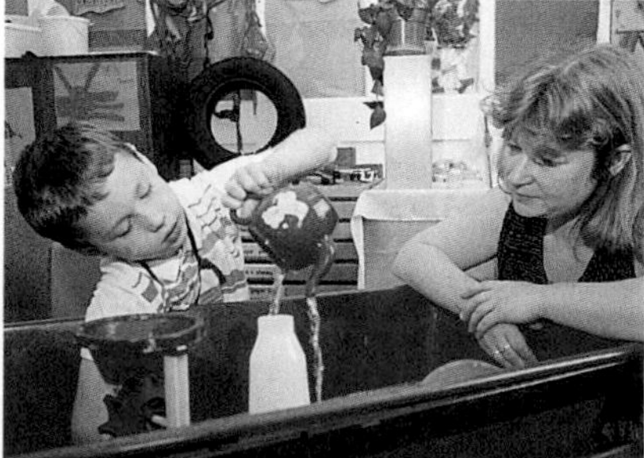

A child with autism may be able to attend a mainstream school. The National Autistic Society can provide a list of accredited schools.

The severity of the condition dictates a child's social and educational needs.

- In some cases, especially for those who have Asperger's syndrome, normal school, with specialised teaching back-up, is an option.
- Children with autism often come across as 'odd', so it is important that teachers are aware of a child's condition, to prevent bullying.
- In more severe cases, placement at a special school will be necessary.
- Some children may need help all of their lives, either being cared for by parents or in institutions with staff who are trained to deal with their behavioural problems.
- With access to developmental training, a good number of ASD sufferers find a place for themselves in society, excelling at jobs requiring little interaction with others, such as computing and data inputting.
- Many children with Asperger's syndrome enter mainstream school and, with the right support, progress to further education and employment.

BIRTHMARKS

WHAT ARE BIRTHMARKS?

Birthmarks are non-malignant lesions of the skin, sometimes present at birth, sometimes appearing a few weeks or months later. They either contain pigment cells or blood vessels. Some disappear while others remain for life.

- Birthmarks can develop from an overgrowth of one or more of the components that make up skin, such as blood vessels, lymph vessels or pigment cells.
- There are two types of birthmarks: pigmented marks, which are usually brown in colour and are caused by a localised abnormality of pigment in the skin; and vascular birthmarks, which are red or even bluish, and are due to problems with the skin's blood vessels.
- While certain types of birthmarks may run in families, there is no proven genetic or chromosomal link.

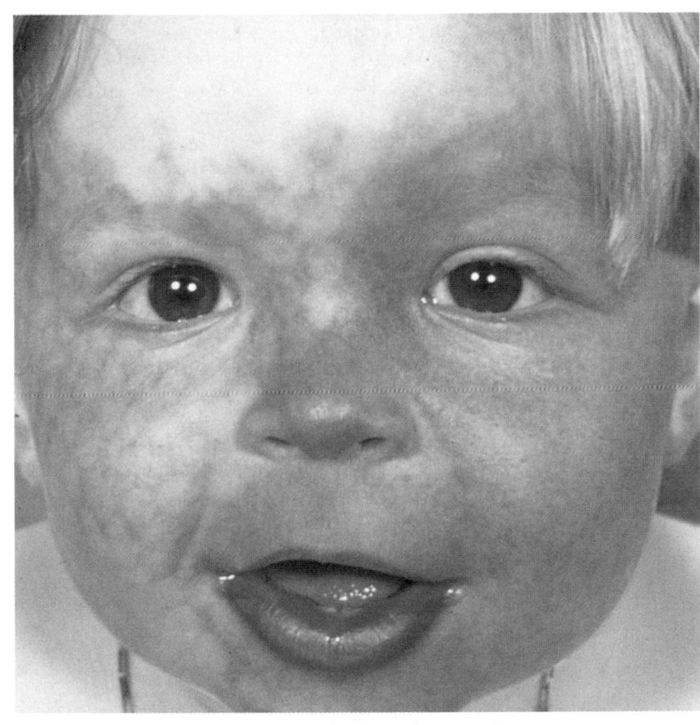

Vascular birthmarks, such as this port-wine stain, are due to an overgrowth of blood vessels. Laser treatment is available if the lesion is disfiguring.

Types of birthmark

Vascular birthmarks

Blood vessels in the skin may overgrow to produce a red, purple or bluish lesion. The birthmark may either be flat or raised.

- Strawberry naevi marks come in all shapes and sizes and mainly appear on the head and neck. They can grow for up to 18 months and then reduce in size between two and three years. Most are gone by the age of five. Plastic surgery may be needed if they remain after this time or if they interfere with vision.
- Stork bites take the form of red or purple V-shaped mottled marks on the back of the head or neck. Similar marks on the forehead or eyelids are called angel kisses. They often fade by the time the baby is six months old.
- The port-wine stain affects about three in every 1000 births. It is so called because it looks as if a glass of port has spilt over the skin, leaving a dark red/purple patch. They can be found anywhere on the body and are not raised. They do not fade, growing darker and sometimes larger over the years.

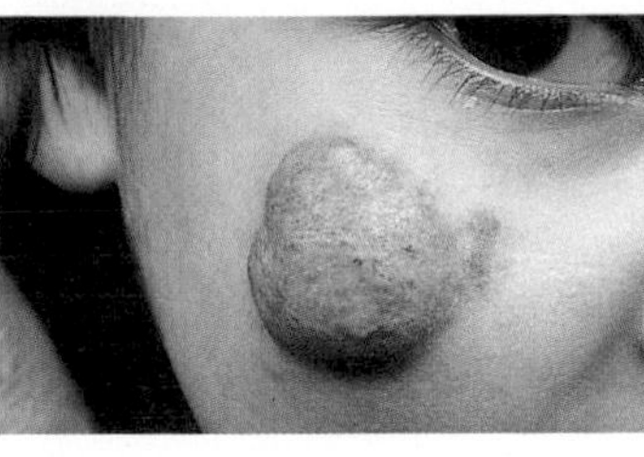

Strawberry naevi marks feature in up to 10 per cent of babies in the first year of life. Often they are not present at birth but appear later.

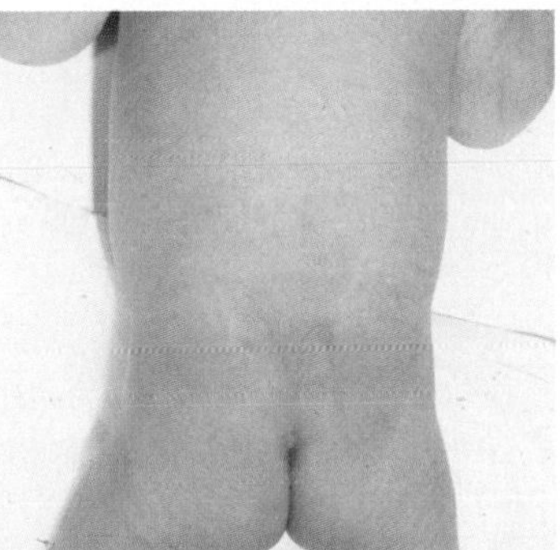

Mongolian blue spots at the base of the back are common in dark-skinned infants. They have no clinical significance and they usually fade after the baby's first year.

Pigmented birthmarks

Pigmented birthmarks are caused by abnormalities of skin cells that produce melanin. This substance normally gives skin its colour.

- The Mongolian blue spot is a pale blue/black patch often found over a baby's lower back, but it sometimes extends to the buttocks; they can also appear on the shoulders. They commonly affect the pigmented skin of black and Asian babies, but they are completely harmless, and almost always fade by adulthood.
- Café-au-lait spots are brown, oval patches seen anywhere on the body. These never fade, and may multiply as the child gets older.
- Moles can be flat, raised or hairy; they can be found anywhere on the body and vary in size. Moles can turn malignant at any time in life, but this is very rare during childhood.

Treatment

The majority of birthmarks are small and insignificant, and do not need to be removed; some will disappear. However, a birthmark may need to be removed if it is very large, if it interferes with vision, breathing or swallowing, or is in a place where it can be infected or bleed easily.

Steroid treatment: if the haemangioma (a swelling or discolouration caused by the overgrowth of blood vessels – in birthmarks in, or just below, the skin) is growing very quickly, or is too deep for laser treatment, steroids can be injected into the birthmark and taken by mouth for several weeks.

Surgery: this may be the only option if the haemangioma is too deep for laser treatment, and involves cutting away the affected tissue.

Removing birthmarks: pulsed-dye laser surgery is useful for treating port-wine stains. It is best used in early stages, and younger children respond better to treatment. Short bursts of light burn and seal the blood vessels that cause the birthmark, leaving a small scar.

Deep birthmarks cannot be treated with laser surgery, but over 80 per cent of young port-wine stain sufferers can benefit. However, laser surgery must be performed over several weeks, and is not painless. Often, the birthmark leaves a web of spider veins and excessive tissue-paper-like skin. Laser therapy can be used to treat this effectively.

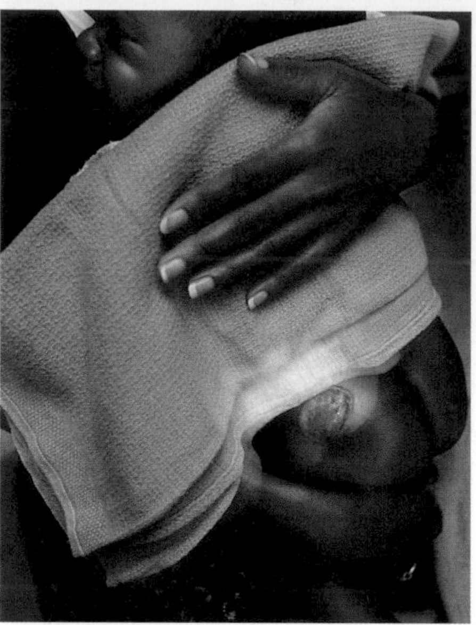

Laser treatment is applied to a strawberry naevi that has broken down. This is an unusual site for a naevi.

Complications

Most birthmarks are completely harmless. However, the location of some haemangiomas may cause problems that need treating.

- Birthmarks may be a problem if they lie close to an eye or other part of the body and stop it functioning properly.
- A lot of large café-au-lait spots may indicate the presence of a rare inherited condition, so it may be wise to seek reassurance from a doctor.
- Port-wine stains may break down, bleed or become infected. Large types are also connected with various syndromes but these are very rare.
- Some birthmarks grow so aggressively that they may break down or start growing into and over the lips or eyes.
- A cluster of several birthmarks may be linked with similar growths in internal organs. These can be very dangerous and should be treated promptly.
- The psychological upset caused by a large birthmark may be considerable; early treatment can help to minimise this.

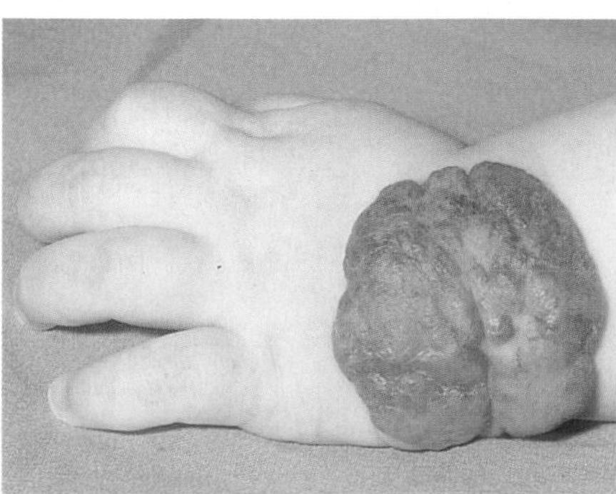

There is a slight risk with some rapidly growing strawberry naevi that the surface might break down and bleed, or that it may deprive the rest of the body of some types of blood cell.

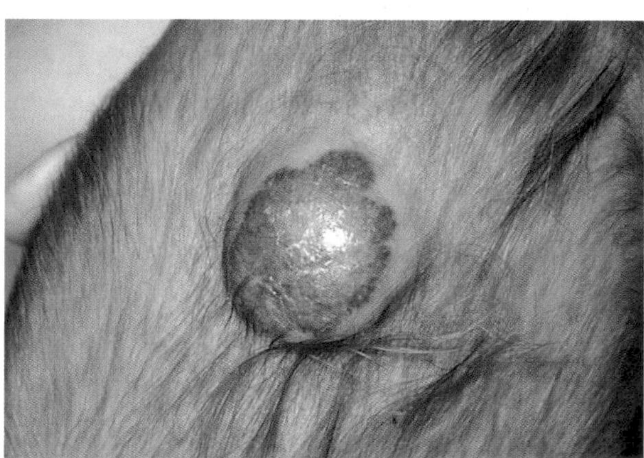

Strawberry birthmarks are most common on the face and scalp. Surgical treatment should be avoided except where it is interfering with the function of a part of the body.

What you can do

You can play an important role in assuring that the correct diagnosis is made, which will then lead to the correct treatment plan.

Strawberry birthmarks are usually noticed sometime after birth, whereas port-wine stains are always present at birth. Strawberry marks grow and then shrink, while port-wine stains gradually get bigger.

Ask yourself:

- When did you first notice the lesion?
- Has it grown?
- Is it shrinking?

CEREBRAL PALSY

WHAT IS CEREBRAL PALSY?

Cerebral palsy is the term used to describe conditions in which children have abnormal movement or posture because the brain has failed to develop properly, or has been damaged in pregnancy, at birth or after birth.

- About one in 400 babies are affected, which means there are around 1800 new cases every year in Great Britain.
- As an affected child grows, the condition does not deteriorate, but the nature of the physical difficulties may change.

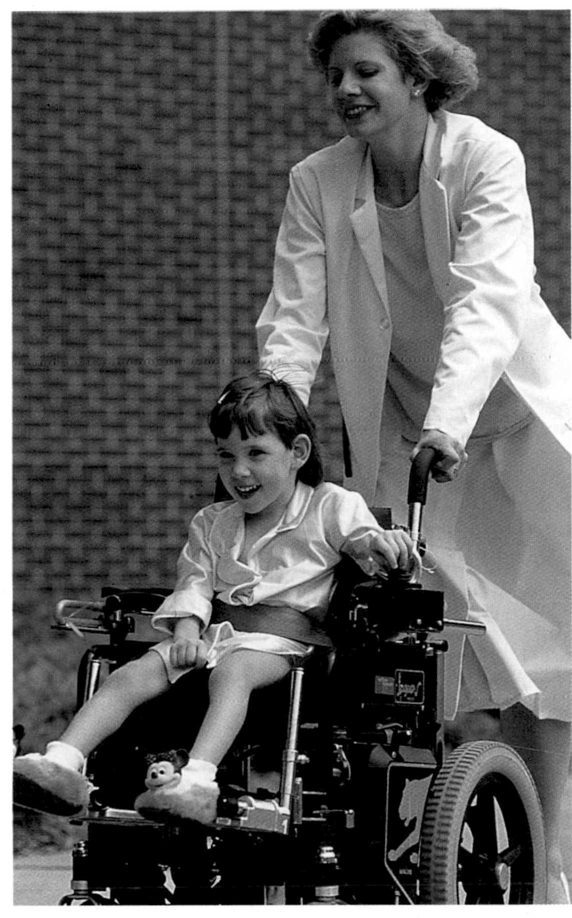

Using a wheelchair helps children with severe cerebral palsy to maintain their independence. Extra help and support is available to parents from specialist organisations.

What are the causes?

For years, cerebral palsy was associated with difficult births. It is now known that in about 80 per cent of babies with cerebral palsy, the damage to brain tissue occurs in the first three months of pregnancy. Causes include:

- **Infection:** rubella (German measles) in particular can lead to cerebral palsy if a mother contracts the condition in the first three months of pregnancy.
- **Premature delivery:** the immature brain can be damaged by severe jaundice or bleeding in the brain.
- **A traumatic delivery:** a baby can be deprived of oxygen during a difficult birth, which can cause cerebral palsy.
- **Illness:** later in childhood, cerebral palsy can result from another condition, such as meningitis (inflammation of the membranes surrounding the brain) or encephalitis (inflammation of the brain tissue).
- **Brain damage:** cerebral palsy can also develop if the brain is damaged following a head injury.
- **Genetic disorder:** very rarely, cerebral palsy is due to a genetic disorder.

Types of cerebral palsy

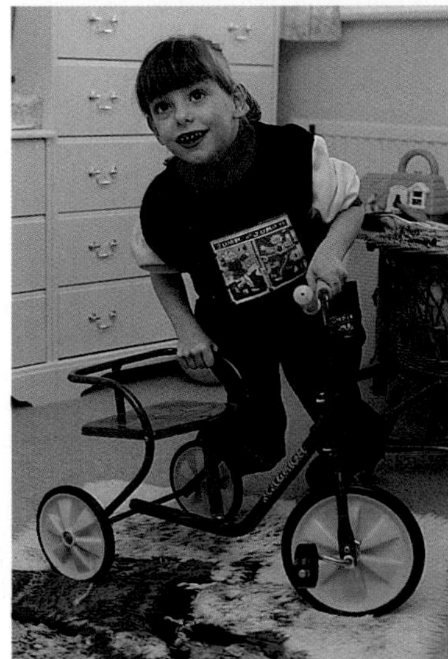

There are three different types of cerebral palsy, each one producing symptoms of varying severity. Sometimes a child may have two or more types, which makes a specific diagnosis difficult.

1 Spastic: about eight in 10 affected children have spastic (meaning stiff) cerebral palsy. This mainly affects the muscles that bend the arms and legs. As a result, these children are unable to straighten their limbs properly.

Despite some children with cerebral palsy being unable to straighten their limbs, many can lead a full and active life.

Sometimes only one side of the body is affected, but in about one in 10 children, all four limbs are in spasm – this is known as quadripatetic cerebral palsy. The arms seem abnormally bent, the legs are often crossed over and there is a distinctive facial appearance.

2 Ataxic hypotonic: this type of cerebral palsy results in problems with balance and causes general unsteadiness.

3 Athetoid: children with athetoid cerebral palsy are prone to involuntary body movements and may suddenly grimace or make writhing movements. These children may also have slurred speech and have difficulty hearing, although their intellect may not be affected.

Signs and symptoms

People with cerebral palsy usually have a unique collection of symptoms.

- In a newborn baby, the only sign of cerebral palsy may be floppiness due to lack of muscle tone. Other, more obvious, symptoms will appear as a child begins to grow and develop.

- There may be a delay in reaching developmental milestones. A child with cerebral palsy may not be able to sit up, walk or talk when expected. Some children have obvious learning difficulties.

- Once an affected child is mobile, movements are often awkward and abnormal and limbs can become stiff and contracted.

Effects on intelligence

Many children with cerebral palsy have perfectly normal intelligence and are able to integrate into mainstream education with no trouble at all. However, about six out of 10 children do have a degree of learning difficulty.

- As they grow, it becomes apparent that they are not reaching milestones and are failing to communicate properly with their parents and with other children.

- For these children, education is particularly important so that, in years to come, they are able to be as independent as possible.

- Special schools are available for children who have very severe learning difficulties. These schools offer one-to-one coaching and appropriate therapy provided by a multi-disciplinary team of experts who will assess the individual needs of each child.

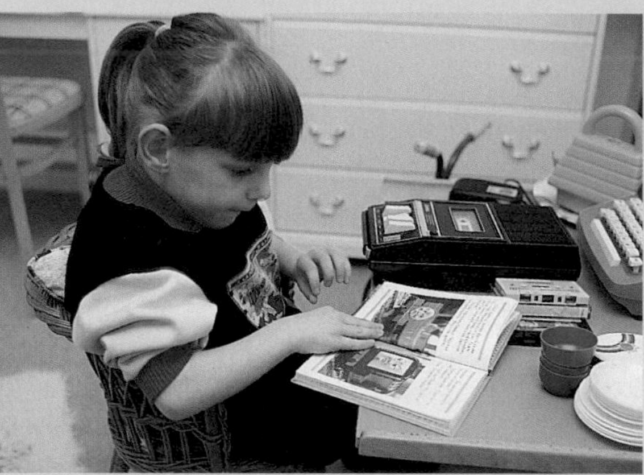

Some children with cerebral palsy may benefit from specialist education, but many have average or above average intelligence.

Therapy and treatment

Care for a child with cerebral palsy focuses mainly on improving mobility by keeping the muscles supple. It is important, too, that support is provided both for those with the condition and their carers.

- **Physiotherapy:** depending on how badly affected the limbs are in terms of spasticity (stiffness), regular physiotherapy can help to loosen up stiff joints and improve walking. Parents can be taught simple exercises that can then be carried out on a regular basis. Swimming in particular is extremely therapeutic.

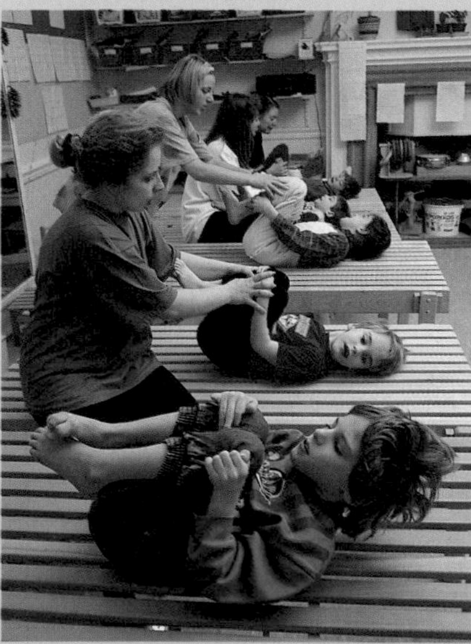

Physiotherapy is used to help with movement problems. Good patterns of movement can be developed through exercise, manipulation and massage.

- **Drugs:** medication may be prescribed to affected children – some drugs are effective in relieving symptoms. For example, antispasmodic drugs, such as diazepam and baclofen, sometimes help to relieve uncomfortable limb contractures. Some children with cerebral palsy have epilepsy, which medication can also help to control.

- **Specialist help:** your GP will be able to put you in touch with other medical services and organisations that are able to offer support. A doctor or health visitor will be able to offer advice about problems that may be encountered with sleeping or constipation, but for more specific problems you'll be put in touch with a specialist. For free confidential advice regarding cerebral palsy, contact Scope on 0808 800 3333 or email cphelpline@scope.org.uk.

Complications

Other difficulties may arise because damaged brain cells are involved.

- **Behavioural difficulties:** children with cerebral palsy sometimes feel frustrated and miserable, especially if they are unable to join in with certain activities. These frustrations can sometimes manifest themselves as outbursts of anger, withdrawal and even depression.

- **Hearing and vision impairment:** some children may have a squint, be short-sighted or have varying degrees of deafness.

- **Language and speech difficulties:** these often arise if a child has learning difficulties and, as a result, delays in developing communication skills. Hearing impairment can also contribute to speech problems.

- **Epilepsy:** this is quite common and about four out of 10 children with cerebral palsy will experience epileptic fits.

CHEST INFECTIONS

WHAT IS A CHEST INFECTION?

Any infection of the lower respiratory tract is termed a chest infection. It is common for this to occur during early childhood because the immune system hasn't matured.

- Chest infections can be caused by any of a number of viruses or bacteria, although in children the cause is nearly always a virus. Chest infections often result from the spread of an infection down the airway following a previous problem, such as a cold. Later, a secondary bacterial infection may attack the build-up of mucus.

- The severity of the symptoms of a chest infection depend on the virus or bacterium responsible and the part of the airway infected. Generally infections involve a fever and over-production of mucus in the chest as a response to irritation by the infecting organism. This causes wheezing, breathlessness and a general feeling of ill-health.

- The most common chest infections are croup, bronchitis and bronchiolitis. Chest infections tend to be more serious the lower down the airway they attack, and the most serious of all is pneumonia, which attacks the alveoli, the air sacs at the base of the lungs.

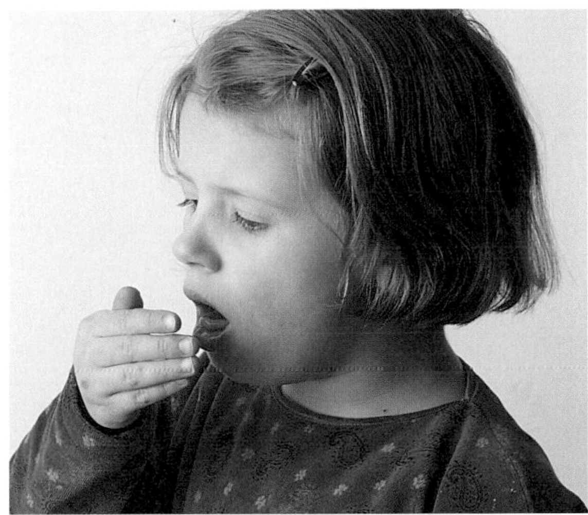

In children, primary chest infections are almost always contracted by contact with infected mucus. This may happen when an affected child sneezes or coughs near another child.

Treatment at home

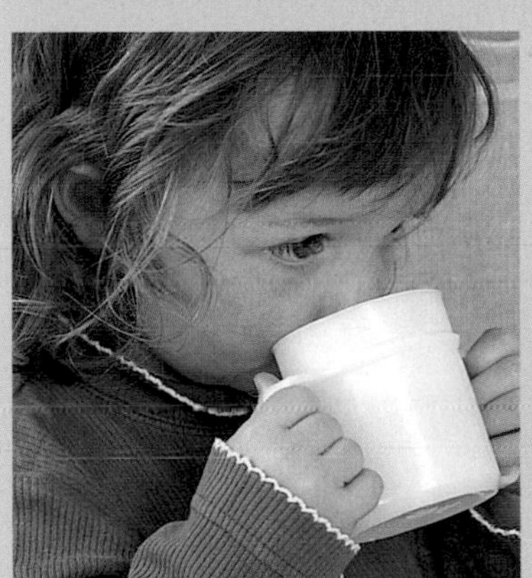

Make sure your toddler drinks plenty of fluid. This will help to prevent her becoming dehydrated.

Since the majority of chest infections in children are caused by viruses, treatment of the symptoms is usually the only option.

1. If your child has a temperature of 37.8°C (100°F) or more, give children's paracetamol – not aspirin – and follow the dosage instructions carefully. Ask your pharmacist or GP if you are unsure.
2. Keep the air in your child's room moist with a humidifier or place wet towels over a radiator.
3. Give your child small, frequent amounts of fluid to prevent dehydration.
4. If necessary, lie your child over your knee and pat her back gently to encourage the mucus to be brought up.
5. Let your baby or child sleep in a sitting position to make her breathing more comfortable.
6. Don't give babies and small children over-the-counter remedies without first checking with your pharmacist or GP.
7. Make sure that you keep your child away from other children for at least a week to avoid spreading the infection. Stress the importance of good hygiene and frequent hand-washing to your family.

When to call the doctor

You should call your GP without delay if your child has any of the following symptoms:

- She has difficulty breathing or breathing is rapid.
- Her temperature rises above 39°C (102°F) or has been high for more than 24 hours.
- There is any tinge of blue around the lips.
- There is any drooling or difficulty in swallowing.
- She is not feeding or is bringing up all her feeds.

Are antibiotics helpful?

- Many parents feel cheated if their child is not prescribed antibiotics for a chest infection, but the majority of chest infections in children are caused by viruses, on which antibiotics have no effect. However, sometimes a secondary, 'opportunistic' infection may set in, requiring antibiotics.
- Occasionally, busy GPs prescribe antibiotics for chest infections even when they are unnecessary because some parents believe, wrongly, that their children need them. Unfortunately, indiscriminate use of antibiotics reduces their effectiveness when they are really needed.

Croup

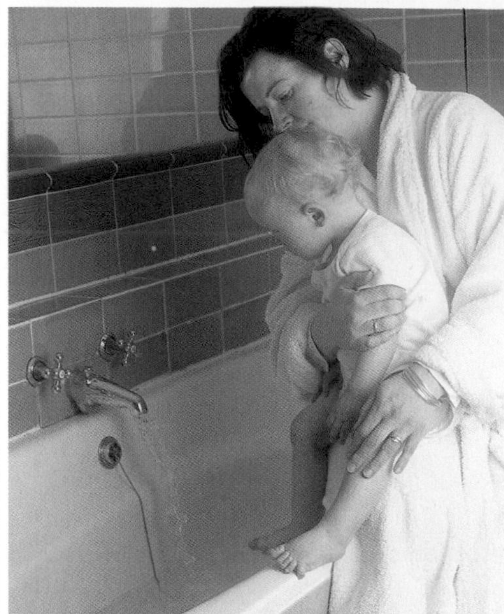

To treat croup, sit with your child in a moist atmosphere, such as a hot, steamy bathroom, or place wet towels on a hot radiator.

Croup affects the upper part of the airways of the chest, and causes a characteristic and worrying cough. It is caused by a number of viruses, including those that also result in colds and flu.

- The hacking cough is often described as sounding like a seal barking. The voice is hoarse, with a sore throat and raised temperature, and there may be a crowing sound as a breath is taken.

- Croup usually lasts for two to three days, but mucus and a cough may continue for several weeks.

IMPORTANT: croup can sometimes be severe and the onset quite sudden. If your child is distressed and her condition is not eased by steam after 15–20 minutes, seek medical help or take her to the nearest accident and emergency department.

Bronchitis

In children, bronchitis is a less serious problem than it is in adults, and rarely becomes chronic.

- Bronchitis is characterised by a cough, over-production of mucus and wheezing. The wheezing is caused by a swelling of the mucus membranes lining the bronchial tubes, which are already clogged by mucus, making the airway narrower and breathing difficult. There is also a fever, sickness and a colouration of the phlegm that is brought up if a secondary bacterial infection sets in.

- Recurrent or persistent bronchitis may be a sign of underlying asthma.

Bronchiolitis

Bronchiolitis is a serious infection. Sometimes affected babies and toddlers may need to go to hospital because their bronchioles are so small that they can easily become blocked.

- Bronchiolitis usually appears in near-epidemics during the winter, and is more severe in babies under one year old.

- The condition usually starts as a cold, with a raised temperature. After a few days, the virus travels down the airways, causing a higher fever, over-production of mucus and swelling of the mucus membranes, which causes wheezing and breathlessness. In severe cases, the child may have serious breathing difficulties – rather like those of an asthma attack – and start to turn blue as a result of oxygen deprivation. This is a medical emergency.

- In less serious cases, bronchiolitis usually clears up in seven to10 days.

Bronchiolitis is caused by the respiratory syncytial virus (RSV). In severe cases, an infected baby may need to be hospitalised.

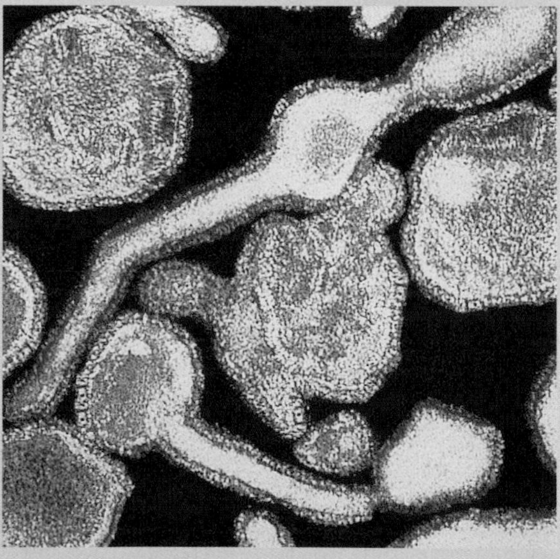

Pneumonia

Pneumonia is the most serious chest infection. Young children and babies are especially vulnerable to this infection because their immune systems have not matured.

- The pneumonia infection attacks the small air sacs (alveoli) and the tissue of the lungs, causing a build-up of fluid. This then prevents oxygen from passing through the lungs into the bloodstream.

- Symptoms of pneumonia will vary, depending on its cause. For example, if a child contracts viral or bacterial pneumonia, she will develop a cough, chest pain (especially when inhaling), fever and loss of appetite.

- Pneumonia can be diagnosed by a blood sample or a chest X-ray. Mild cases can be treated at home. Severe cases will require hospitalisation.

CHICKENPOX

WHAT IS CHICKENPOX?

- Chickenpox is a mild but highly infectious disease caused by a herpes virus called varicella.
- Coughing and sneezing passes the virus from one child to another, as does direct contact with the rash.
- Chickenpox affects children of any age, and varies in severity from a few spots and a slight fever to lots of spots, which make the child very miserable. It is most severe in babies less than 12 months old, in adolescents and in adults.
- The incubation period – from being in contact with the illness to becoming ill – is 10 to 21 days. The illness lasts for up to 10 days with the rash appearing on day one or two, and disappearing around the eighth day. The child is infectious for 24 hours before the first spots appear and until all the spots are covered with scabs.

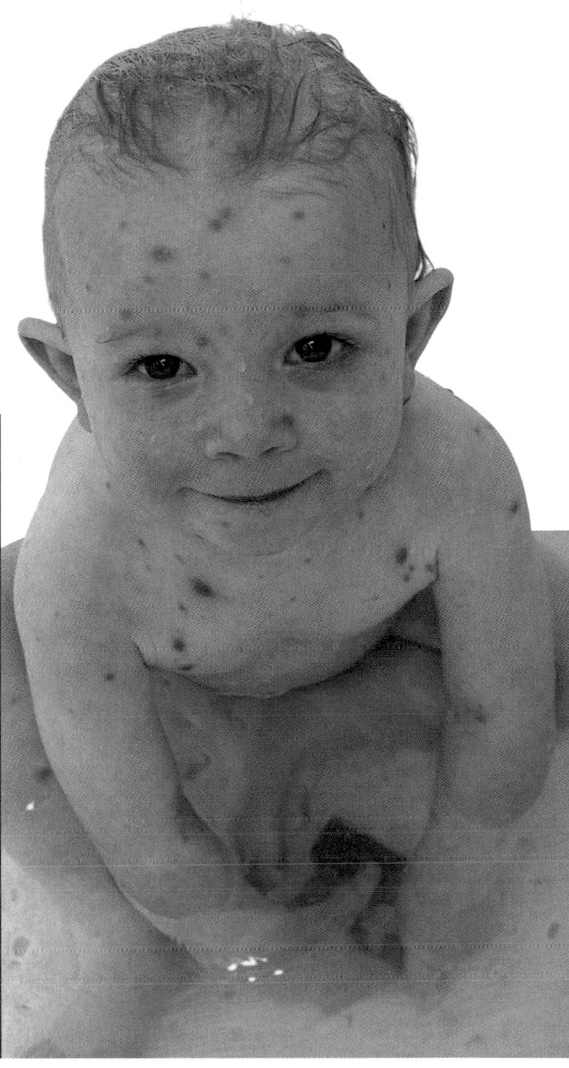

When to call the doctor

Ring the doctor if your child has:

- Fever of over 39°C (102°F) for over 48 hours
- Persistent cough and difficulty breathing
- Severe earache
- Painful sore throat
- Unexplained bruising
- Severe headache, drowsiness and vomiting after the chickenpox has begun to clear
- Infected spots – redness around pus-filled spots with pain and soreness
- Problems with his immune system and you suspect chickenpox

If your child has a rash, it can be very alarming, and many children are taken to see the doctor to have chickenpox confirmed. It is not a difficult rash to recognise, and if you're confident that this is a chickenpox rash, it is best to keep your child at home.

Chickenpox in adults can be life-threatening. Vulnerable adults – such as pregnant women (especially those who have never had chickenpox before), those with leukaemia or people on long-term treatment with steroids – are likely to be at your doctor's surgery. If you feel that your child needs to see a doctor, it's best to tell the receptionist that your child has chickenpox and she will put you into a side room to protect adults from infection.

Signs and symptoms

The first symptoms are:

- Low fever – over 37°C (98.4°F)
- Headache
- Tiredness
- Aching muscles
- Sore throat

A day or so after the above, the distinctive rash appears.

1 The rash starts on the trunk and spreads to the scalp, face and neck, initially sparing the arms and legs.

2 The spots are very itchy, flat and red.

3 After a day, these spots become raised and then form a blister, which may turn yellow and then ooze and crust. There are fresh crops of spots over the next three to five days.

4 Eventually, each spot dries up and scabs over. These scabs drop off and leave tender, healing skin underneath. Over the course of the disease, different parts of the body will show the different phases of chickenpox, with some red flat areas, some areas of new blisters, areas where sores are crusting over and scabbing, and areas of healing.

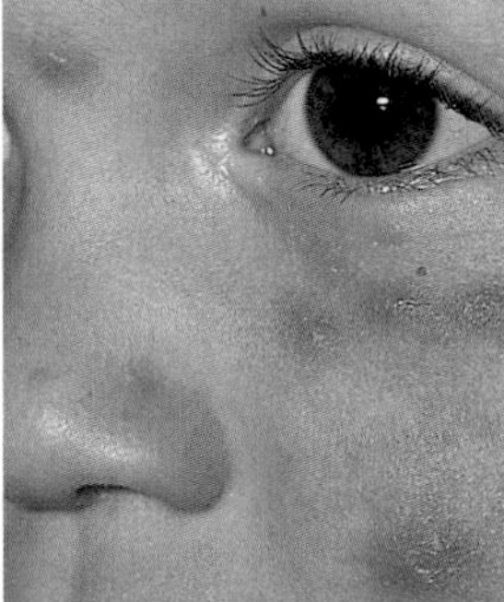

RIGHT: These spots on the face are in their second day. They are becoming raised, but have not yet blistered. The spotty stage rarely lasts for more than two weeks.

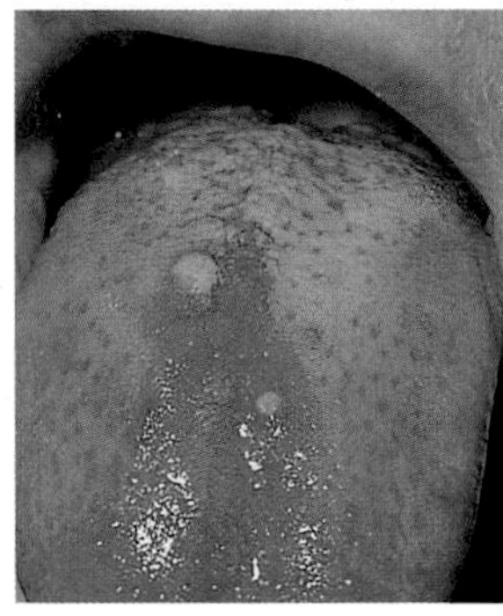

LEFT: Chickenpox spots can appear on the eyelids, in the ears and on the tongue. Although distressing and irritating, they will usually leave no scars.

Nursing a child with chickenpox

Your child will probably have a slightly high temperature during the first week or so. Use a child thermometer regularly to check it. Paracetamol syrup should help to lower it and keep him more comfortable.

How to relieve the symptoms

- Apply calamine lotion.
- Apply ice briefly to any very itchy spots.
- Calendula tincture or gel rubbed on to itchy spots can cool irritation.
- Camomile infused into bath water soothes itchy skin.
- Tepid oatmeal or sodium bicarbonate baths help – wrap a handful of uncooked oatmeal in a flannel and whirl it around in the child's bath; also rub the flannel gently over itchy areas.
- Hot baths will make the itching worse – give your child tepid baths once a day and do not scrub the sores.
- Once the chickenpox is fully healed and there are scars, apply vitamin E oil twice a day. You should also be very careful to protect your child's skin from the sun in the early days after chickenpox as the new skin will burn much more easily.

1 Make sure your child is given plenty to drink so he does not dehydrate. Drinking will help soothe the sore throat that often accompanies chickenpox.

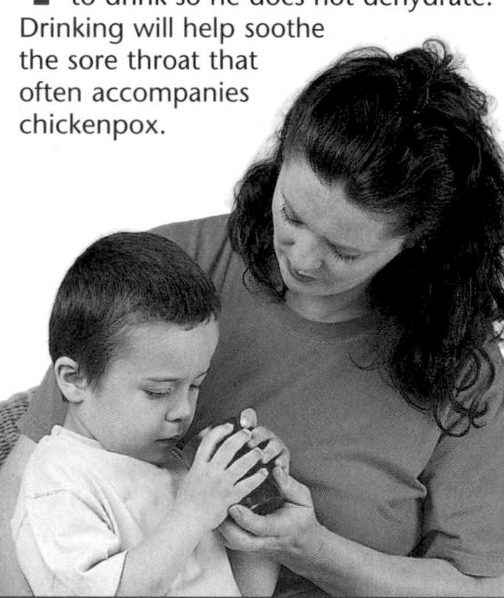

2 Calamine lotion on the very itchy spots is helpful, and if the itching is very troublesome your doctor may prescribe an antihistamine syrup. You can reduce the damage done by your child's scratching and the risk of infection by keeping his nails clean and short.

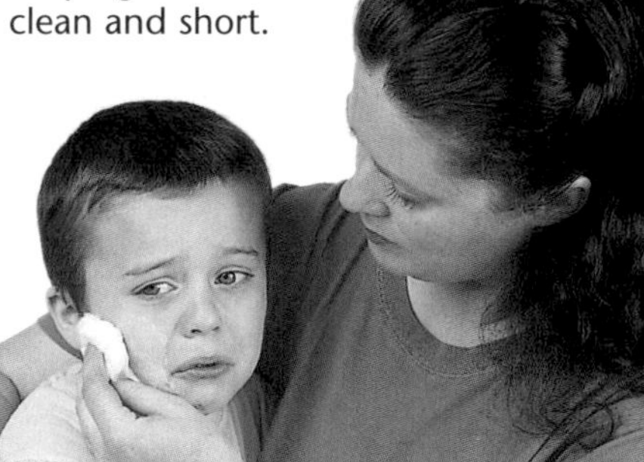

Back to nursery

Children are contagious from 24 hours before the rash appears until the last of the blisters has dried and scabbed over. Scabbed lesions are not infectious so keep your child at home while he has chickenpox. Inform the nursery so they can alert other parents.

3 Regular paracetamol syrup will help to keep your child's fever down and this will make him feel less miserable. Aspirin should never be used in young children because it has been linked to a serious disease.

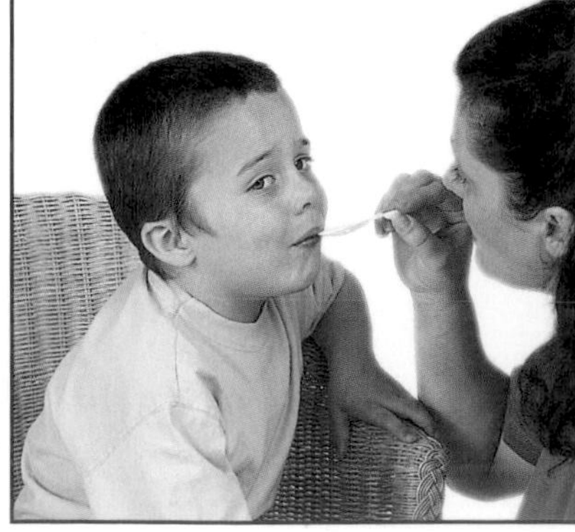

Complications

Healthy children with normal immunity are extremely unlikely to develop complications in chickenpox. They may arise in children with reduced immunity, such as leukaemia or HIV sufferers.

- **Shingles** is a very painful condition linked to chickenpox. It can cause nerve pain that lingers for months or even years and is difficult to treat. Shingles is not contracted directly from someone with chickenpox. A person who has had chickenpox can develop shingles, often many years after having had the chickenpox infection. In a non-immune person, contact with shingles can cause chickenpox.

- **Chickenpox pneumonia and haemorrhagic chickenpox** may be severe or even fatal but are both extremely rare.

- **Chickenpox encephalitis** is when chickenpox affects the brain, causing it to swell. The child will become confused and unsteady on his feet about three to 10 days after the chickenpox rash appears. Antiviral drugs are used to treat it and most people make a full recovery.

CLEFT LIP & PALATE

WHAT IS CLEFT LIP AND PALATE?

Cleft means split or separation. A cleft lip is an opening in the upper lip that can affect one or both sides of the lip; a cleft palate is an opening in the roof of the mouth.

- This part of the face develops in the womb at about six weeks into a pregnancy, and failure of the different parts of the face to fuse together creates the cleft. The cleft may be tiny, creating a small dent in the lip line, or big, causing a complete separation extending into the nose and through the gums and soft palate.

- A baby can have a cleft lip and a normal palate, a cleft palate and a normal lip, or both cleft lip and palate.

- The majority of children with a cleft are normal in every other aspect of their anatomy, intelligence and abilities.

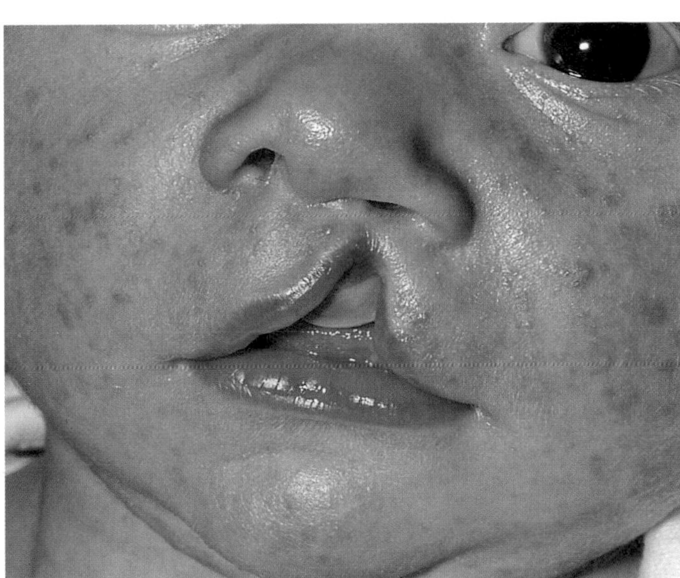

A cleft lip occurs when the tissue in the lip fails to fuse together during the unborn baby's development. It is the most common birth defect of the head and neck, affecting one in 700 babies in the UK.

Causes of cleft lip and palate

If a developing baby's lip or palate fail to fuse in the uterus, a cleft will form. There are three reasons why this happens:

1 Congenital deformity: although clefts can appear in families with no previous history of the problem, there is almost certainly a genetic element. If a parent has had a cleft, the chances of the child having one are much higher. Similarly, if one child has a cleft, another child born to the same parents has a much higher chance of being affected than a child in the general population.

2 Maternal drugs: certain drugs taken in early pregnancy may affect a baby's development and lead to a cleft lip and/or palate.

3 Syndromes: in some cases, a cleft lip and palate may be associated with a syndrome. A syndrome is a known collection of physical abnormalities that occur together.

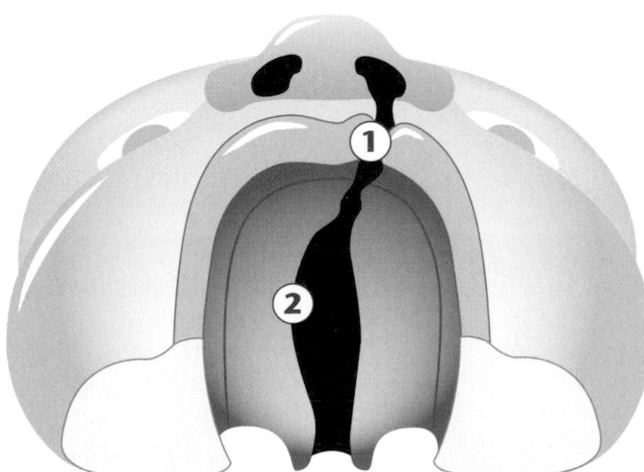

① CLEFT LIP
This affects the top lip and can range from a small hole in the lip to a wider gap, dividing the lip in two.

② CLEFT PALATE
A cleft palate is a hole in the middle of the roof of the mouth. This can affect both the soft and hard palate.

Diagnosing the conditions

- If there is a family history of cleft lip or palate, a high resolution ultrasound scan may pick up some clefts but, if there is a small, unsuspected cleft lip, it may not be identified.

- Cleft palate may be seen in the womb using ultrasound scanning. Spotting it depends upon the size of the cleft and the level of suspicion.

- Part of the examination before a baby is discharged from hospital is to place a finger into her mouth to check that the palate is intact. A cleft lip will be obvious at birth.

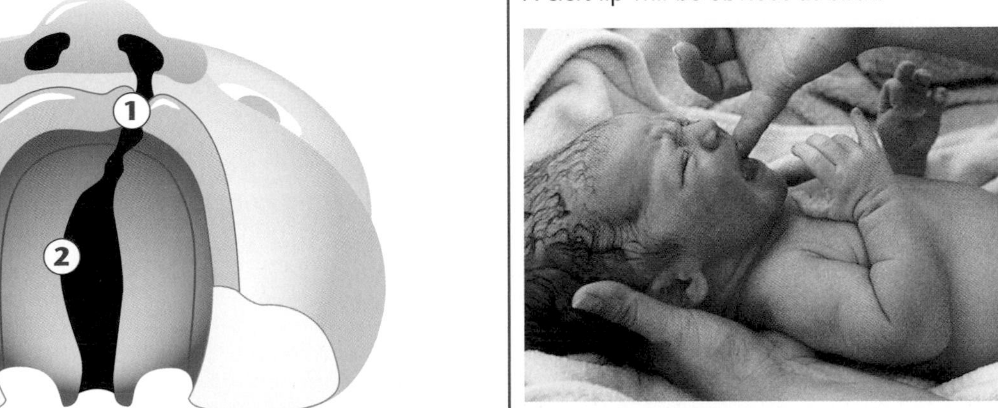

Shortly after the birth, a doctor will press his finger against the roof of your baby's mouth to check for signs of a cleft palate. Damage to the palate will be corrected by surgery.

Treatment

Cleft lip and palate are corrected by surgery. The amount of surgery required will depend on the severity of the cleft. If a child has a severe cleft through the lip and the hard and soft palate, he will need three operations:

1 **Cleft lip repair:** this is done very early on, sometimes within the first few days of birth and certainly within the first three months. The baby will be under a general anaesthetic and the operation takes about one-and-half hours.

2 **Soft palate repair:** the soft palate is repaired when the baby is older, usually at around the age of six months.

3 **Hard palate:** this area involves the teeth so surgeons will usually wait until the permanent teeth are through and then perform a bone graft at between 10 and 12 years.

4 **Further surgery:** sometimes a child will need a touch-up operation to improve the appearance of scars. As a teenager, he may need nasal surgery to improve his breathing and also his appearance. As he grows, his jaw may need to be aligned, and he may need final lip and nose surgery once his face has reached maturity at 17 to 21 years.

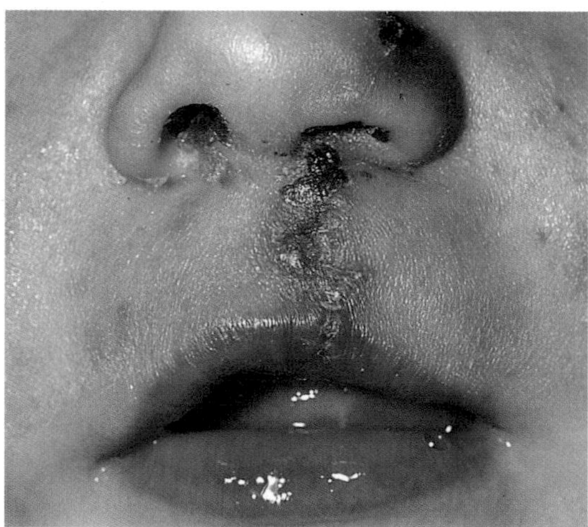

Surgery on the cleft lip is carried out before a baby is three months old. It will leave a scar, but should cause no further discomfort. The cleft palate is treated at a later stage.

Complications

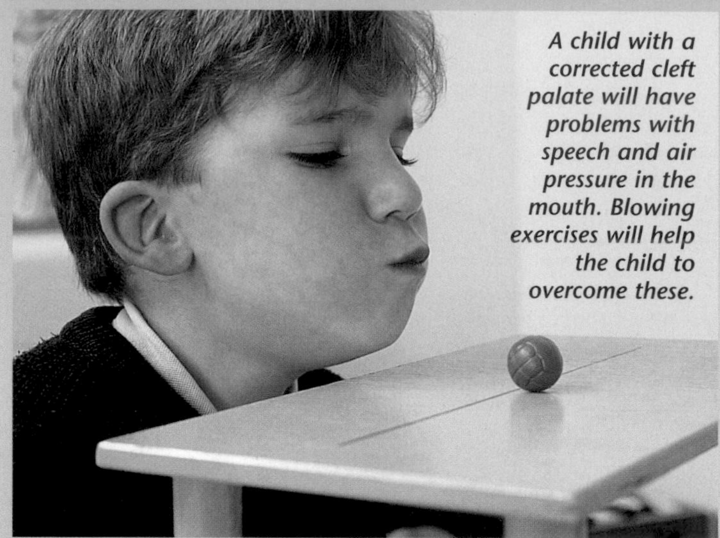

A child with a corrected cleft palate will have problems with speech and air pressure in the mouth. Blowing exercises will help the child to overcome these.

Feeding: if there is a large cleft palate, a baby will have problems forming a seal around a breast or bottle and won't be able to suck properly. The baby may be a very slow feeder and may be upset by milk coming out through his nose. There are special bottles and teats designed for babies with cleft palates.

Hearing and ear infections: hearing loss is frequently associated with children with cleft palate; it is essential that all children with cleft palate have full hearing tests. There is a high incidence of middle-ear infection and glue ear, which can reduce hearing. This is because the eustachian tube, which maintains an air-filled middle ear, lies just above the soft palate and may be affected by the cleft. A grommet can be inserted to correct the condition.

Dental problems: if the cleft palate involves the gum line, a child's teeth may be absent or crooked. Once the permanent teeth arrive, the child may need a brace. As he grows, an operation, called an alveolar bone graft, may be needed to put some extra bone into the gum.

Speech: all children with this condition will have had their palates and lips repaired by the time they start to talk. They can have problems with pronouncing some sounds, giving their speech a nasal tone. This can usually be treated with speech therapy. In about 20 per cent of cases a child needs an extra operation to reduce the amount of air going into the nose.

Disfigurement: the skills of surgeons nowadays make this a much less likely outcome than even 20 years ago.

Informing your child's carers

If your child has a cleft lip or palate, inform his carers and teachers so that they can look out for potential problems that could affect his progress.

- It is important for carers to be aware of, and understand, the condition. A child who looks different is often treated differently, and presumed to be less able than his peers. This can affect self-esteem and confidence if it is not nipped in the bud at every opportunity.
- A child may be reluctant to speak and find it difficult to make friends. He may also be absent from school to have surgery. If teachers are aware of this, they can ensure the child does not lose touch with schoolwork, and make the child's peers more understanding of his condition.

Useful address

For advice and information on cleft lip and palate, contact:

CLAPA (Cleft Lip And Palate Association)
235–237 Finchley Road
London NW3 6L5
Tel: 020 7431 0033
Email: info@clapa.com
www.clapa.com

COELIAC DISEASE

WHAT IS COELIAC DISEASE?

Sufferers of coeliac disease react badly to gluten, a protein found in wheat, rye, barley and oats. This causes damage to the lining of the small intestine and stops it from working properly. Not only does this cause pain, bloating and diarrhoea, but it stops the absorption of certain important nutrients, which may slow your child's growth.

How could my child get it?

The exact cause of coeliac disease is not yet known, but there is a 10 per cent chance that, if a parent or other family members have it, so will the child.

The incidence of coeliac disease in infancy and childhood is much lower than it used to be. This may be because mothers are encouraged to delay weaning for longer and also because gluten-containing foods are not now recommended for babies under six months. However, although there is less overt coeliac disease in childhood, children who are genetically predisposed to gluten sensitivity may develop coeliac disease at a later stage in life when exposed to gluten.

Symptoms

In babies:
- Diarrhoea
- Constipation
- Swollen tummy
- Failure to gain weight
- Loss of appetite and vomiting
- Thin, floppy muscles

In childhood:
- Diarrhoea or constipation
- Anaemia
- Short stature
- Irritability and fatigue

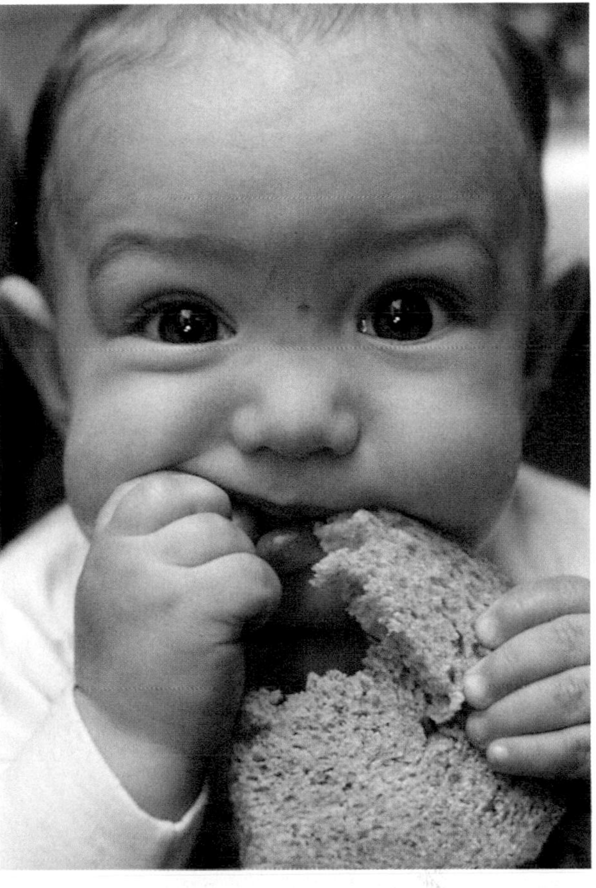

RIGHT: Coeliac disease is a lifelong condition. However, by removing gluten – including bread – from the diet, many coeliacs can recover within weeks.

BELOW: This is the small intestine of a coeliac sufferer. The wall of the intestine becomes very flat and begins to waste away, making it difficult to absorb food.

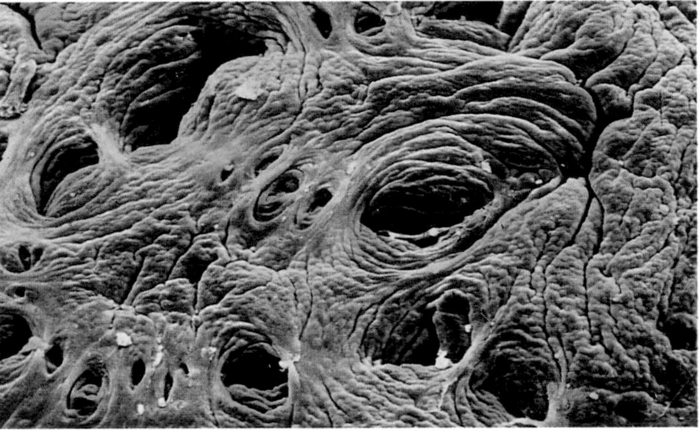

What problems does it cause?

The condition makes itself known in children between nine months and three years of age after the introduction of cereals in the diet. In the short term, nutritional deficiencies cause a number of problems:

- **Anaemia:** blood needs iron and folic acid to have its normal red pigment – neither are properly absorbed, leading to fatigue and listlessness.

- **Low levels of fat-soluble vitamins:** vitamins A, D, E and K are lost through diarrhoea. Vitamin D is needed for the absorption of calcium, vitamin E for nerve development and vitamin K for normal blood clotting.

- **Lack of calcium:** this causes a thinning of the bones, called osteoporosis, in adulthood.

- **Lack of calories:** diarrhoea, vomiting and poor absorption of nutrients lead to weight loss, or a failure to gain weight.

NOTE: there is also an increased risk of other auto-immune diseases, including type 1 diabetes and thyroid problems.

Testing for coeliac disease

Many parents are tempted to treat their children themselves by removing gluten from the diet without waiting for medical investigations. The problem with this is that the tests for coeliac disease may then be negative because the children have been on a gluten-free diet; it is better to go to see your doctor first if you suspect that your child may have coeliac disease. Tests include:

Biopsy: a tiny piece of the lining of the small intestine is cut away using a tube (introduced through the mouth) called an endoscope. Under a microscope, the normal lining of the small intestine looks like a deep-pile carpet, with lots of hair-like protrusions, called villi, on the surface. With coeliac disease, the villi start to flatten out and the lining looks more like kitchen lino than carpet. The biopsy should be repeated after some time on a gluten-free diet, and again after a gluten challenge to be absolutely certain of coeliac disease.

Blood tests: there are two tests that have a high chance of showing a gluten allergy: the endomysial antibody test and the antigliadin antibody test. Although the blood tests are very accurate, they are not foolproof; specialists prefer to biopsy the gut to confirm the diagnosis.

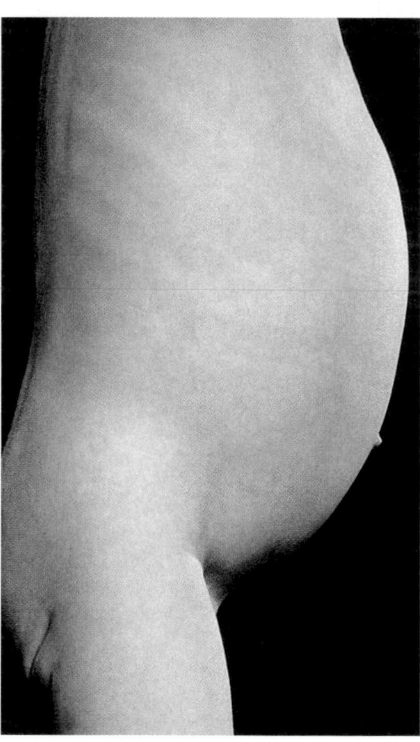

ABOVE: Coeliac disease can cause the stomach to become very swollen. If undetected, it can also lead to anaemia and osteoporosis in the long term.

Changing your child's diet

It is difficult to know which foods contain gluten, and the advice of a trained dietitian is invaluable. Here is a guide to the foods to avoid and to what is acceptable on a gluten-free diet:

Foods to avoid:

- Any flour made from wheat, oat, barley or rye
- Breakfast cereals
- Bread, cakes, pastries, biscuits, and puddings
- Most commercially available soups and sauces
- Semolina
- Oats – many brands also contain gluten
- Pasta, macaroni and spaghetti
- Couscous – this contains semolina
- Stock cubes
- Baking powder
- Soy sauce
- Suet

Foods that are allowed:

- Special gluten-free variations of rice cakes, bread, biscuits, spaghetti and flour can be prescribed by the family doctor
- Unprocessed meat
- Vegetables and fruit
- Fish
- Rice
- Eggs
- Potatoes
- Millet, corn and buckwheat
- Sago and tapioca
- Plain cheese

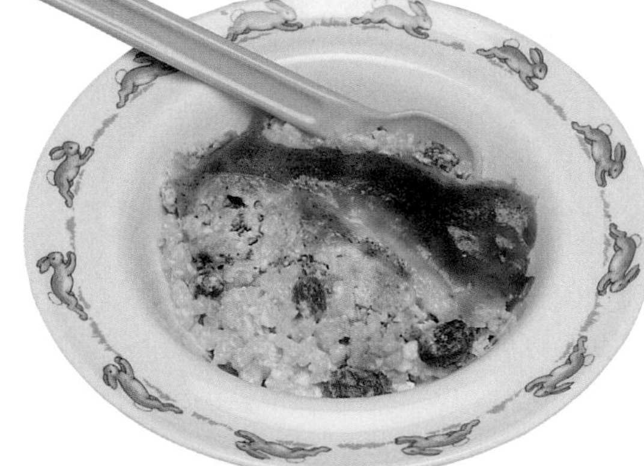

RIGHT: A coeliac sufferer must adhere to a very strict diet. Rice pudding or sago are gluten free.

Controlling coeliac disease

Controlling the symptoms is the lifelong aim for the coeliac sufferer. On the plus side, avoiding gluten in food will almost always heal the damaged intestine, and there is usually no need for any other treatment. If your child is a sufferer, take note of the following:

- Keep to a strict gluten-free diet.
- Monitor treatment. Once a gluten-free diet has been started, your child should be checked regularly with visits to a specialist clinic.
- Make sure that your child sees a dietitian regularly.
- Add vitamins and extra minerals as recommended by your health-care team.
- Regular blood tests will check the diet is effective.
- A gut biopsy may be performed again if the child remains unwell.

Useful address

The Coeliac Society is a national group offering help and support to sufferers. It also provides a 'food list', which is a directory of gluten-free brand names and natural foods.

Coeliac UK
P.O. Box 220
High Wycombe
Buckinghamshire
HP11 2HY

Helpline:
0870 444 8804
www.coeliac.co.uk

COLIC

WHAT IS COLIC?

Doctors have classified colic as persistent and vigorous crying for at least three hours a day, on more than three days of the week, over a period of three weeks or more.

Colic is a common cause of crying in babies. It affects breast-fed and bottle-fed babies equally, and seems to be more common in first-born children. Babies tend to suffer from it only in their first three months of life, so it is often referred to as three-month colic.

The crying usually starts once the baby is around three weeks old. All babies cry from time to time, but crying caused by colic can be particularly distressing for the parents. Most babies with colic are happy and content when they are not crying and are otherwise well.

Colic has no lasting effect on the baby. Most babies will have grown out of it by the time they are four months old, and the crying usually stops as suddenly as it began. During the night, the baby stops screaming and only cries for the usual reasons, such as hunger or thirst.

Sometimes rhythmically stroking your baby's back or tummy can help to ease colic as it could be a sign of trapped wind. Alternatively, giving your baby a dummy (pacifier) can help to satisfy his need to suck and stop the crying. A warm bath may also help to calm him down.

Causes

It is not fully understood what causes colic. The main theory is that colic is a problem with the baby's digestive system, possibly caused by an allergy to milk, painful spasms of the baby's gut, or trapped wind caused by an intake of air. It could also be due to the immaturity of the baby's gut, which is still developing and finding it difficult to cope with food.

Feeding problems may also be a trigger (for example, not latching on to the mother's breast properly, rushed feeds or a poor milk supply from the mother). Colic has also been linked to tension between the parents, anxiety of the mother or agitated handling of the baby.

Symptoms and signs

Colic attacks are usually worse in the late afternoon or evening and can be a very distressing time for a parent. If your baby is suffering from one or more of the following symptoms, he may have colic:

- Cries incessantly in a high-pitched tone for long periods of time (a bout of crying can last for several hours).
- Is not willing to settle.
- Goes red in the face during a crying episode.
- Wakes from a short sleep with a startled cry.
- Pulls his knees up to his stomach, as if in pain.
- Has a tense and swollen stomach, clenched fists or arched back.
- Fails to respond to the usual means of comforting, such as cuddling, feeding and nappy changing.

When to call the doctor

Persistent crying should always be checked by your doctor, especially if it is accompanied by other symptoms. The many possible causes include discomfort or pain, and the crying may be a sign of an illness that needs to be treated. In particular, you should ring the doctor if your baby shows any of the following symptoms:

- Brings up an excessive amount of wind
- Is fretful throughout the day
- Vomits or possets a lot
- Has diarrhoea or constipation
- Refuses feeds
- Has a fever or a rash
- Stops gaining weight
- Starts to cry a great deal
- Is still experiencing colic after the age of five months

Easing colic

There is no cure for colic but there are ways to make your baby more comfortable.

- Keep your baby in an environment without loud noises or bright lights and make sure he follows a regular feeding and sleeping routine.

- Hold him in a position that puts gentle pressure and warmth on his stomach, such as lying face down across your lap or against your shoulder. Rub and stroke your baby's back and tummy regularly.

- If you are bottle-feeding, talk to your health visitor or doctor, as your baby could be allergic to infant milk. Try switching to a different formula, possibly one free of cow's milk proteins. You could also try giving your baby small amounts of milk more frequently or feeding him more slowly, to stop him swallowing large amounts of air.

- If you are breast-feeding, the crying could be triggered by something in your diet. Perhaps noting down everything you've eaten or drunk in the last 24 hours could produce a link. Common culprits include dairy products, caffeine, citrus fruits and gas-forming foods.

- When breast-feeding, keep your baby in an upright position and let him finish one side first, so that he receives enough hindmilk to aid his digestion.

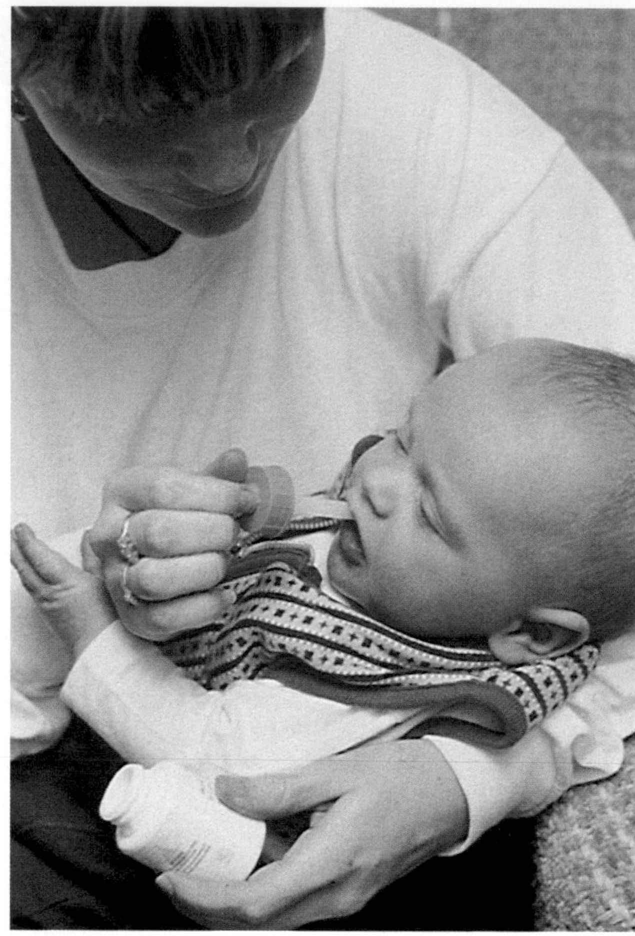

ABOVE: Most colic drops can be given from birth, but read the instructions carefully. They should not be given at the same time as other medicines.

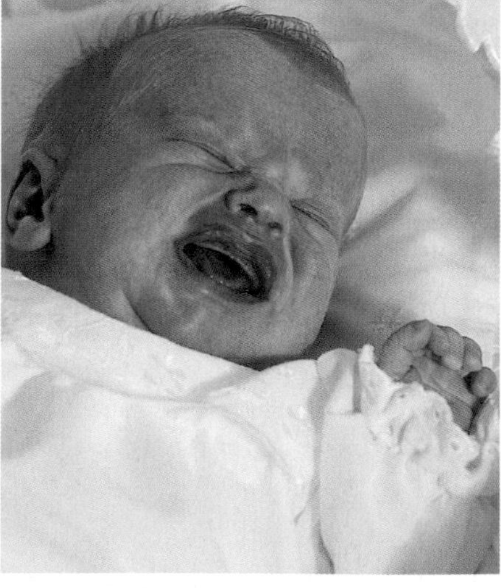

RIGHT: When your baby cries, first check that he is not hungry, thirsty, too hot or too cold or in need of a nappy change. Keep him in a soothing environment.

Easing the symptoms

Your baby should have been diagnosed with colic before you give him any over-the-counter preparations that are available from pharmacies.

1 Colic drops contain drugs that help break down the tiny air bubbles in the baby's stomach. This allows swallowed air to be brought up more easily, easing any stomach pains and getting rid of trapped wind. The medicines can be given with your baby's feed or by syringe or spoon.

2 Gripe mixtures can help to settle your baby's stomach by getting rid of wind. Colic doesn't usually need medical treatment, but your doctor can prescribe medicines that stop gut spasms, such as dicyclomine. However, these shouldn't be given to babies under six months because of possible side-effects.

Useful address

Cry-sis is an organisation formed to help parents cope with colicky and crying babies.

BM Cry-sis
London WC1N 3XX
www.cry-sis.com

Helpline: 020 7464 5011

When it gets too much

Coping with a colicky baby can be very stressful and may reduce parents to a state of despair, particularly as they often lose a lot of sleep during this trying time.

It is important to remember that the crying is only temporary and the bouts of colic will eventually cease.

Make sure you give yourself regular breaks and share the crying times with someone else. Above all, never punish a crying baby. If you are losing patience, put your baby in a cot or pram and close the door, to allow yourself time to calm down. If you are finding it hard to cope, ask your GP or health visitor for advice.

CONSTIPATION

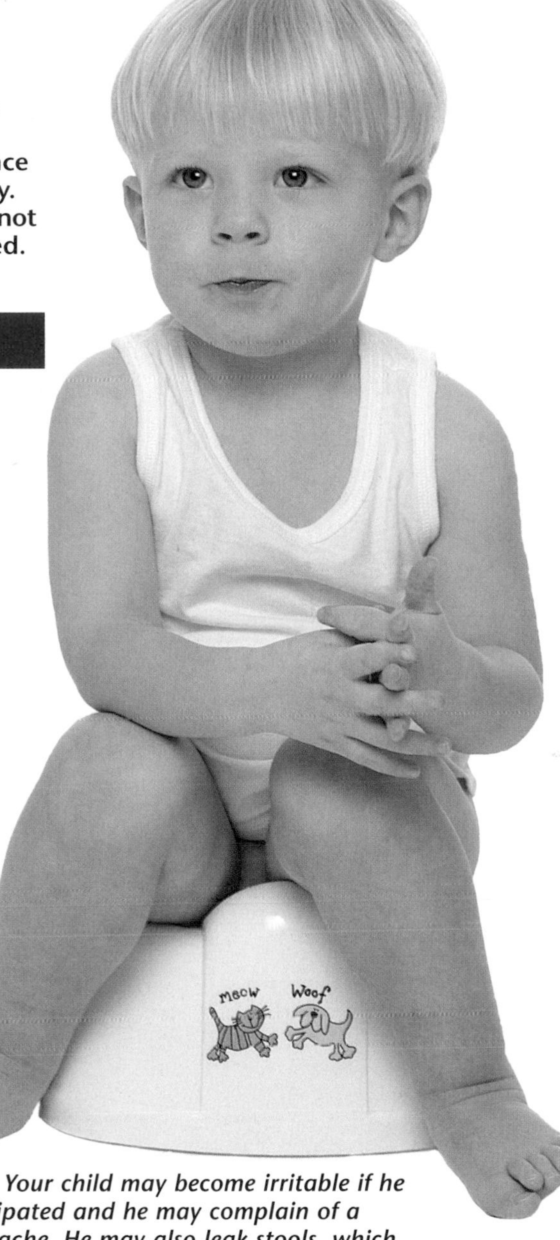

WHAT IS CONSTIPATION?

Constipation means the passage of infrequent, hard stools. Almost everyone experiences this at times and children are no different. Parents may feel it is normal to open their bowels every day and think they are constipated if this does not happen. If their child passes a painless, soft motion once every three days, they may worry. However, this is normal and does not mean that the child is constipated.

What causes constipation?

- Babies can become constipated at times of change, such as moving from breast to bottle milk, and when they are being weaned on to solid foods. Bottle-fed babies are more prone to constipation – breast-fed babies rarely suffer from it. Breast-fed babies may pass one motion every week because so much of the breast milk is absorbed through the gut that there is little left to be expelled.
- Children can suffer from brief bouts of constipation and this tends to happen at times of change. Your child may develop a vicious cycle where he passes a painful motion that frightens him enough to withhold the next. He may then tear the anal tissue, which makes the pain worse and therefore the withholding worse.

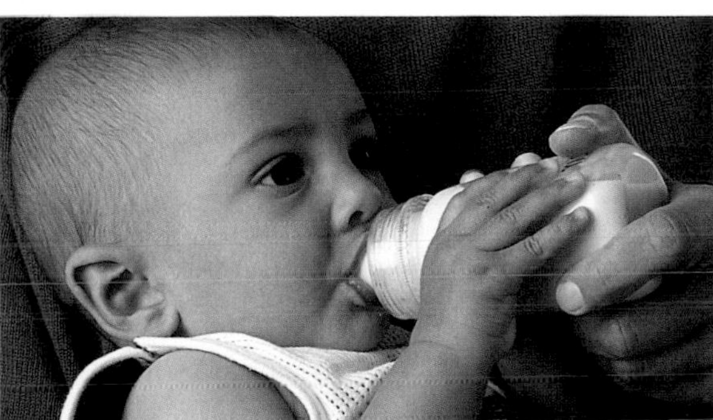

LEFT: If your baby is straining or crying before she passes a hard, pellet-like motion, she may be constipated. Your baby is more likely to become constipated when she first makes the change from breast to bottle milk.

ABOVE: Your child may become irritable if he is constipated and he may complain of a tummy ache. He may also leak stools, which can cause him to soil his underwear.

When to see the doctor

Occasional bouts of constipation are nothing to worry about. However, you should contact your doctor if:

For a baby:
- Your baby has not passed a stool in the first 24 hours after birth – she may have Hirschsprung's disease, a rare congenital abnormality of the bowel.
- There is blood in your baby's motions – she may have developed a small tear in her anus, which is quite common when she is passing hard stools.
- Your baby seems irritable and is off her feed.

For a child:
- Your child has increasing pain around the anal area when passing stools.
- He has increased abdominal pain.
- Your child is experiencing vomiting as well as constipation.
- Your child's stools are bloody.
- Your child is soiling his pants regularly.
- The constipation lasts for more than three days.

What your doctor will do

- If your child or baby is experiencing pain when passing stools, your doctor may give lactulose syrup to soften the motions. This will make them less painful to pass.
- Sometimes quite high doses of a stimulant laxative, such as senna, are given to restore the urge to defecate, which may not have returned after the bowel is cleared.
- Your doctor may prescribe a short course of glycerol suppositories for your child if the constipation is not responding to these mild measures.

Other causes of constipation in children

Not only can life changes cause constipation in your child, he may also become constipated because he is worried about something, or there may be a physical problem preventing him from passing motions. If you are concerned, discuss it with your GP.

- **Toilet training:** this can be a traumatic time for your child and may lead to him withholding his motions and to chronic constipation. It is important never to punish your child for accidents. Consider giving up until a later date and letting his bowels settle down.
- **Starting or changing school:** your child may be embarrassed about asking where the toilets are and therefore hold on to his stools. It is very common for children not to drink enough water during school hours and a change in their diet may trigger constipation.
- **Illness:** any illnesses that are associated with fever may lead to constipation. Other illnesses that may cause constipation are cystic fibrosis, an underactive thyroid and anal abnormalities.

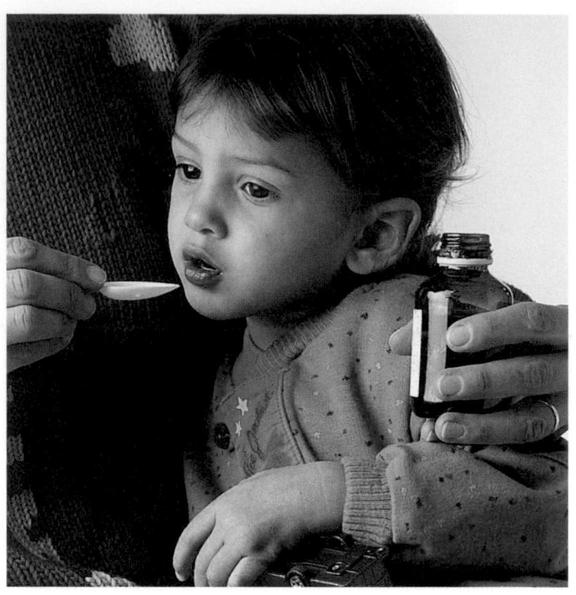

Your doctor may prescribe lactulose syrup for your constipated child. This works by softening the stools, which enables your child to pass a motion.

Treating constipation at home

For babies:

Constipation can be treated at home by paying special attention to your baby's diet. Do not give her any medication without your GP's instruction.

- Make sure the formula feed is being made up correctly and is not too concentrated.
- Try giving your baby sterile water between feeds.
- Add sieved fruit or vegetables to your baby's diet if she is weaned.
- Moving your baby's legs when she is passing a stool may help.

For children:

Try not to make a fuss of your child. He will sense your anxiety, which may make matters worse. Constipation usually settles with simple methods.

- Increase your child's fluid intake, especially of real fruit juices.
- Frequent exercise often moves the bowels!
- Increase your child's fibre intake. Fibre absorbs fluid, which increases the softness of the stools.

A diet rich in fibre can help to combat constipation. Fibre is present in fruit juices, pulses, vegetables and most fruits.

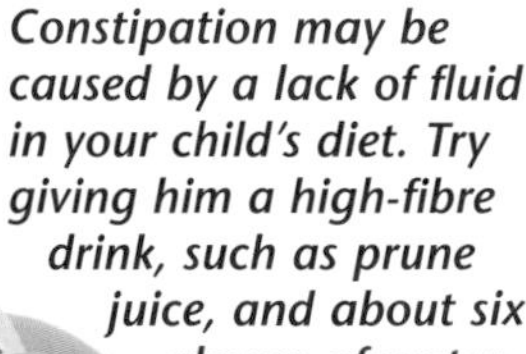

Constipation may be caused by a lack of fluid in your child's diet. Try giving him a high-fibre drink, such as prune juice, and about six glasses of water a day.

Avoiding constipation

In babies:

- Do not start your baby on solids too early, i.e. before your baby is four months old.
- Once on solids avoid too much baby rice, banana and apple and give your baby more plums, apricots, peaches, spinach and beans.
- Avoid changing your baby's formula milk too often.
- Offer cooled boiled water before each feed.

In children:

- Some foods may cause constipation, so you should try to cut these out of your child's daily diet:

White bread
Fruit squash (high in sugar)
Biscuits

- Do not give your child too much sugar or too much processed and 'junk food'.

COUGHS & COLDS

CATCHING COLDS

Children frequently get colds. In fact, some children have up to 10 colds a year, mainly during the autumn and winter months.

- Colds are caused by over 200 different viruses. Every time a child catches a cold virus, she develops resistance to that particular type.
- Children often catch a cold and then infect the rest of the family. Cold viruses spread in tiny droplets in the air, usually when a person coughs or sneezes, and pass quickly around schools and nurseries.
- Children are most at risk of recurrent colds if they are regularly exposed to smoky environments, are under stress or have enlarged adenoids (which lie at the back of the nose and form part of a child's natural defence against germs).

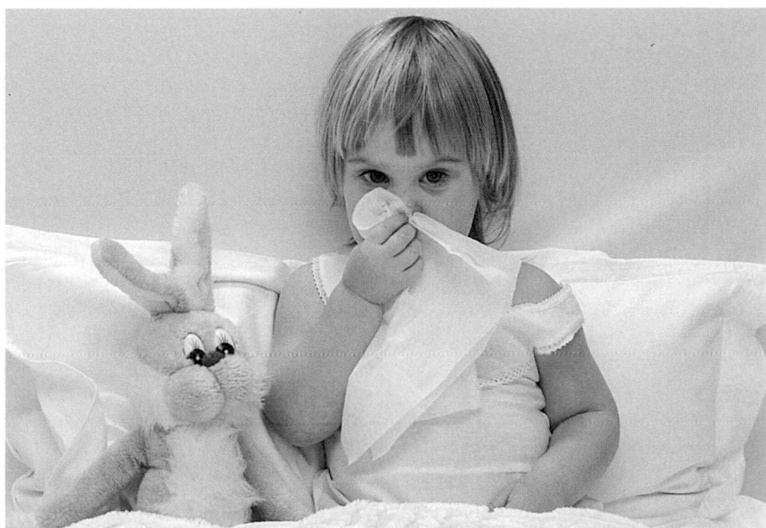

Children are more prone to colds than adults because their immune systems are not yet mature. Colds are most common in the winter – more time is spent indoors, which helps the virus to spread.

Symptoms

Colds rarely last for more than a week. The symptoms vary, but include:

- A runny or blocked nose
- Watery eyes
- Sneezing
- A sore throat
- A slight fever
- Occasional vomiting
- Occasionally, a headache or a cough

NOTE: if a cold starts very suddenly, with a high temperature, shivering and general aches and pains, your child may have flu, which can be much more severe than a cold and may need medical supervision.

When to call the doctor

Consult your GP if your child has any of the following symptoms:

- A persistent or hacking cough or wheeziness
- Earache (a younger child may simply pull at the affected ear)
- Difficult, fast or noisy breathing
- Drowsiness (it may be harder to wake your child than usual)
- A temperature over 39°C (102°F) for more than 12 hours or a lower fever for 48 hours or more
- Persistent vomiting or diarrhoea
- A severe sore throat causing swallowing difficulties or a refusal to eat
- Dislike of bright light
- Neck pain
- A rash

Over-the-counter remedies

If your child has mild symptoms, it isn't worth making an appointment to see your GP. A doctor won't prescribe antibiotics for a cold, as these medicines only work against bacteria, not viruses. Instead, you can buy children's cold remedies over the counter from pharmacies.

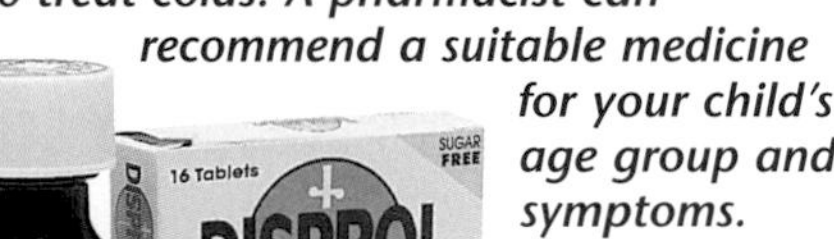

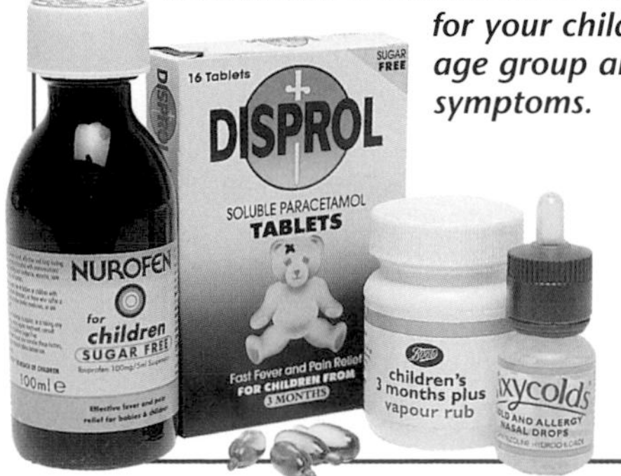

There is a range of medicines available to treat colds. A pharmacist can recommend a suitable medicine for your child's age group and symptoms.

- Junior paracetamol or ibuprofen can help to bring down a high temperature and soothe a sore throat (aspirin isn't suitable for children).
- You can also buy glycerine, lemon and honey syrup to soothe your child's sore throat.
- If your child has a blocked nose, she may find it difficult to breathe or eat. A pharmacist can recommend a suitable decongestant, such as junior syrup or nasal drops.
- You can buy inhalant capsules containing decongestant oils, such as eucalyptus. Sprinkle these on your child's pillow at night.
- An older child can try placing her face over a bowl of hot water containing a decongestant oil. By inhaling, she may be able to clear her blocked nose, but she must be supervised at all times.

Home nursing

A cold is not a serious illness and is best treated by bed rest and plenty of loving attention from you.

- Make sure that your child has a drink every hour or so to prevent dehydration, especially if she has a fever – a temperature above 37.2°C (99°F).

- Raising the head end of the cot or bed with a couple of books can help your baby breathe more easily. If your child is over one year old, an extra pillow may help.

- Teach your child to blow her nose. Press your finger over one of her nostrils and show her how to snort through the other one. Use moist cotton wool or a tissue and throw it away immediately. Wash your hands thoroughly afterwards to stop the virus from spreading. If your child's nose is dry or sore from constant blowing or mopping up a runny nose, smearing petroleum jelly around her nostrils may help.

- Your child should stay away from other children, especially young babies, so that the virus doesn't spread. However, make sure that she doesn't get bored – play games or buy her a new toy or a book.

- Don't forget to give your child lots of cuddles and reassurance.

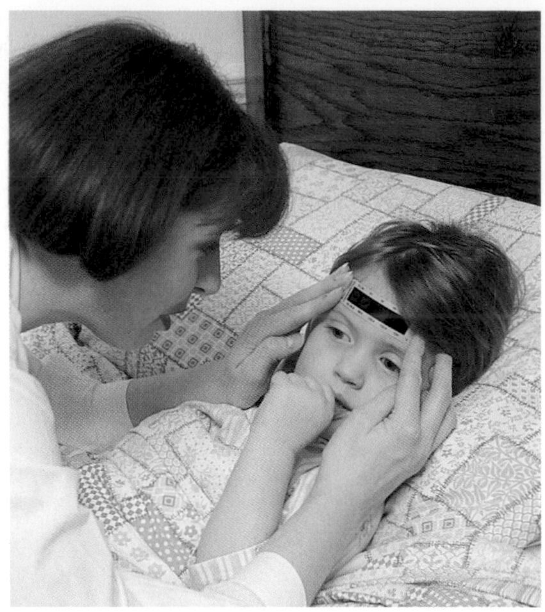

Check your child's temperature regularly. Don't dress her in extra clothes or make the room too hot. If she has a high fever, try to lower it by sponging her body with warm water.

When your child has a cough

There are two types – chesty coughs and dry coughs – and these should be treated differently.

- **Chesty coughs:** a chesty cough may sound rattly, and your child may bring up mucus from her lungs. Expectorant medicines are used to loosen and break up the mucus so that it is easier to cough up.

- **Dry tickly cough:** a dry tickly cough may sound hollow, doesn't produce any mucus and may be accompanied by a sore throat. It is often aggravated by dust and can be very irritating, especially at night. Dry coughs don't usually need treating, unless your child is finding it difficult to sleep. A sugar-free junior linctus will help to soothe your child's throat and make it less tickly. For children aged over one, you can also buy junior cough suppressants, which stop the urge to cough (some contain a mild anti-histamine, which helps a child to sleep at night). A persistent dry cough may be a sign of asthma.

NOTE: consult a pharmacist before giving your child cough medicine.

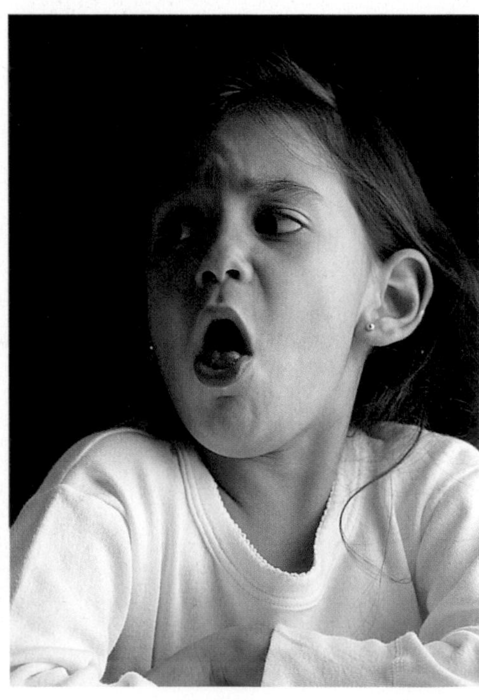

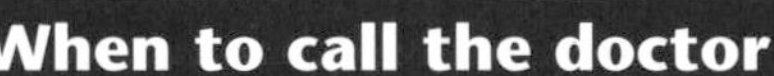

When to call the doctor

Coughs have many causes, including chest infections and asthma. See your GP if your child experiences any of these symptoms:

- Breathing difficulties or wheezing
- A persistent dry cough with no other symptoms
- A cough triggered by exercise
- She brings up coloured or blood-stained mucus
- Repeatedly vomits after coughing
- A cough which lasts for more than three to four days

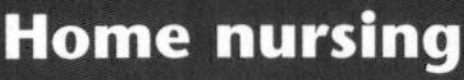

Home nursing

- Give your child plenty of fluids to drink. A teaspoon of honey in warm water can help to loosen mucus and soothe a sore throat.

- For a chesty cough, rub your child's back to break up the mucus.

- Make sure your child doesn't panic while she is coughing, as this will make the cough worse.

- Encourage your child to lie on her side at night so the mucus doesn't dribble into her throat.

In children, most coughs follow on from a cold. The cough will either be a dry cough or a chesty cough and each will need to be treated differently. If the cough does not clear after a few days, consult your GP.

CRADLE CAP

WHAT IS CRADLE CAP?

Cradle cap is a scalp condition which is most common in young babies, and is related to dandruff. It varies in severity and appearance, ranging from patches of dry, flaky skin to a greasy, yellowish-brown crust that covers the whole scalp like a cap, hence the name.

What causes it?

The cause is unknown but it's thought that cradle cap arises as a result of hormonal changes that stimulate the over-production of oily secretions from the scalp. It is not the result of poor baby care or hygiene, and cannot be prevented.

Cradle cap commonly appears during the first few weeks of life, but can affect older babies, too. It usually disappears spontaneously within a few months, but can continue for longer in severe cases, or even clear up then recur.

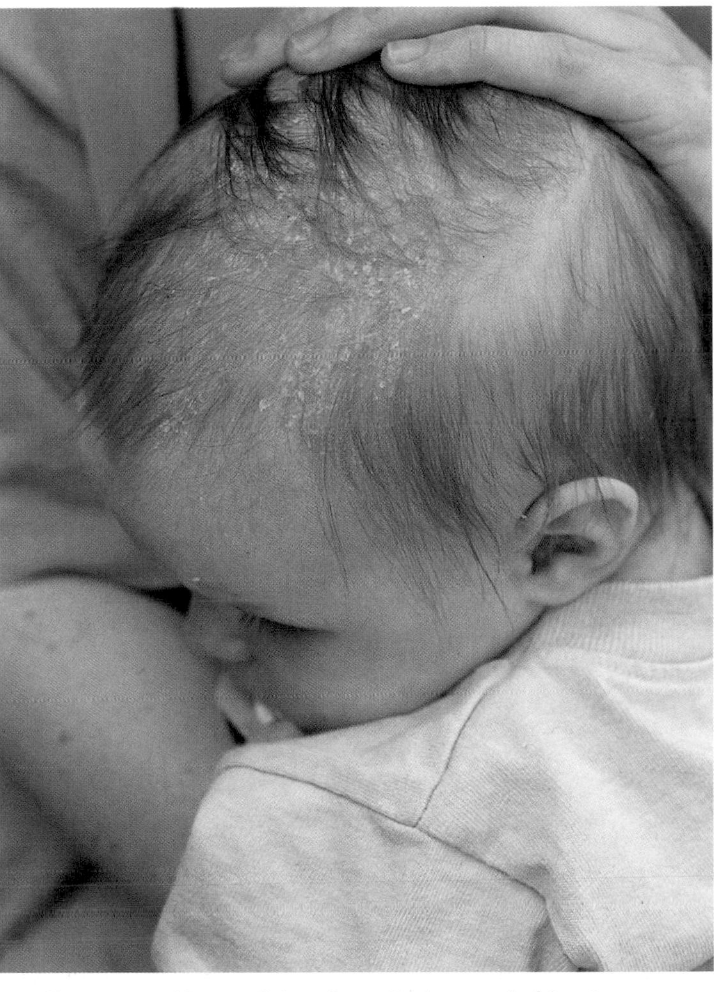

Cradle cap is a skin condition that affects most babies. It causes dry, flaky skin on the scalp, or, in more severe conditions, forms greasy crusted scales that can spread to the face, neck and ears.

When to see the doctor

Cradle cap is unsightly, but harmless. However, it is advisable to consult your GP if:

- The condition appears distressing or irritating to your baby.
- Your baby's cradle cap doesn't improve after five days following home treatment (see overleaf).
- The condition worsens or spreads.
- The scales are oozing or become infected.
- Your baby has red, scaly areas elsewhere on his body.

What the doctor may do

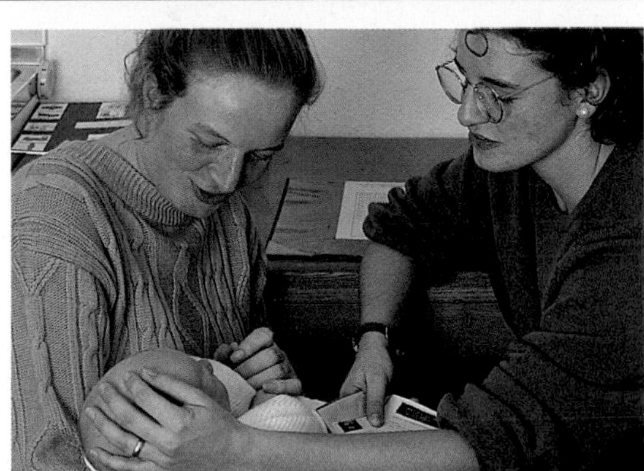

If the condition does not improve, consult your GP. She may recommend a special shampoo, a hydrocortisone cream or an antibiotic cream, depending on the severity of the cradle cap.

If you are concerned, consult your GP, who will be able to recommend a variety of treatments to ease your baby's cradle cap.

- Your GP might prescribe a special hypoallergenic shampoo for you to use on your baby. Follow the instructions carefully.
- You may be advised to leave the lather on your baby's scalp for 20 minutes before rinsing. This can be difficult, so have some toys ready to distract your baby.
- In severe cases, a mild hydrocortisone (steroid) cream may be prescribed, often to be used in conjunction with a special shampoo.
- If the scales on your baby's scalp have become infected, your GP may prescribe an antibiotic cream.
- If the condition persists or worsens, or if your baby appears to have seborrhoeic dermatitis (see page overleaf), your GP may refer you to a dermatologist.

Treating cradle cap at home

Home treatment is usually all that is needed to alleviate cradle cap, and the condition should eventually clear up on its own. Below are four tried and tested methods of treating the condition yourself. Use one option or a combination.

Brushing: (BELOW) try to brush or comb out the flaky scales, but stop if your baby is becoming distressed. Don't attempt to loosen the scales if they won't come away easily.

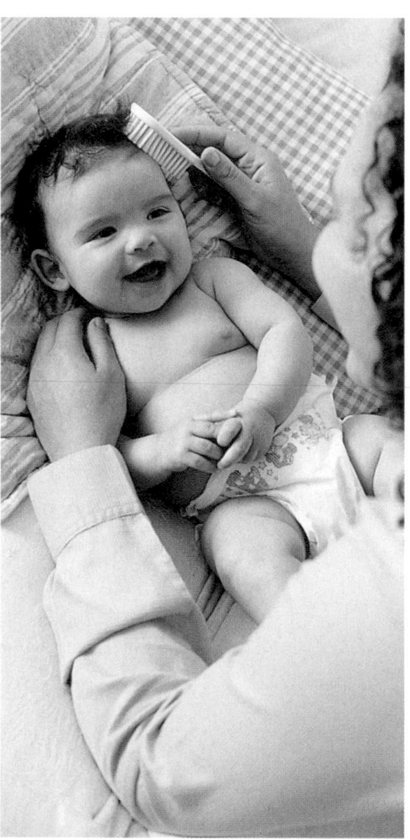

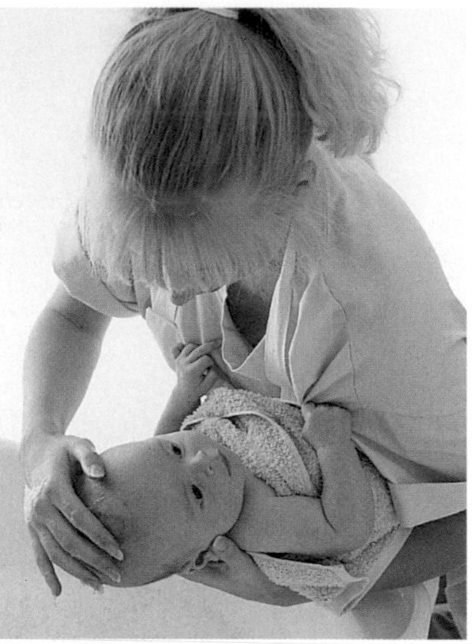

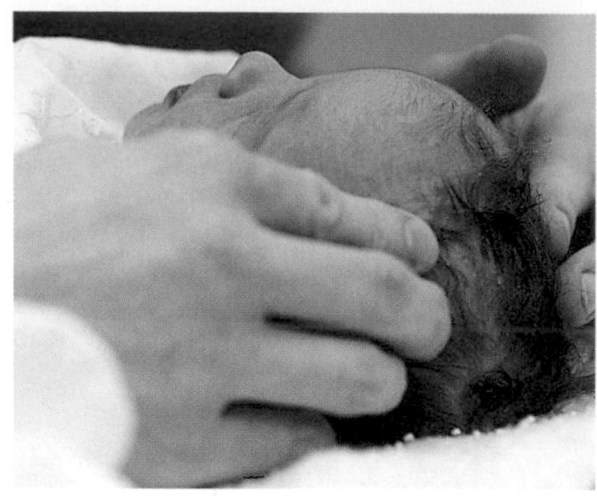

Washing: (LEFT) using a no-tears baby shampoo, gently wash your baby's hair and scalp. Do not use medicated or anti-dandruff shampoo except on the advice of your GP.

Rubbing: (ABOVE) before you put your baby to bed, rub a little baby oil, olive oil or petroleum jelly into his scalp to soften the scales, and leave it on overnight.

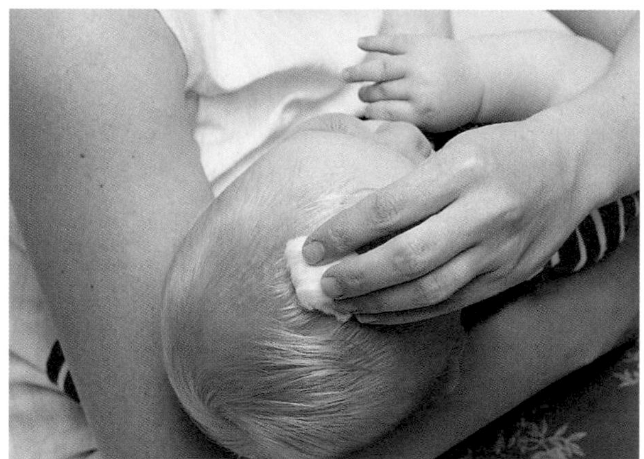

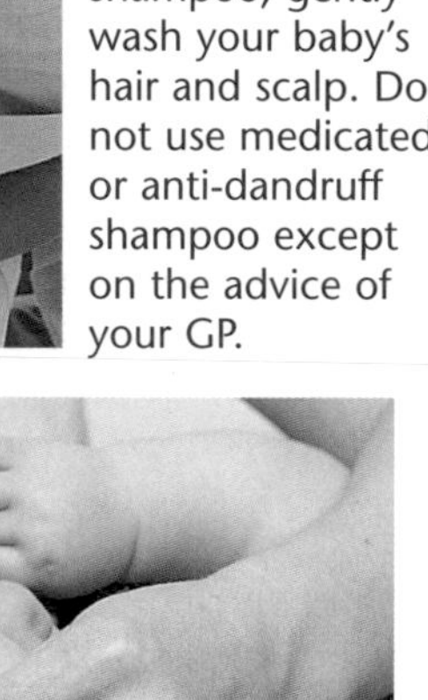

Wiping: (LEFT) often the simplest and gentlest method of treating cradle cap is to take a piece of cotton wool, dampen it slightly and carefully run it over your baby's scalp. Repeat this treatment two or three times, using a fresh piece of cotton wool each time you wipe your baby's head.

Could it be seborrhoeic dermatitis?

Seborrhoeic dermatitis is a type of eczema that occurs in places on the body where sebaceous glands are most prolific. In babies, these include the scalp, eyelids and greasy areas, such as around the nostrils, ears and groin.

- Unlike the more common form of childhood eczema, known as atopic eczema, seborrhoeic dermatitis is not characterised by extreme itchiness, and it responds well to treatment.

- The symptoms include: a scaly, blotchy rash, often in the skin creases of the nappy area, but also on the scalp, face, ears, neck and chest, and in the armpits; slight itchiness, although this does not always occur; and cradle cap, accompanied by scaly areas on the forehead, in the eyebrows and behind the ears.

- You can help treat the condition, which usually clears up by the age of two, by using emulsifying bath additives and creams, such as aqueous cream, instead of soap-based products and baby oils. You will find these at your local pharmacy and in some supermarkets, or you may be able to get them on prescription.

- If the condition still does not improve, consult your GP, who may decide to prescribe a mild steroid cream.

Important

- If the cradle cap is particularly stubborn, repeat the home treatment for 10 consecutive days. If you do not see an improvement after this period, consult your health visitor or GP.

- Never try to remove the scabs that form on your baby's scalp as these can leave scars.

CROUP

WHAT IS CROUP?

Croup is one of the most common causes of respiratory illness in young children, affecting up to 6 per cent of children under six years old every year.

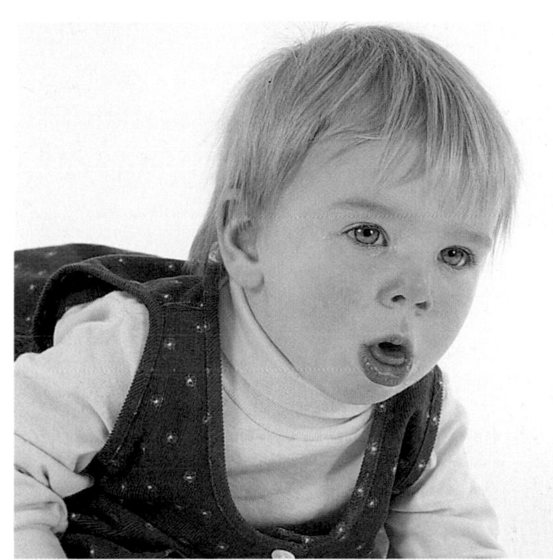

- Otherwise known as acute laryngo-tracheobronchitis, croup is an infection of the airways. There is progressive obstruction of the airway caused by inflammation and swelling of the tissues lining the larynx (voice box), trachea (windpipe) and bronchi (large airways in the lungs).

- Croup is caused by a virus, so antibiotics are ineffective and the illness has to run its course, with treatment aimed at alleviating the symptoms.

- The majority of cases of croup do not need medical treatment, but of those seen by GPs, up to 30 per cent are admitted to hospital.

One of the main symptoms of croup is a harsh 'barking' cough. Other symptoms include a sore throat and, in extreme cases, difficulty breathing.

How croup is contracted

The viruses responsible are normally present in the environment.

- It is usually caused by the parainfluenza virus.

- Children are more susceptible than adults as they have an immature immune system.

- The virus may be caught by droplet infection from person to person.

- It can occur in babies as young as two months, and is common up to the age of six years, occurring more frequently in boys than in girls.

- It tends to occur during late autumn and early winter, when the viruses are more prevalent.

Symptoms

The symptoms of croup are varied, but the main ones to look out for are respiratory problems and a harsh cough.

- The symptoms usually begin with a cold that lasts for one to four days. The child will have a runny nose and sometimes a slight fever with a temperature above 37.2°C (99°F).
- The child gradually develops a hoarse voice and a characteristic cough, which sounds like the barking of a seal.
- A baby may be miserable and reluctant to feed.
- On breathing in there is a harsh, rasping noise, known as stridor.
- An older child may also complain of a sore throat, and find it difficult to swallow.
- As is often the case with respiratory illnesses, the symptoms tend to be worse in the evening and at night, and often become worse for several nights before getting better.
- In a more severe case, the child will be breathing hard, and flaring the nostrils with each breath.

When to call the doctor

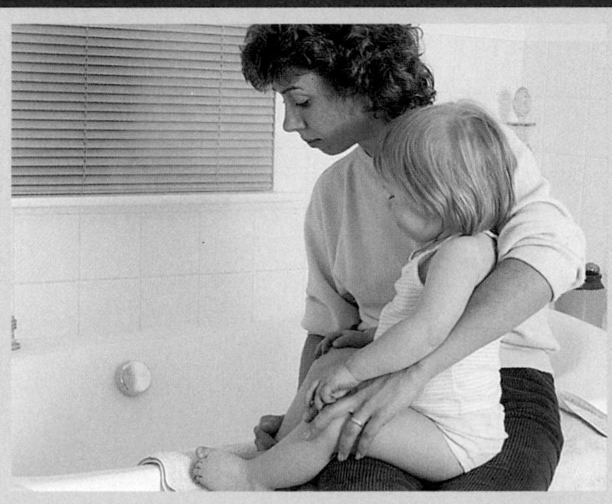

You should call a doctor immediately if your baby has any of the symptoms of croup listed above, or if a toddler or older child has any of the symptoms below.

1. Looks very pale and has dusky (blue tinged) lips and nails.
2. Is breathing very hard and sucking in the muscles between the ribs and under the rib cage, or there is stridor.
3. If the symptoms don't improve after at least 20 minutes of breathing steamy air or your child is fighting for breath.
4. If your child is becoming increasingly agitated or increasingly lethargic.

While you are waiting for help, take your child into the bathroom, close the door and turn on the hot taps as steam can alleviate the symptoms.

Home nursing

Most cases of croup are mild, and can be treated at home. However, severe cases can be life-threatening, so if you are in any doubt at all you must seek medical help – whatever the time of day or night.

- Encourage your child to sit up to help him to breathe, comfortably propped up with pillows. The head of a baby's cot can be raised by placing a folded towel under the mattress.
- A warm, steamy atmosphere will alleviate the symptoms and is most easily achieved by taking your child into the bathroom, closing the door, and turning on the hot water in the sink, bath and shower.
- Stay with your child until the symptoms subside, and afterwards ensure he sleeps in a room where you can hear him during the night if he happens to wake up.
- Make sure your child is sitting comfortably and keep him calm, for example by reading a story or talking to him.
- Offer him regular sips of clear fluids to drink, such as water or diluted squash – not milky drinks as these thicken the mucus in the throat, making breathing more difficult.
- Try to appear calm, even though you may not be feeling it. If your child senses you are anxious, this may heighten his anxiety and make his breathing difficulties worse.
- Give regular infant paracetamol to ease the sore throat and any fever.

Medical treatment for croup

A device called a nebuliser is usually prescribed to help a young child inhale medication for breathing difficulties.

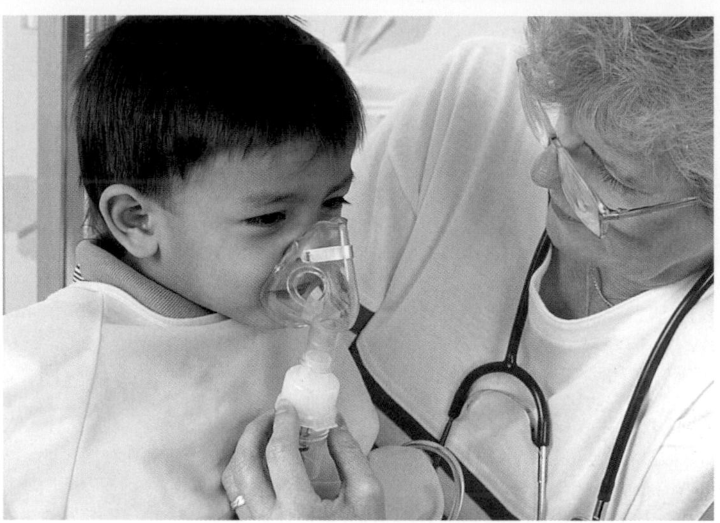

- A nebuliser administers steroid medication, which the child inhales via a face mask or mouthpiece.
- After this treatment, the doctor will assess its effectiveness and decide whether it is necessary to admit the child to hospital for observation and further treatment. If not, you should continue to treat your child at home, but don't hesitate to call the doctor if the attacks get worse and more frequent.

If your child suffers from croup, your doctor may show you how to use a nebuliser to administer medication that can soothe the symptoms. She will monitor its effectiveness.

- The symptoms of a croup attack will gradually subside over a few days. However, although seemingly cured, in some cases children may go on to develop an ear infection or a chest infection. These can be treated by your GP with antibiotics.

Recurrent croup

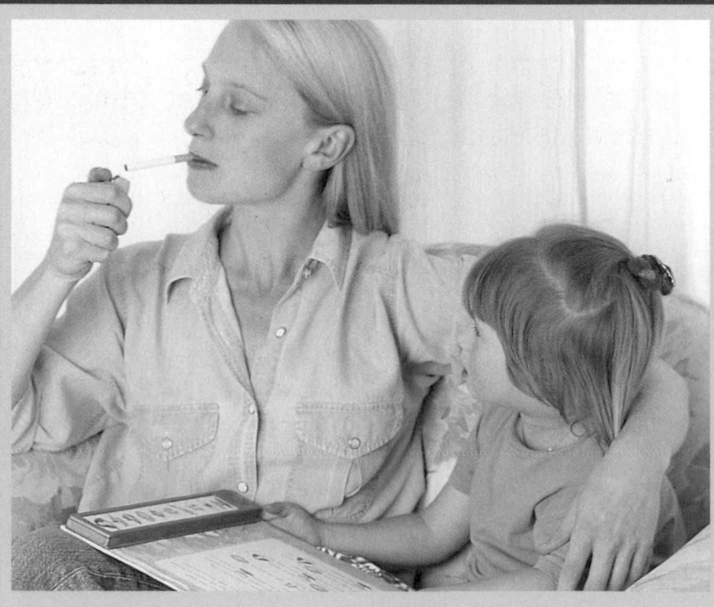

Some children do suffer recurrent attacks of croup for a few years. Medications used to prevent asthma are ineffective for croup and at the moment there is no known way of preventing it. However, there are ways in which you can help.

1 Some success has been claimed in treating croup with natural, homeopathic remedies.

Do not smoke anywhere near to your child if she suffers from croup. This is because the smoke from tobacco can exacerbate the condition and any other respiratory illnesses.

2 Breast-fed babies are thought to be less prone to developing respiratory illness, such as asthma, croup and pneumonia, than bottle-fed babies.

3 Don't allow smoking in the household or anywhere near your child as this can irritate your child's respiratory system.

CYSTIC FIBROSIS

WHAT IS CYSTIC FIBROSIS?

Cystic fibrosis is an hereditary disease caused by an abnormal gene. The condition affects the exocrine glands in the body (including the sweat and sebaceous glands) resulting in chest problems and possibly causing the body to have difficulties absorbing nutrients from food.

Cystic fibrosis is the most common life-threatening hereditary disease in the UK. More than 7,500 people in the UK have it, and currently three sufferers die every week. However, life expectancy levels are increasing all the time.

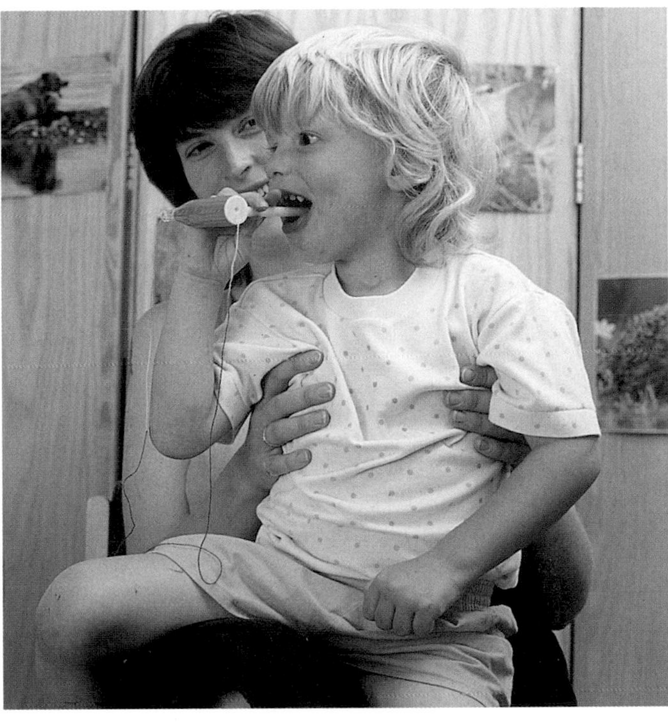

A child may have cystic fibrosis if both her parents carry the defective gene. One in 25 people carry the disease. If cystic fibrosis is suspected, a sweat test will be carried out. The disease produces high levels of salt in the sweat.

The effects of cystic fibrosis

A person with cystic fibrosis lacks a protein that regulates the passage of salts and water across the cells that line the surfaces of the lungs and digestive system. This results in the production of thick, sticky secretions and a build-up of mucus.

- The build-up of mucus in the lungs limits their ability to clear bacteria. This can lead to repeated infections and inflammation, which progressively damages the lung tissue. Complete respiratory failure can result and a lung transplant may be the only chance of survival.
- Blockages can occur in the lower intestine, producing abnormal stools.
- Pancreatic damage can lead to poor production of insulin and diabetes is common in adults with cystic fibrosis. It may also cause malnutrition because food is not digested properly.
- As life expectancy increases for people with this disease, osteoporosis is becoming a common complication of cystic fibrosis in older people.

Symptoms

A newborn baby may have a swollen stomach and may not pass any stools for a few days after birth. Other signs that emerge later include:

- Frequent chest infections
- Poor weight gain
- Malnutrition
- Abnormal stools that have an unusual smell

How is the cystic fibrosis gene detected?

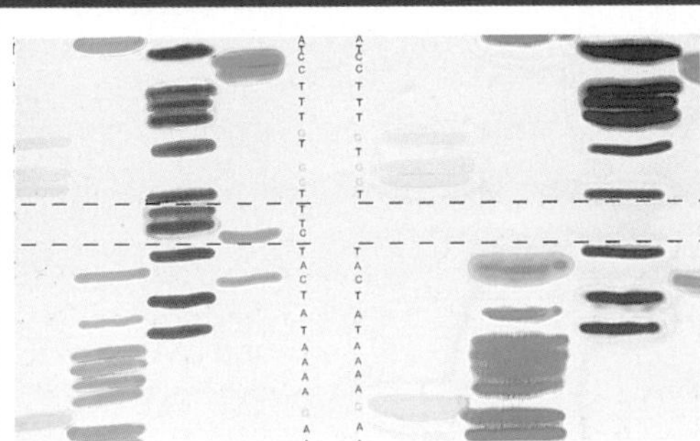

Here, the DNA (represented by coloured bands) of a healthy person is compared with a cystic fibrosis sufferer. In cystic fibrosis, part of the DNA sequence is missing – seen within the dotted line to the right-hand side.

Screening will be offered to couples who have a family history of cystic fibrosis. The disease cannot be passed on unless both partners are carriers. A child born of parents who are both carriers of the faulty cystic fibrosis gene has a one-in-four chance of having the disease. Cystic fibrosis can be detected using the following methods:

1 A mouthwash test is used to detect whether someone is carrying the cystic fibrosis gene.

2 Antenatal testing is offered at an early stage in pregnancy to mothers who are at high risk of passing on the disease, for example, if they have relatives with cystic fibrosis.

3 Newborn babies can be tested for cystic fibrosis by means of a heel-prick blood test. A third of babies born in the UK are currently tested in this way.

4 Ultrasound scans may reveal blockages in the bowel of the unborn baby, which can indicate the presence of cystic fibrosis.

Caring for a child with cystic fibrosis

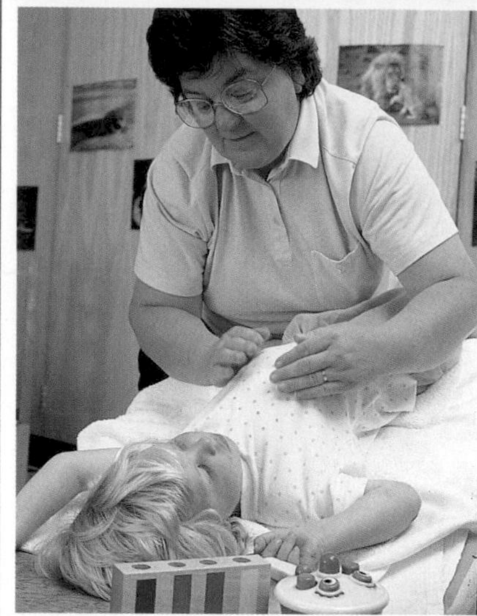

Tapping your child's chest and back daily will help to dislodge some of the build-up of mucus from her lungs.

The most immediate concern for people with cystic fibrosis is to try to unclog the mucus blocking their lungs in order to reduce infections and tissue damage. This is attempted by means of:

1. **Breathing exercises:** these exercises should be taught by a physiotherapist and consist of breathing control, deep breathing and a technique called huffing.

2. **Daily physiotherapy:** this can involve tipping the sufferer upside down to release mucus and unclog the lungs and airways, and percussion – tapping the chest area to dislodge mucus.

3. **Regular physical exercise:** trampolining is highly recommended for children who are strong enough, because it exercises the lungs and chest muscles and the jumping motion can help to shift and disperse mucus. Swimming, running and walking can also be highly beneficial.

4. **Controlled diet:** medical supervision of food intake is important because the effects of cystic fibrosis can vary. To reduce the risk of malnutrition, it's important that people with cystic fibrosis have a diet that is sufficiently high in protein, calories and extra vitamins if required.

5. **Enzyme supplements:** pancreatic damage means that people with cystic fibrosis usually have to take enzyme supplements with every meal.

Types of treatment available

There is currently no cure for cystic fibrosis. However, new drugs are helping to counteract some of the symptoms of the disease and reduce any damage to the internal organs.

- Mucus-thinning drugs such as Pulmozyme® can help to clear internal blockages.
- Bronchodilating drugs can reduce obstruction to the airways to make breathing less constricted. Sometimes a nebuliser may be used.
- Antibiotics can be sprayed directly on to the lungs to treat any infection.
- Anti-inflammatory agents can reduce the risk of tissue damage.
- Surgery may be necessary for babies with cystic fibrosis who are born with severe intestinal blockages.

Useful address

The Cystic Fibrosis Trust

This provides further information and support for people with cystic fibrosis and their families.

11 London Road,
Bromley,
Kent BR1 1BY.

Tel: 020 8464 7211
www.cftrust.org.uk

Quality of life and life expectancy

Modern drugs and advances in medical treatment and care have dramatically improved life expectancy and the quality of life for people with cystic fibrosis.

- In 1964, the average life expectancy of cystic fibrosis sufferers was just five years. Today it is 31. However, many people with cystic fibrosis live longer than this.
- Longer life expectancy and better treatment of symptoms has enabled many people with cystic fibrosis to lead active lives, take further education and build a career.
- Improved medical treatment has enabled some women with cystic fibrosis to give birth. An increasing number of women with the disease are giving birth happily and remaining in good health to care for their children.

The outlook for people with cystic fibrosis is improving. With specialised treatment and care, many can be expected to live well into their 30s.

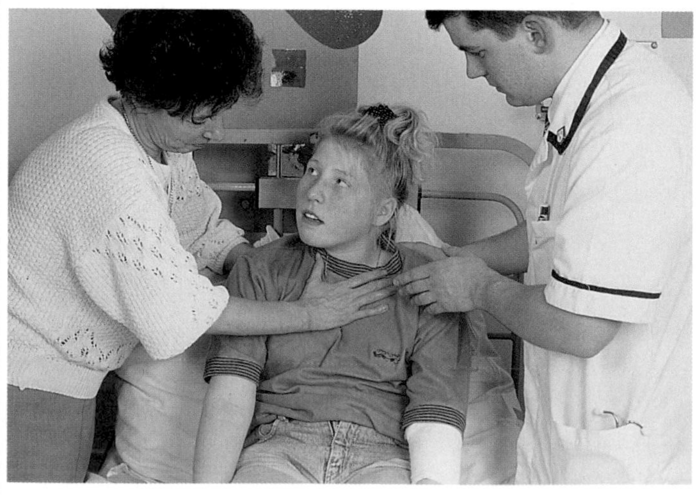

DIARRHOEA IN BABIES & CHILDREN

WHAT IS DIARRHOEA?

Diarrhoea is the frequent and sometimes explosive passage of loose, watery stools that may be green, slimy and foul smelling.

- Diarrhoea is extremely common. In fact, by the age of five years the majority of children will have experienced a bout of diarrhoea.

- Generally, this is a minor problem that can be treated at home. Sometimes, however, it can become more serious. This is more common in babies under two, who can become dehydrated very quickly.

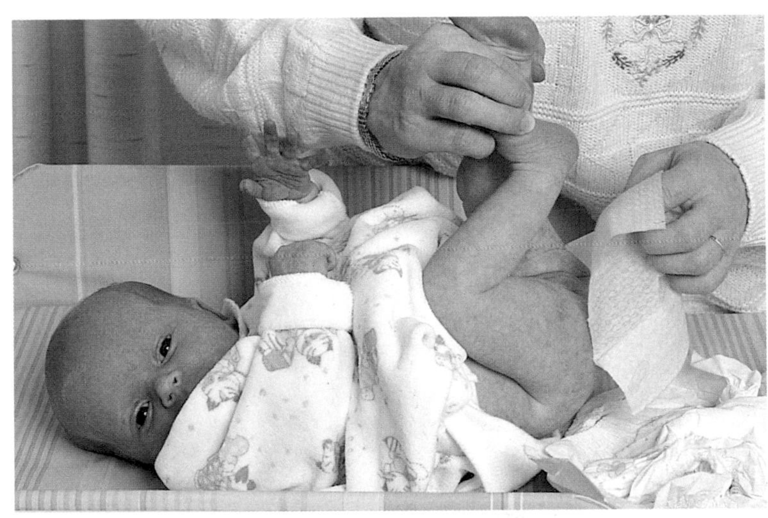

Diarrhoea is common in babies, although the condition is usually mild. However, it can lead to dehydration so should be closely monitored.

What causes diarrhoea?

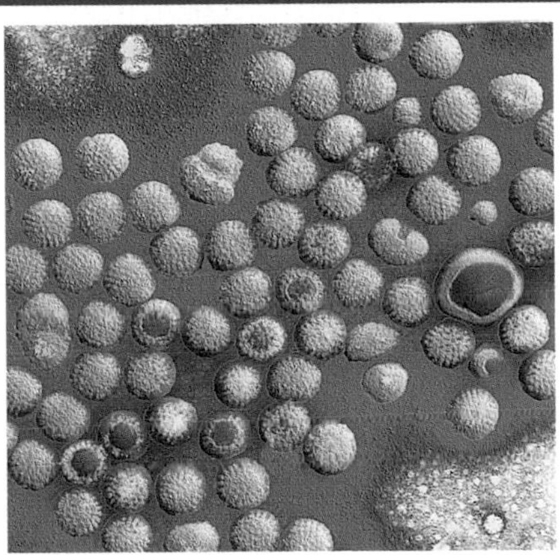

This is the most common virus to infect people and is called rotovirus. It often causes diarrhoea.

Damage to the lining of the intestine results in food not being digested and this causes diarrhoea. The damage can have a variety of causes:

- The most common cause in babies is a viral infection, often a rotovirus, or a form of E. coli.

- An acute viral or bacterial infection can lead to inflammation of the small intestine (gastroenteritis), which is usually accompanied by vomiting and a fever. Gastroenteritis is highly contagious.

- Certain antibiotics can cause diarrhoea.

- Some fruit juices contain sorbitol, a sugar that is not absorbed in the intestines. Sorbitol draws water from the walls of the intestines, and so can either aggravate diarrhoea or even trigger the problem when excessive amounts are consumed.

Associated symptoms

A baby or child who is suffering from diarrhoea may also:

- Vomit
- Have a raw, red nappy rash around the anus
- Be generally unwell, lethargic and have a slight temperature, if the cause is an infection
- Be dehydrated. This is a serious problem and if your baby starts to lose weight or shows signs of dehydration (see overleaf), you should contact your GP straightaway.

NOTE: breast-fed babies have loose, yellow, inoffensive stools. This is normal and should not be confused with diarrhoea.

What you can do

Check your child for other symptoms of illness and closely monitor his wellbeing.

1 If your baby or child is feeding and drinking well, he probably has a mild case of diarrhoea that will clear up in a few days. Make sure he has plenty of fluids.

2 If your baby is listless, off his food, colicky, vomiting and generally unwell, seek medical advice. Watch for signs of dehydration which can develop rapidly.

3 If you are breast-feeding, make a note of what you have eaten in the last few days. Your baby may be intolerant to an ingredient that has been passed through your milk.

4 If you have recently changed from formula to cow's milk, or introduced a new food to an older child, try changing back again to see if the diarrhoea stops.

Signs of dehydration

Dehydration can occur quickly and may cause your baby or child to:

- Be unusually quiet, unresponsive and drowsy.
- Have a dry mouth and tongue, and reduce the elasticity of his skin.
- Cry persistently, but shed few tears or none at all.
- Pass dark, yellowish urine infrequently (less than every eight hours).
- Lose body weight – if your baby has lost an excessive amount of weight, he may be severely dehydrated and you should contact your GP immediately.

Treating diarrhoea

Diarrhoea can usually be treated at home, but in serious cases hospitalisation may be necessary.

- If your child is well except for the diarrhoea and is not vomiting, stop all juices and high-fat foods and ensure that he drinks plenty of fluids. Do not give anti-diarrhoea medicines. These may lessen the frequency with which stools are passed but will not increase intestinal re-absorption of water.
- If your child has diarrhoea and is vomiting, contact your GP. You may need to start 'oral rehydration'. Your GP will advise you how much you should give. Continue giving bland foods and/or formula milk. Continue breast-feeding as breast-milk contains essential antibodies.
- If the diarrhoea worsens and is accompanied by vomiting and/or signs of dehydration, seek medical help immediately.

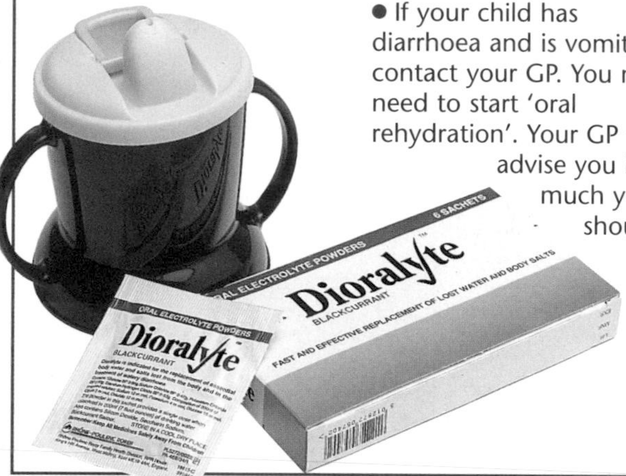

If your child has prolonged diarrhoea, your GP may prescribe oral rehydration solutions. They contain salts, sugar and minerals to replace those that have been lost.

Caring for a baby or child with diarrhoea

A child or baby with diarrhoea is likely to feel listless and unwell and will need some basic home nursing.

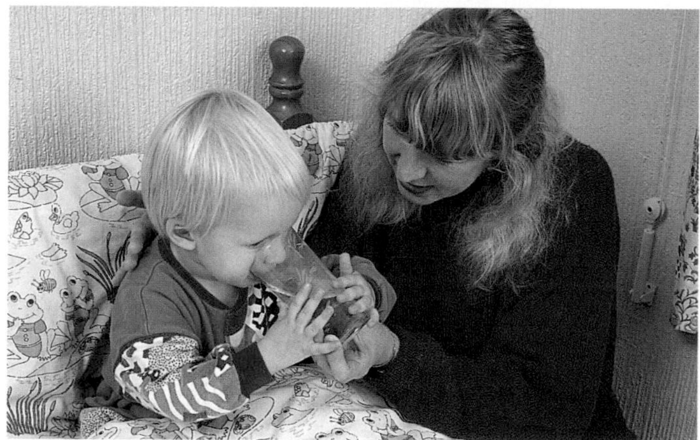

Give your child frequent drinks of water at room temperature to avoid him becoming dehydrated.

- Keep your child warm and away from other children in case the diarrhoea has been caused by an infection.
- Change any soiled nappies immediately to avoid a severe nappy rash. Cover the bottom with a petroleum cream to safeguard the skin.
- If you are breast-feeding, continue to do so, letting your baby suckle little and often for comfort and nourishment. Some of the breastmilk will be absorbed.
- Weigh your baby regularly to monitor any weight loss.
- Seek medical help if the condition persists for more than 48 hours, worsens or your child won't take fluid.

Preventing diarrhoea

No preventive measures against diarrhoea are completely effective, but the following can reduce the chances of the condition occurring:

1 Breast-feed: diarrhoea caused by an infection is rare in breast-fed babies and, if it does occur, the symptoms are usually less severe and less prolonged.

2 Guard against food intolerance: introduce new foods one by one to check for any intolerance or allergic reaction.

3 Treat infections: an infection in another area of the body can spread to the intestines if untreated.

To prevent diarrhoea, make sure you sterilise feeding bottles, teats and dummies correctly.

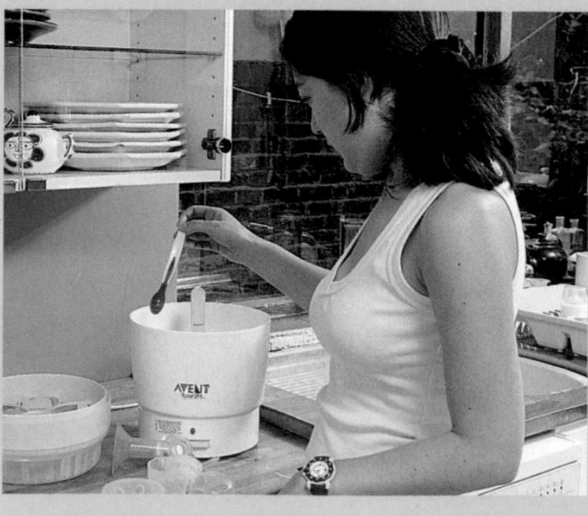

DOWN'S SYNDROME

WHAT IS DOWN'S SYNDROME?

Down's syndrome is a genetic condition that causes a number of distinctive physical characteristics and a degree of learning disability. The extent of any learning difficulties varies from person to person and it is impossible to predict at birth what the abilities (and disabilities) of the baby will be.

The chance of having a baby with Down's syndrome increases as the mother gets older. The reason for this is not known. However, it must be remembered that more babies with Down's syndrome are born to younger women because of the higher number of births to these women. On average, around two Down's babies are born every day in the UK.

Signs of Down's syndrome

Experienced doctors and midwives can diagnose Down's by recognising subtle characteristics at birth. A blood test is then taken to check the number of chromosomes. The common signs include:

- Eyes slanting upwards and outwards, with the eyelids having an extra fold of skin, which appears to exaggerate the slant.
- The back of the head may be flatter than average.
- The tongue may appear too large for the mouth, which can inhibit feeding.
- Looser muscles and joints than other babies.
- Babies with Down's may have a single crease that runs across the palm of the hand (this can also be present in babies who don't have the condition).
- Lower birthweight and slower growth rate than other babies.

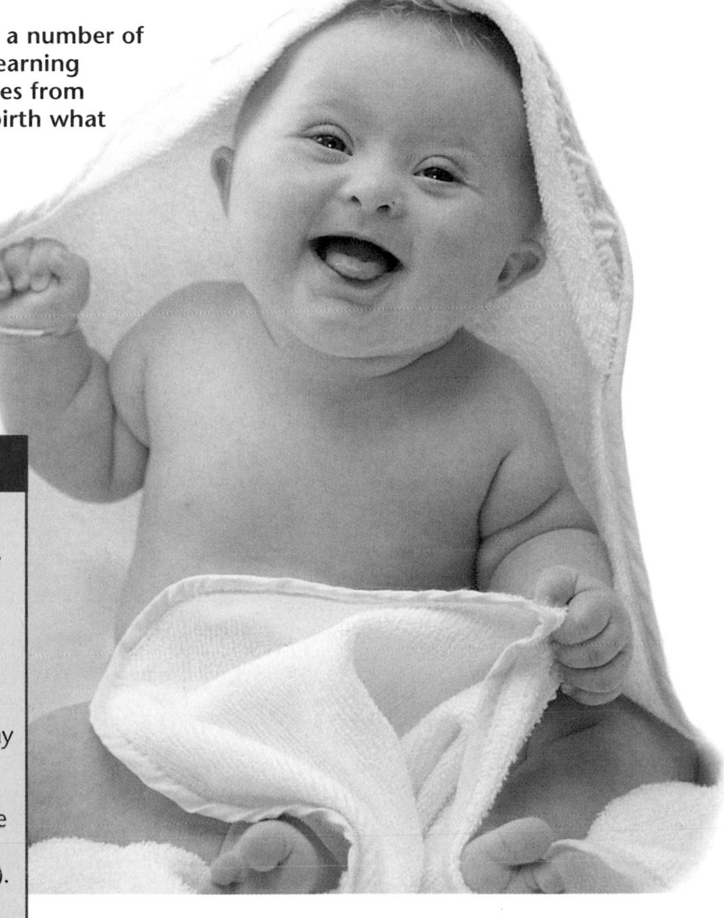

Approximately 750 babies are born with Down's syndrome in the UK each year. Although all babies are different, Down's syndrome babies share similar features, such as slanting eyes and a large tongue.

Why Down's syndrome occurs

Down's syndrome is caused by the presence of an additional chromosome, but it is not known why this extra chromosome occurs. It can come from either the mother or the father.

- Chromosomes are tiny particles that are present in every cell in our bodies. They carry the 'blue-print' for all the characteristics we inherit and influence everything about an individual, such as sex and eye colour.
- There are 23 pairs of chromosomes in each cell, giving 46 chromosomes altogether. One chromosome in each pair comes from the mother, the other from the father. Chromosome pairs are numbered from one to 23 and each pair will be responsible for a different aspect of our physical and psychological make-up.
- Down's syndrome is caused by the presence of an extra chromosome, making 47 chromosomes in total. The most common form of Down's syndrome is known as Trisomy 21. Instead of existing as a pair, there are three chromosomes in number 21.
- Nothing can be done before or after pregnancy to prevent or cause Down's syndrome. Mothers throughout the world give birth to Down's babies, regardless of their race, colour or quality of life.

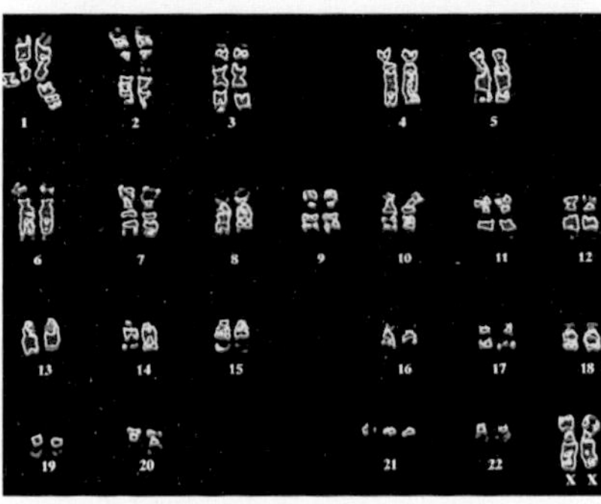

Every cell has 23 pairs of chromosomes – a total of 46 chromosomes. Trisomy 21, Down's syndrome, is when a baby is born with an extra copy of chromosome 21.

Looking after a Down's syndrome baby

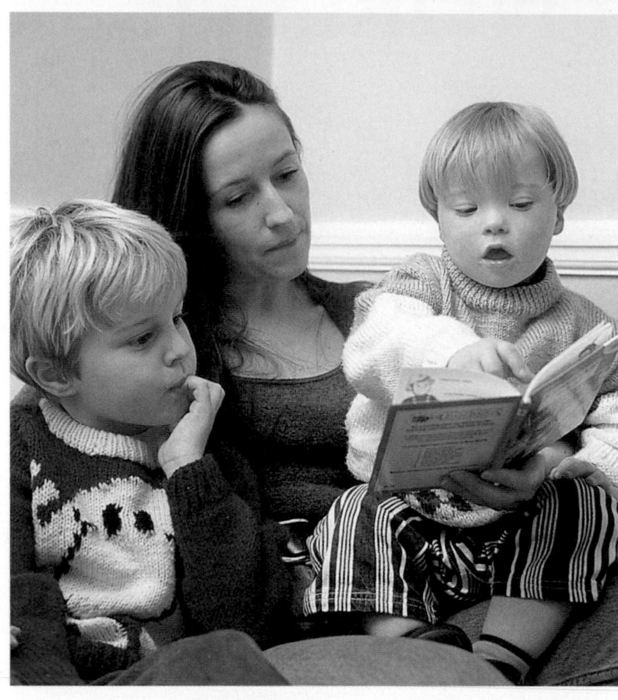

- Babies with Down's syndrome do need extra love and attention as they take longer to reach their developmental milestones. For example, more patience may be required when breastfeeding; he may take longer to learn to feed himself; he may not start walking until he is three; he may need additional support when he goes to school.

A child with Down's syndrome will need extra care and support from the whole family. You may find that an older child becomes more compassionate if he has a sister or brother with Down's syndrome.

- If you are a parent of a baby with Down's syndrome, remember that he is a baby first and foremost. He has his own unique personality and his own path in life to follow. You can help by being as supportive as possible, just as you would for any other child.
- He may not have been the baby you were expecting and you may feel sorrow, anger, shock, guilt or shame. You may feel your world has changed irrevocably for the worse. This is all very normal. The overwhelming majority of new parents of a baby with Down's come to love their baby as much as any other.

Health issues

There are a number of health problems associated with Down's syndrome. Although some are serious, most are easily treated with timely and appropriate medical intervention:

- **Chest and ear problems:** children with Down's syndrome are prone to chest and ear infections. They may need hearing tests.
- **Thyroid problems:** there is a higher chance of an underactive thyroid gland. Regular blood tests are taken to detect this.
- **Heart problems:** 40 per cent of all babies born with Down's syndrome will have a heart defect. However, many of these are treatable, if detected early. Your baby will be examined by a paediatric cardiologist and undergo heart tests.
- **Leukaemia:** children with Down's syndrome have higher rates of leukaemia than usual.

Down's in adulthood

Children with Down's syndrome can and do grow up to live long and fulfilled lives. Like everyone else, provided they are given the right support and opportunities to be independent and develop skills, Down's syndrome children can thrive. They are able to overcome many everyday challenges: in school, further education, work, living independently in a home of their own, and sustaining relationships.

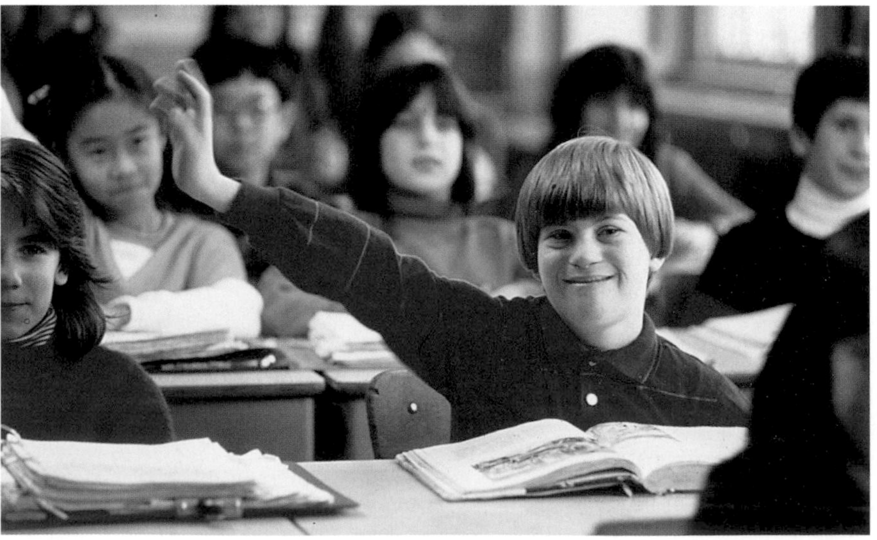

Many Down's syndrome children lead full lives, attending school and finding employment.

Useful address

For help and support contact:

The Down's Syndrome Association
Langdon Down Centre,
2a Langdon Park,
Teddington TW11 9PS

Tel: 0845 230 0372
Email: info@downs-syndrome.org.uk
www.downs-syndrome.org.uk

The Association can put you in touch with other parents of Down's syndrome children.

DYSPRAXIA

WHAT IS DYSPRAXIA?

Dyspraxia is a common childhood complaint in which a child has difficulty coordinating his movements. However, the reason for the condition is unknown.

- Many normal children go through a clumsy stage, but most grow out of it. In children with dyspraxia, however, the tendency towards clumsiness persists and interferes with everyday life and with progress at school.

- Behavioural problems are common in children with the condition.

- Dyspraxia affects about one in 20 children, and is more common in boys.

- Dyspraxia is also known as Clumsy Child Syndrome, Developmental Coordination Disorder, Minimal Brain Dysfunction and Motor Learning Difficulty.

- Early diagnosis is important to reduce the chances that a child will have behavioural or educational problems.

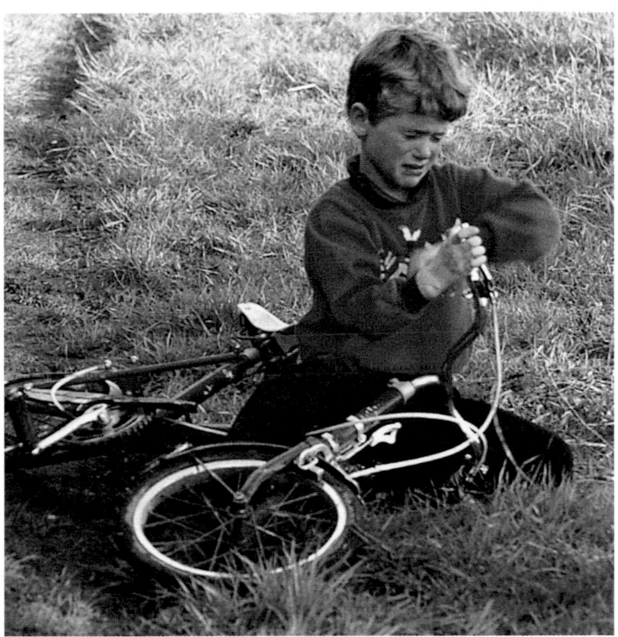

Dyspraxia causes clumsiness and a lack of co-ordination in a child. This makes skills such as learning to ride a bike difficult to achieve.

What causes dyspraxia?

The cause is unknown, but research has found that:

- Dsypraxia could be due to an immature neurone development in the brain rather than brain damage. It is thought to arise from failure of the neurones to form precise pathways during the brain's development, resulting in messages not being properly transmitted to the body.

- Some parents of dyspraxic children had similar problems, which suggests there could possibly be a genetic link.

Effects on the child

Children may be ostracised by their peers because they are different and, if their dyspraxia is not recognised and addressed early, they may not achieve their full potential. Children may be:

- Passive – not wanting to get involved in any fine or gross motor tasks.
- Frustrated because they find it difficult to relate to new skills.
- Tired because they have to make a great effort to perform everyday tasks.
- Shy, anxious, stubborn and unco-operative.

Symptoms

The symptoms and severity of dyspraxia can vary. If your child is experiencing any of the following signs, she may have dyspraxia:

- Reaches her developmental milestones late
- Slow to learn to dress and feed herself
- Clumsiness
- Confused about which hand to use
- Poor posture
- Has difficulty throwing and catching a ball
- Is slow to learn to speak, and speech may be incoherent
- Messy when eating and drinking
- Is sensitive to touch
- Falls over often
- Has a poor short-term memory and forgets tasks learnt the previous day
- Has poor drawing abilities
- Cannot hop, skip or ride a bike
- Has difficulty reading and writing
- Fails to answer simple questions even though she knows the answers
- Has a poor sense of direction

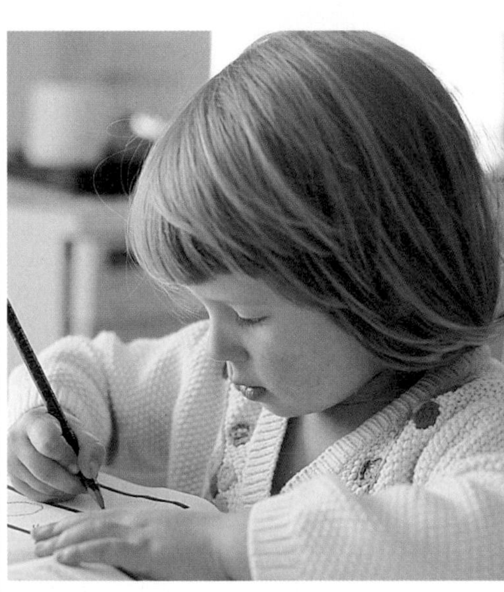

A child with dyspraxia is normally bright and intelligent, but will tend to have problems with reading and writing.

Helping your child

You should encourage your child to pursue activities that help her to develop skills.

- Choose activities that your child wants to do.
- Try to maintain your child's motivation by encouraging her to do a variety of fun and challenging activities.
- Never assume that your child knows what is expected of her. Always make the rules and the goal clear.
- Do the tasks with your child so that she can imitate your actions.
- Always keep to set routines.
- Do not tell your child what to do, it is better to ask her what needs to be done next.
- Communicate with your child's pre-school teacher frequently.
- Praise your child for the effort she puts in, not the end result.
- Emphasise what your child can do, not what she cannot.
- Provide plenty of time for your child to complete a task, and try to be patient.

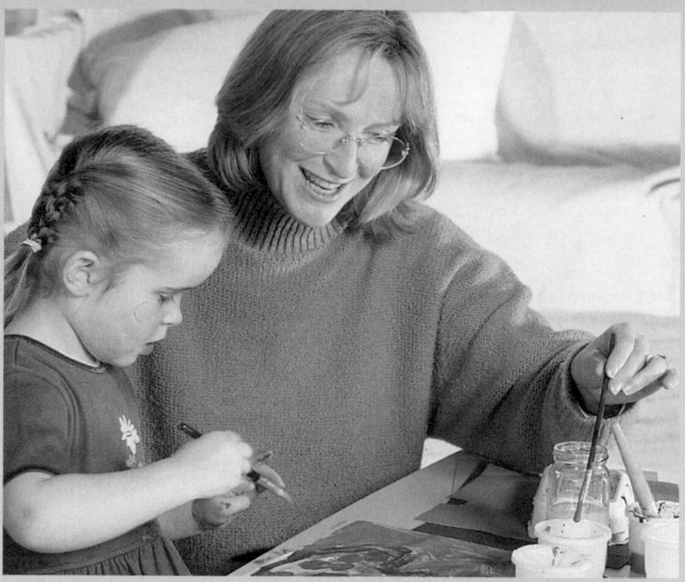

Taking part in activities such as painting, drawing, sewing, tracing and playing musical instruments can help to improve a dyspraxic child's visual skills and hand-eye co-ordination.

Professional treatment

If your GP suspects that your child has dyspraxia, he will be referred to a paediatrician or a local child development centre. A specialist will assess your child and identify the cause of his problem. The recommended treatment will depend on which of your child's faculties are most affected:

1 Speech: articulation may be immature or even unintelligible. A speech therapist will help to prevent delayed or impaired speech.

2 Movement: occupational therapists will help your child to develop strategies to enable him to learn certain skills. Different therapists use different strategies, but they will often break a skill down into its small component parts. Each skill is then learnt separately before being put back together into a whole skill.

3 Thought: a child psychologist may be able to help your dyspraxic child to plan and organise his thoughts. The psychologist will also aim to find ways to build your child's confidence and self-esteem.

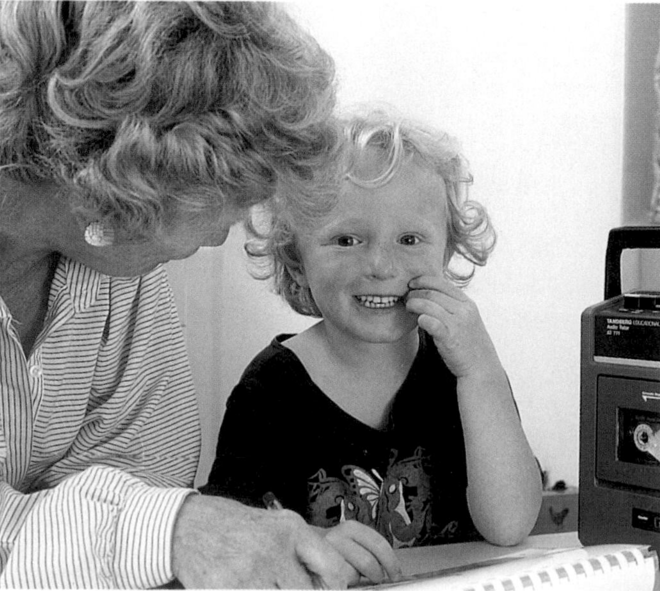

A specialist will set your child tests to assess his levels of co-ordination and identify the main areas of concern.

Outlook

There is not a cure for dyspraxia, but the earlier your child is treated the greater the chance for improvement.

- A lot of the skills that are taken for granted will never be automatic to a dyspraxic child and he may have to be taught these skills.
- The impact of motor planning difficulties will lessen as a dyspraxic child gets older.
- Motor planning is needed to help your child learn new skills. Once a skill is learnt, less motor planning is needed and therefore the dyspraxia is less of a problem.

Useful address

The Dyscovery Centre,
4a Church Road,
Whitchurch,
Cardiff, CF14 2D2

Tel: 029 206 28222
www.dyscovery.co.uk

EARACHE

WHAT IS EARACHE?

Earache in children can be caused by a middle ear infection, a foreign body in the ear, an infection in the outer ear canal or referred pain (where the problem is based somewhere else, for instance in the teeth). Children often have earache when they have a cold. The difficulty is distinguishing between an earache that will pass of its own accord in a few days and one that needs to be treated by a GP.

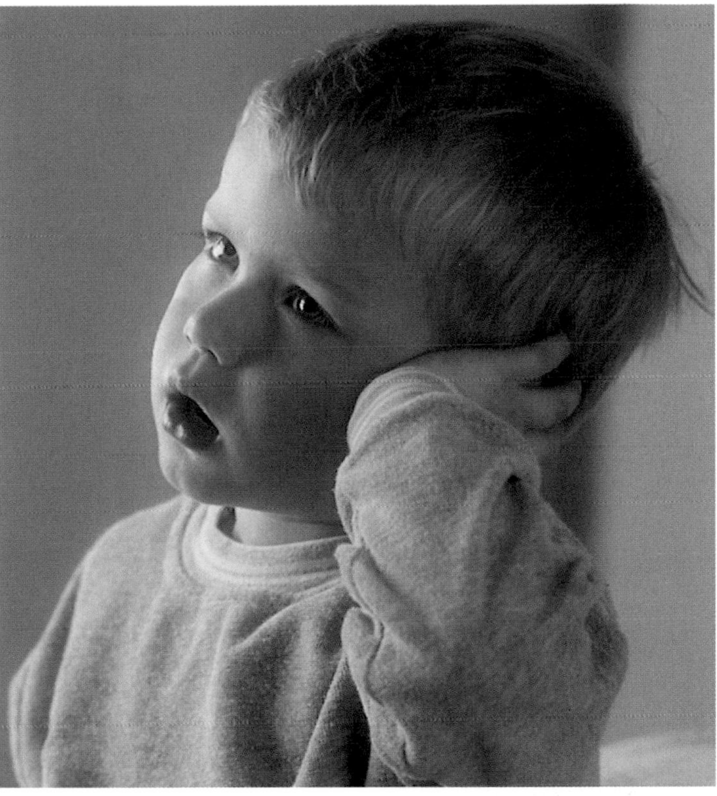

Signs that your child has earache are if he tugs at or keeps touching his ear. He may also be irritable.

Middle ear infection (otitis media)

The most common cause of earache in children is otitis media, or middle ear infection, following a cold. If the pain is severe, the doctor will probably see that the ear drum looks dull, red and bulging, and it may even pulsate. As pressure builds, the ear drum may burst, with a profuse, even blood-stained, discharge from the ear. There may be some temporary deafness.

Symptoms of otitis media

Under two years old:	Older children:
• Fever	• Fever
• Vomiting	• Ear pressure or a feeling of fullness in the ear
• Diarrhoea	• Severe earache
• Irritability	• Deafness
• Difficulty feeding	
• Not sleeping	

When to call the doctor

Earache can be so painful – and otitis media is potentially very serious – that GPs usually do all they can to see your child the same day. It is important to seek medical help if:

- There is fluid coming from the ear canal.
- Your child has a temperature over 38°C (100.4 °F), which does not go down with pain relief.
- Your child has severe earache that paracetamol or ibuprofen does not relieve, or if symptoms persist for more than 24 hours.
- Your child develops pain and tenderness over the skull behind the ear about 10 days after the initial earache, as this could indicate mastoiditis.
- Your child has other worrying symptoms, e.g. severe headache or profuse vomiting.
- Your child is not drinking enough, i.e. if he has not passed urine for over eight hours or his nappies are dry all day or overnight.

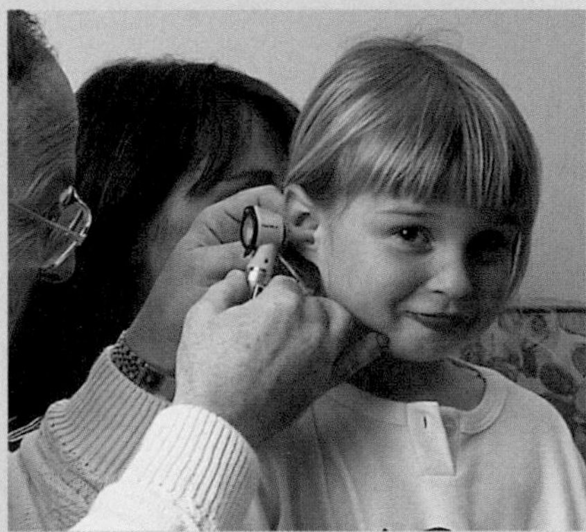

The doctor will look into your child's ear using a special instrument called an auroscope. If your child has otitis media that requires treatment by antibiotics, the ear drum will look red and bulging and will probably pulsate.

What you can do at home

There are several things you can do at home to ease the pain of otitis media:

- Give your child infant paracetamol or ibuprofen both to alleviate pain and reduce fever.
- Apply heat to soothe his ear – for instance, a hot water bottle filled with warm water.
- Raise your child's head when sleeping as the pressure on the ear drum when lying down could increase pain.
- Do not get his ear wet in the bath. Your child should not go swimming until the infection has totally cleared up.
- Consult your doctor before flying.

What causes earache?

The middle ear is a small cavity filled with tiny bones, lying behind the ear drum. Children are more prone to earache because their ears are less developed.

When the thin membrane of the ear drum vibrates in response to sound waves, the bones in the middle ear transmit the sound signals to the inner ear. The eustachian tube connects the middle ear to the nose and this ventilates and equalises pressure to the middle ear. Otitis media is an infection that produces pus in the middle ear. Children have smaller eustachian tubes than adults and are more prone to bugs tracking along the tube to the middle ear.

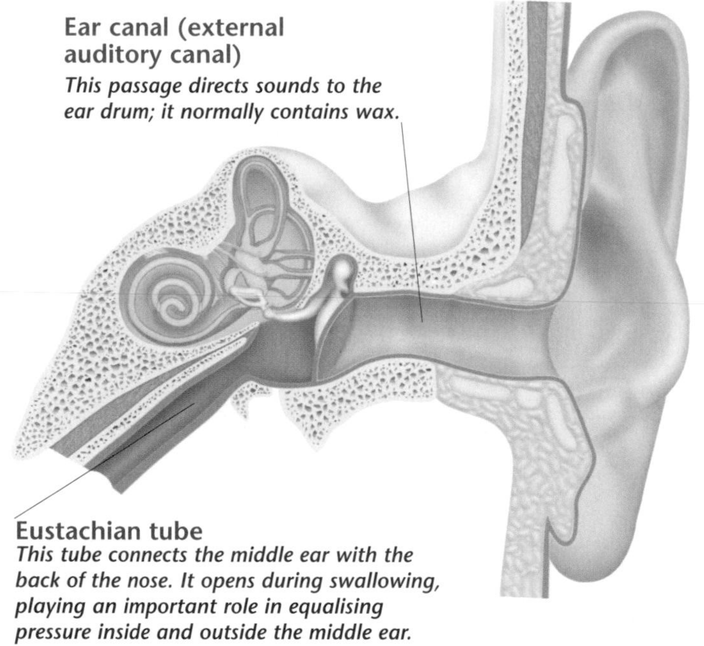

Complications of otitis media

It is important to monitor a child with otitis media closely as complications associated with the illness can be serious and prolonged.

- **Perforated ear drum:** this will take four to six weeks to heal and your GP will want to see the child at six weeks to confirm that the ear drum has healed.
- **Deafness:** after the infection, fluid can remain in the middle ear causing temporary deafness. Short-term deafness following otitis media may last several weeks before gradually improving. Long-term deafness may be caused by glue ear. Sometimes both operations are performed.
- **Glue ear (chronic secretory otitis):** if fluid remains in the middle ear, it can become thick and gluey causing deafness. It can be corrected by an operation either to remove the adenoids (glands at the entrance to the eustachian tubes) or to insert grommets (tiny plastic tubes) into the middle ear to rebalance pressure. Sometimes both operations are performed.
- **Recurrent otitis media (chronic suppurative otitis media):** the ear constantly discharges and there is a persistent perforation of the ear drum.
- **Mastoiditis:** the mastoid bone is in the part of the skull that lies behind the ear. Before antibiotics, an infection in the mastoid was a rare, but serious, complication of otitis media, developing about 10 days after the initial ear infection.
- **Intracranial abscess:** this is very rare.

Preventing earache

Unfortunately, if you suffered from frequent earache as a child, your own child is at greater risk. Most children get ear infections when they catch colds from other children, and this can't always be avoided. But there are some precautions you can take.

- Wrap up your child in cold, windy weather and get him to wear a hat.
- Children who are breastfed have fewer incidences of otitis media.
- Your child is more likely to have problems with glue ear and deafness if subjected to a very smoky environment.

Although covering up ears in cold weather will not prevent infection, it might ensure the condition doesn't get worse.

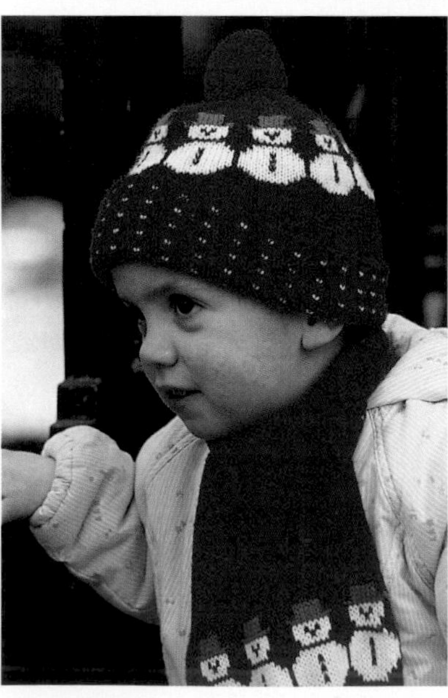

Otitis externa

This is an infection of the outer ear canal, between the eardrum and the external opening of the ear. Otitis externa is not commonly seen in children. The symptoms include a discharge from the ear and itchiness and pain, especially on touching the ear canal. Any dead skin, pus and wax need to be removed and then the ear should be packed with special dressings until the infection dies down. Sometimes, antibiotic drops into the ear canal are enough to cure it. Oral antibiotics can increase the risk of diarrhoea, rashes and vomiting. Your doctor will advise you about the best treatment.

ECZEMA

WHAT IS ECZEMA?

Eczema, or dermatitis, is a common condition in which the skin becomes inflamed, itchy, dry and scaly. In children, the main form is atopic eczema.

Atopic eczema affects around one in eight babies and usually starts before the age of six months, varying in severity from just a few patches of dry, itchy skin to a red, sore, weeping rash. Eczema is often inherited and has been linked to other allergic conditions, such as hayfever or asthma. Most eczema comes and goes, and the flare-ups have many triggers, such as pet fur, stress, heat, house dust mites and some foods. In severe cases, the flare-ups can be extremely distressing and interfere with family life.

Half of all babies with eczema grow out of it by the time they reach five years old and, in most children, the condition will clear up completely by the time they reach their teens. However, it may reappear later in life at times of stress.

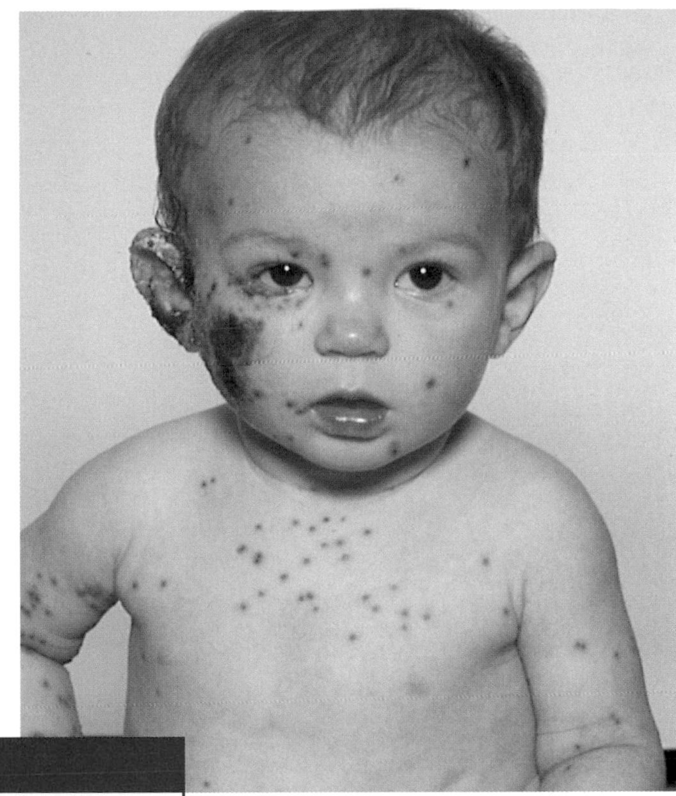

This child has a fairly severe form of eczema that has made his skin red, sore and inflamed.

Signs and symptoms

One of the first signs of eczema is a dry, flaky patch of skin on the face, usually appearing when your baby is three to six months old.

- Your baby may rub his face against his bedding and find it difficult to sleep. As his fingers become more co-ordinated, you may notice scratch marks on his skin.
- Once your baby becomes more mobile, the eczema may spread to other parts of his body, such as his hands and feet, the inside of his elbows and backs of his knees. In some cases, it can occur all over a child's body.
- The worse the eczema, the itchier it gets, and once it is scratched, the skin becomes sore and inflamed. This can lead to weeping and crusting and even the risk of an infection.

When to call the doctor

Occasionally, your child's eczema will flare up without an obvious trigger. Take him to the doctor if:

- His eczema spreads rapidly.
- He finds it difficult to sleep.
- His eczema becomes weepy and crusted or bright red.
- New symptoms develop, such as breathing problems or a fever.

Cradle cap

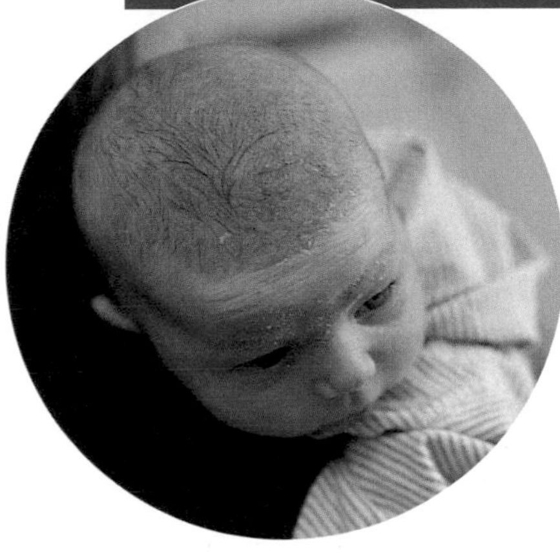

Cradle cap is a form of eczema called infantile seborrhoeic dermatitis.

It is very common in young babies, and varies in severity from a few yellow flakes of skin on the top of the head to a greasy cap of thick crusted scales covering the whole scalp. Sometimes, cradle cap spreads to the baby's face, neck and ears.

Although cradle cap may look unpleasant, it is harmless and shouldn't trouble your baby. It may last just a few weeks or stay for up to 12 months.

The scales can be difficult to remove. You can soften them by rubbing in a little baby oil or olive oil, leaving overnight and then washing your baby's head with a baby shampoo or a special cradle cap shampoo, available from pharmacies. You may need to repeat this several times before the scales come away.

Cradle cap is a mild form of eczema that affects many young babies. Special cradle cap shampoo or baby oil will help to clear the condition.

Reducing the triggers

Eczema can be aggravated by many factors. Fortunately, there are precautions you can take to reduce the risk of a flare-up:

- Avoid using soap or bubble bath – choose a bath emollient or an emollient cleansing bar.
- Change bedclothes often and vacuum beds and carpets to control house dust mites.
- Use anti-allergenic cotton bedding.
- Wash soft toys regularly at high temperatures.
- Keep your child's bedroom cool and turn down the heating overnight.
- Keep your child cool during hot weather.
- Keep household pets away from your child.
- Avoid putting wool or synthetic fabrics next to your child's skin.
- Experiment with different washing powders, as some may make your child's eczema worse – non-biological detergents are less likely to provoke a reaction.

Scratching problems

Babies and young children can't resist the urge to scratch, but unfortunately this makes the eczema worse. Young babies should wear cotton mittens to stop them from scratching themselves. Their fingernails should be kept short and clean. Older children should be taught to pat or rub the itch rather than scratch it. If your child is itchier at certain times of the day, apply extra emollients during these periods.

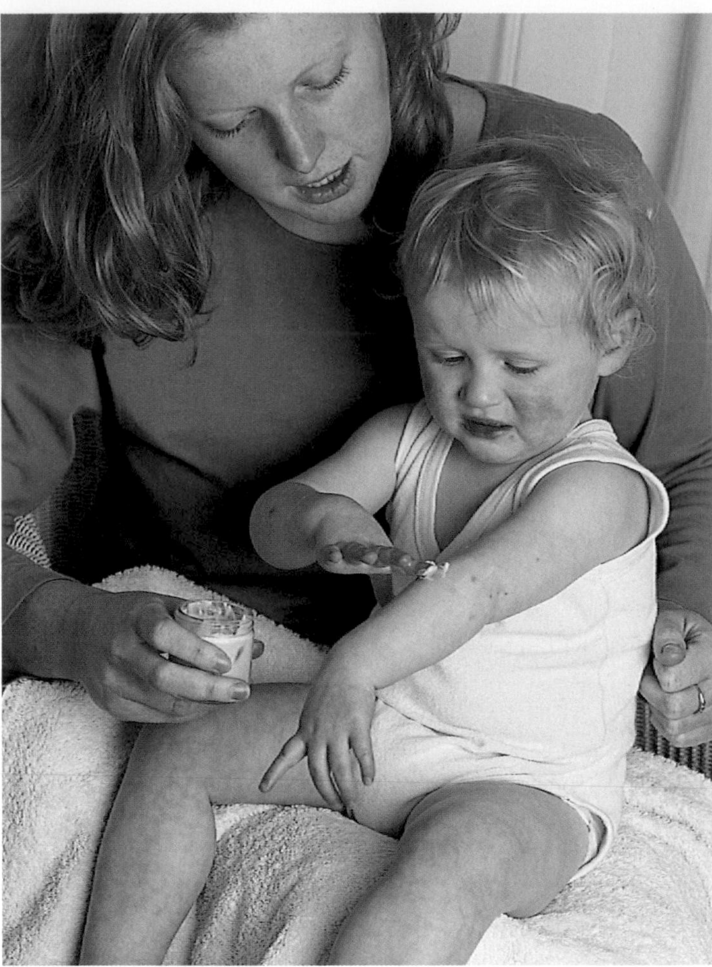

Emollient lotion helps to soothe eczema by moisturising the skin. It is best to allow the emollient to soak into the skin rather than rubbing it in.

Treating eczema

Remedy	***Emollient cream, ointment or lotion***	***Steroid creams and ointments***	***Dietary changes***	***Antihistamine and antibiotic tablets***
What does it do?	Keeps the skin moist and reduces the itching.	Soothes skin inflammation and itching.	A change in diet can reduce eczema that may be triggered by a food allergy.	Reduces more severe forms of eczema.
Procedure	Can be used on all forms of eczema. Apply liberally and frequently to the skin, ideally every half an hour and after bathtime. In severe cases, use wet wrapping to enhance the emollient's effectiveness during the night. Smear a thick layer of emollient on to your child's skin, cover this with a layer of warm, damp tubular bandages and place a layer of dry bandages on top. Then dress your child in loose clothes and ensure the bedroom is not too hot.	A weak steroid cream can keep flare-ups under control. The creams are available over the counter in varying strengths, but should be used under medical supervision only. For babies, the mildest steroid, hydrocortisone, is usually prescribed.	Elimination diets are usually reserved for very young children with severe eczema that hasn't responded to standard treatments. Common culprits include dairy products, citrus fruits, fish and peanuts. Before eliminating any foods from your child's diet, consult a doctor. It can be dangerous for a child to miss out on certain foods, as this could result in nutritional deficiencies.	If the itching is severe and your child has problems sleeping, your doctor may recommend sedative antihistamine tablets or syrup. These should be given at least half an hour before your child goes to bed. If the eczema becomes infected, your doctor may prescribe antibiotic tablets or creams or ointments containing both an antibiotic and a steroid.

ENCEPHALITIS

WHAT IS ENCEPHALITIS?

Encephalitis is inflammation of the brain, an extremely serious condition that can affect both children and adults.

- Encephalitis is the result of an infection, usually caused by a virus.
- The brain tissue itself is inflamed, as opposed to the meninges (the membranes that surround the brain), which occurs in meningitis.
- Sometimes, both the brain and the meninges become inflamed. This condition is known as encephalomyelitis.

If encephalitis is suspected, a brain scan will be taken to detect swollen tissue. This is one of the main symptoms of the condition.

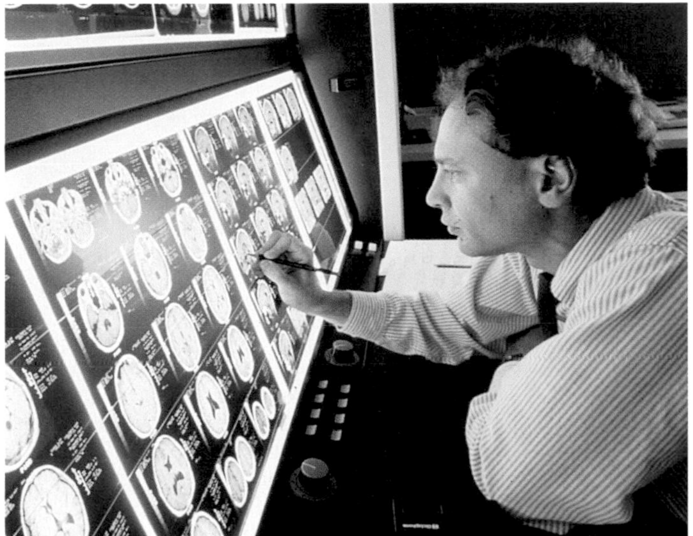

What are the causes?

A range of viruses can cause encephalitis and/or meningitis.

- **The herpes simplex virus:** this is the virus that causes genital herpes. It can be passed by a mother infected with genital herpes to her baby during a vaginal delivery, and therefore a Caesarean section is usually performed.
- **The measles virus:** about one in 5000 children with measles have encephalitis as a complication. The condition usually develops a few days after the rash becomes obvious.
- **Mumps virus:** this is another condition that can cause encephalitis as a complication.
- **The varicella virus (chickenpox virus):** this is usually a comparatively mild form of the illness compared with the other types.

Encephalitis can be caused by the herpes simplex virus. A pregnant woman infected with genital herpes can pass it on to her child during a vaginal birth.

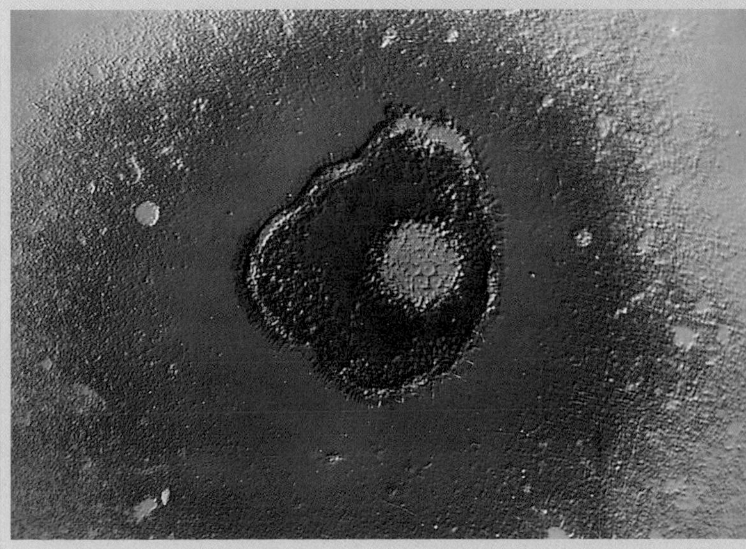

Recognising the symptoms

The symptoms of encephalitis in a child vary greatly; they may be mild or serious and can either appear suddenly or develop over a period of time. The symptoms also depend on the cause – for example, if encephalitis is a complication of measles, the symptoms of measles will be present as well. The symptoms outlined below may be present in affected children.

1. A raised temperature, above 37.2°C (99°F), or vomiting.
2. Headache – if a child is too young to explain that he has a headache, there may be obvious signs of distress, such as persistent crying or rubbing the head.
3. The child behaving strangely, or being consistently irritable or confused.
4. Weakness in one or more parts of the body.
5. Occasionally, the speech is affected and there may be blurred vision and poor balance.
6. Decreased levels of consciousness ranging from unusual drowsiness to unconsciousness.
7. Convulsions – the child may have seizures.

NOTE: fever and headache occur in lots of minor childhood illnesses but if a child also has any of the other symptoms listed above, or if you are worried, you should seek urgent medical advice.

Confirming the diagnosis

If a child has suspected encephalitis, admission to hospital is usually arranged straightaway. The problem is that the symptoms could apply to a range of diseases that affect the brain, for example an infection or a tumour, so investigations need to be carried out to exclude these.

- **Physical examination:** a special series of tests will be carried out, such as testing reflex reactions, to assess the nervous system.
- **Blood samples:** these are taken to look for infection, and specimens of the child's urine and faeces may also be sent to the laboratory for examination under the microscope.
- **Electroencephalography (EEG):** this shows the brain's activity as waves on a graph. In some types of encephalitis, particularly herpes simplex encephalitis, the results are abnormal.
- **Scans:** both MRI (magnetic resonance imaging) and CT (computed tomography) scanning can show up any swelling of the brain tissue.
- **Lumbar puncture:** this will be carried out in most cases because it can distinguish between a viral and bacterial infection, and will therefore exclude bacterial meningitis as the cause of the symptoms. A lumbar puncture involves taking a small sample of fluid from around the spinal cord. The procedure is done using local anaesthetic, so it is not painful. A narrow needle is inserted into the space between the vertebrae in the lower back and fluid is withdrawn using a syringe. The sample is then examined for inflammation or infection.

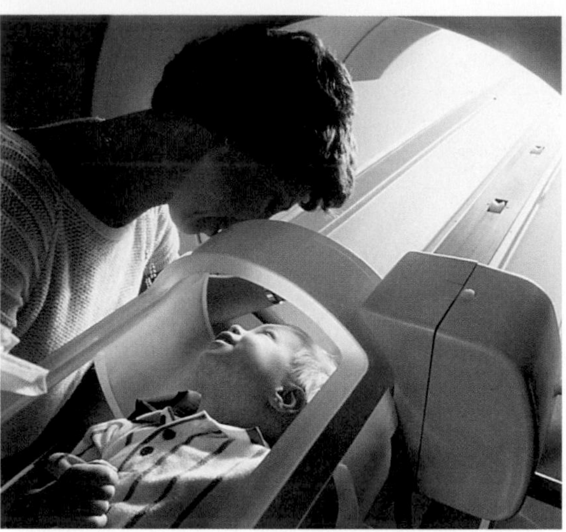

If encephalitis is suspected, a range of investigations will be recommended. MRI scans may be carried out to check for swelling of the brain tissue.

Treatment

The treatment of encephalitis has two aims – to treat the cause of the inflammation and to treat the effects of the encephalitis. Most children with encephalitis improve once the cause is treated.

1 Affected children are usually nursed in a specialist unit. It is important to monitor a child's consciousness and, if he is drowsy, to make sure that his airway is kept clear and that he is breathing easily.

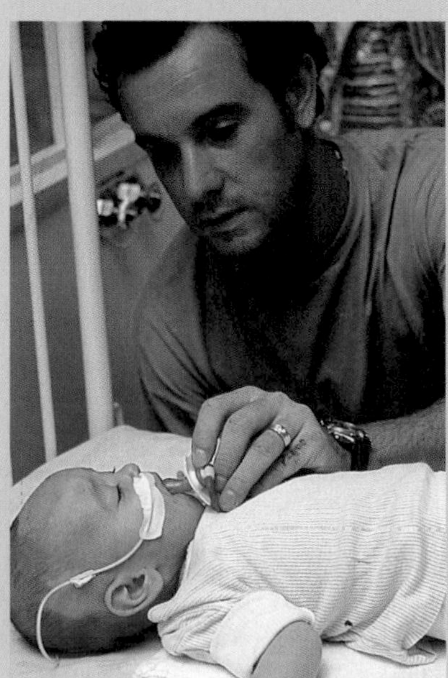

2 Fluids are usually given directly into a vein to keep a child well hydrated, especially if he is unable to drink regularly. If the illness persists for more than a few days, it may be necessary to feed the child with special liquid nutrition into a nasogastric tube (a tube passed down the nose and into the stomach).

3 Rarely, if the brain inflammation is severe, a child may have increased pressure within the skull. In the short term, artificial ventilation (a breathing machine) helps to reduce this pressure.

4 Herpes simplex encephalitis is treated by administering the anti-viral drug aciclovir directly into the bloodstream.

Children with encephalitis are kept in a specialist unit where they can be monitored closely. Certain equipment may be used, such as a breathing machine and a nasogastric tube.

Reye's syndrome

This rare condition may follow a viral infection, typically chickenpox or influenza, and is associated with children under sixteen years taking aspirin. Reye's syndrome causes liver failure and this causes brain poisoning. The brain poisoning is called encephalopathy and, like encephalitis, it has brain swelling as a symptom.

- Symptoms initially include vomiting and signs of a chesty cold. The child becomes drowsy and has convulsions.
- If doctors suspect Reye's syndrome from the symptoms, they will probably carry out a scan – either a CT scan or an MRI scan – which will show swelling of the brain. Blood tests will show that the liver is not functioning properly.
- A child with Reye's syndrome will need to be looked after on a paediatric intensive care unit. There is no treatment, but doctors will provide medical 'support' – such as artificial ventilation to decrease the pressure in the brain – until there are signs of improvement.

ENURESIS

WHAT IS ENURESIS?

Enuresis is the medical term for an inability in children to control urination. Bedwetting at night is known as nocturnal enuresis and can be caused by a range of factors.

- When young children are awake, they gradually learn to recognise signals from the bladder. Thus most children become dry during the day relatively easily.
- When the child is asleep, urinary control has to be carried out subconsciously, and bedwetting continues until the brain learns to recognise the signals from the bladder.
- Nocturnal enuresis is divided into two groups; primary nocturnal enuresis occurs when bladder control has never been acquired; secondary nocturnal enuresis when bladder control has been gained and lost.

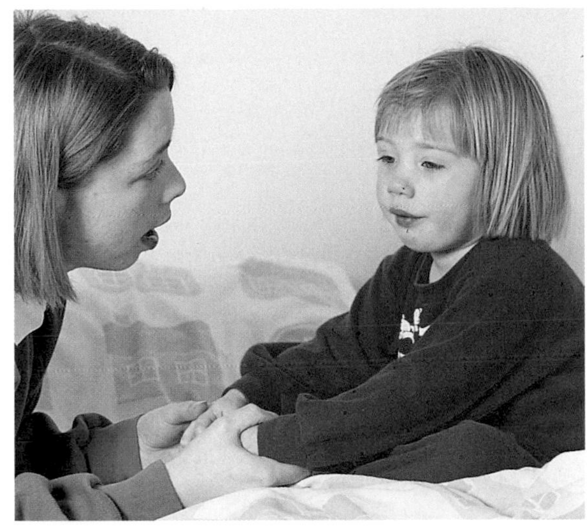

A child who wets the bed may be insecure and upset. Be sympathetic and patient with your child and remember that it is not her fault.

What age group is affected

Enuresis is diagnosed when a child over the age of five, with no other health problems, wets the bed at least once a month.

- Nocturnal enuresis affects about one in six children over the age of five. By age seven only about one in 10 children still wets the bed, and this reduces to one in 20 by the age of 10. Bedwetting can carry on into the teenage years (one in 40) and even adulthood.
- Daytime enuresis is less common, affecting about one in 75 children over the age of five, because children learn to recognise bladder signals when they're awake.
- Boys often take longer than girls to learn bladder control.

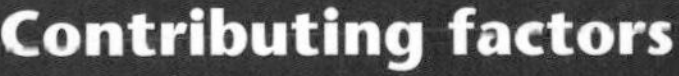

Contributing factors

There may be factors in a child's life that can delay the acquisition of bladder control or trigger secondary enuresis.

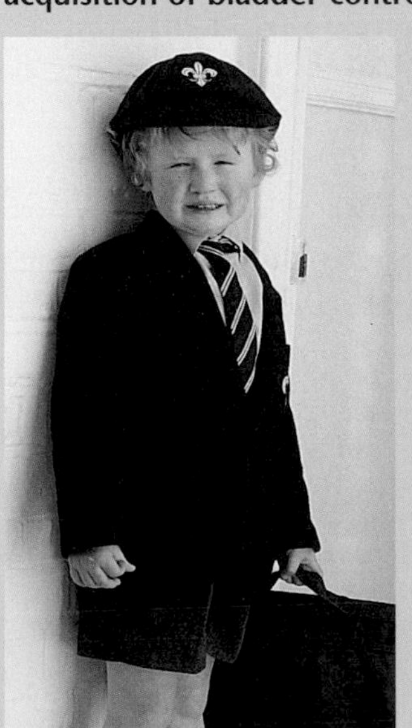

- Children with small bladders are more likely to have accidents at night until their bladders have fully expanded.
- Major changes, such as a new brother or sister or moving home or school, can cause anxieties that may subconsciously trigger enuresis.
- Situations, such as emotional difficulties in the home, can result in psychological problems that may trigger enuresis.

A major change in your child's life, such as starting a new school, can subconsciously trigger enuresis.

The causes of enuresis

Despite a considerable amount of research, the causes of enuresis are not fully understood.

- **Hereditary:** bedwetting can run in families because a deep sleep disorder can be inherited. In very deep sleep, the brain does not respond when signalled by the bladder. The sphincter muscle around the opening of the bladder remains relaxed and the bladder empties involuntarily. Consequently, the bladder develops a small capacity and the sphincter muscle remains weak.
- **Physiological:** although rare, disorders that can result in enuresis include anatomical abnormalities and infections of the urinary tract, and abnormalities of the nerves that control the bladder. Constipation and untreated diabetes can also be a cause.

Keep a potty next to your child's bed, so she will be able to go to the toilet easily if she does wake up during the night.

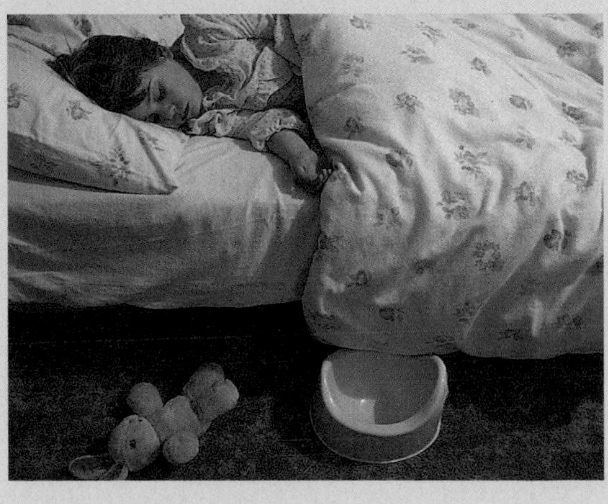

Treating enuresis

In most cases, bedwetting stops without treatment. Medical treatment is unlikely to be recommended for a child under six.

- After the age of six special tests on bladder function may be carried out to establish that the nerves and muscle are working normally.
- Bedwetting alarms are triggered by a few drops of urine and wake the child. They are considered by most specialists to be an effective way of training a child. Alarms are said to cure 70 per cent of cases, only 10 per cent of which return to bedwetting after the alarm has been removed.
- Behavioural therapy, such as praise and reward for dry nights, is often used and is good for your child's self-esteem. However, it is not thought to be as effective as a bedwetting alarm.
- In rare cases medicines can be given, but most children start bedwetting again after a drug is withdrawn. A hormone tablet or nose spray which helps to cut down on urine production may be used.

Helpful measures

There are a number of precautions that can be taken, if your child is happy with them.

- If possible, try to ensure that your child avoids drinking fluids for a couple of hours and empties his bladder before going to bed.
- Protect the bed by using a waterproof mattress or a fitted waterproof mattress cover fastened securely to prevent any danger of suffocation.
- Leave clean night-clothes and sheets near the bed, so that they can be changed if the child wishes to do

Show your child how to make her bed so she feels in more control of the situation.

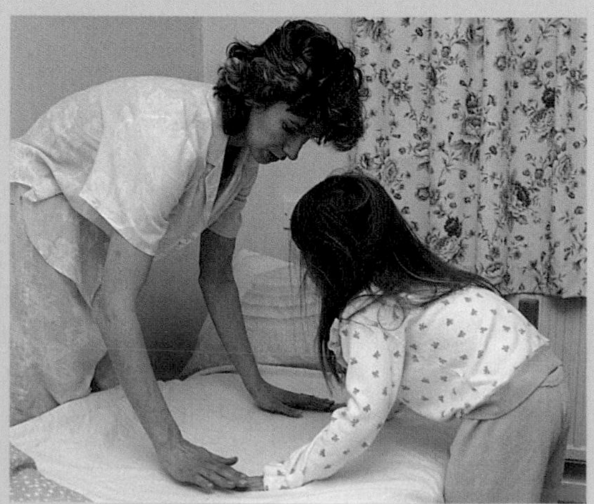

Dos and Don'ts

Children do not wet the bed on purpose. It is not due to laziness or a lack of willpower, and a child should not be disciplined when he has an 'accident'.

✘ Do not scold or punish the child or in any way make him feel that he is to blame.

✘ Do not put a nappy on the child at night, as this may reduce his awareness of the problem.

✘ Do not make the subject a big issue in the family; instead, treat it in a matter-of-fact way. Some children gain pleasure from the attention given as a result of bedwetting, even if the attention is negative.

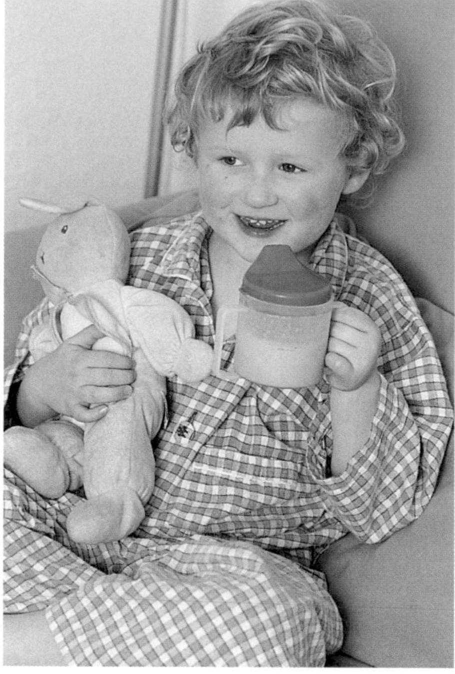

Try to limit your child's drinks from the evening onwards so the need to urinate doesn't occur while asleep. Remember to encourage him to drink plenty of fluid during the day to avoid dehydration.

✔ Do let your child know that bedwetting is very common and is nothing to be embarrassed about. If other members of the family suffered from enuresis in the past, tell the child about their experiences.

✔ Do praise your child for going through the night with a dry bed, but don't over stress the praise, as this can reinforce the idea that bedwetting is a cause for shame or embarrassment. Some parents ask their child to keep a chart, offering a small reward for dry nights.

✔ Do praise your child in other areas of his life, to help him feel better and more positive. Bedwetting can cause a child to develop low self-esteem.

Who can help

If bedwetting becomes a problem and you feel you need help, it is almost certainly available somewhere near you.

- Many districts have enuresis clinics, which specialise in the treatment of bedwetting.
- Your health visitor should be able to offer advice and in some areas there are specialist nurses and doctors who can visit people at home.
- ERIC (The Enuresis Resource and Information Centre) offers support and advice via a telephone helpline, plus a pen pal service with older children who have successfully stopped bedwetting. Tel: 0117 960 3060; email: info@eric.org.uk; website: www.eric.org.uk

EPILEPSY

WHAT IS EPILEPSY?

An epileptic seizure occurs when an upset in the electrical activity of the brain causes disturbance of the normally ordered signals that pass between the brain's neurons (nerve cells). Epilepsy is diagnosed when such seizures occur regularly.

- About one in 200 people in the UK suffers from epilepsy and this makes it the second most common neurological condition after migraine.

- Fits (convulsions) are one of the main features of epilepsy. In babies and young children fits can also be caused by a high temperature – these are generally known as febrile convulsions.

- Epilepsy can affect anyone of any age. Boys and men tend to be slightly more prone to epilepsy than girls and women, although the reason for this is not known.

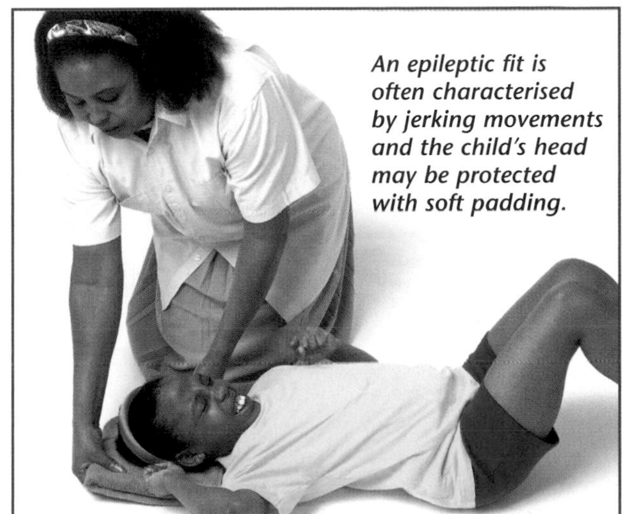

An epileptic fit is often characterised by jerking movements and the child's head may be protected with soft padding.

What causes epilepsy?

Every person's brain has the capacity to undergo a change in brain chemistry that produces a seizure. Some people have a low seizure threshold and this means that seizures may occur more frequently.

1 In six out of every 10 cases the reason why a person has epilepsy is unknown. It can develop at any age, but in most cases seizures start to occur during infancy. After adolescence the chances of epilepsy developing are reduced, but the incidence rises again after the age of 65.

2 Epilepsy may run in families. If either or both parents have a low seizure threshold, this may be passed on to some or all of their children.

3 Epilepsy occasionally develops as a result of brain damage or other structural abnormality of the brain. This may be the result of a difficult birth, a blow to the head, a tumour, a brain infection, stroke or meningitis.

4 Most seizures have no obvious trigger. But some people are able to distinguish factors that result in seizures, including excess alcohol, stress, lack of sleep and illness.

5 A temporary lack of oxygen or glucose may trigger an epileptic seizure.

6 A few people are photosensitive and react to flickering patterns of light, such as those that may be seen when watching television or playing video games.

Symptoms

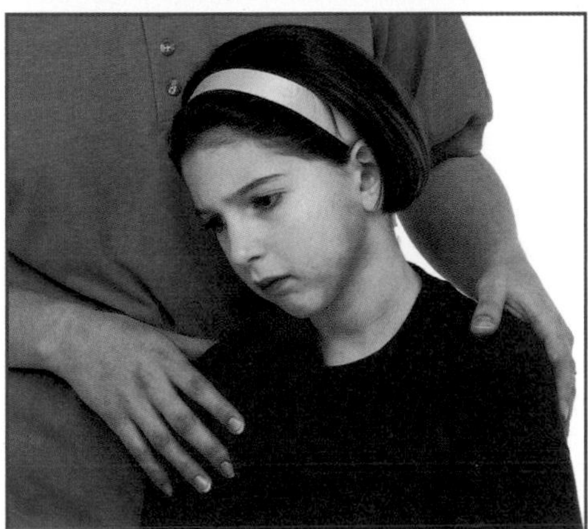

Many seizures occur without warning. Some forms of epilepsy cause the child to go into a trance-like state. Parents should comfort and reassure the child.

Usually when a person is having an epileptic seizure, her brain sends out abnormal signals that cause the muscles of the body to stop moving or to relax and tighten rapidly.

- A seizure may last a few seconds or several minutes. There are over 40 kinds of seizure and every epileptic person experiences epilepsy in a way that is unique to them.

- Some people experience an 'aura' before a seizure. This may be a strange feeling or an unusual smell or taste.

- During a seizure the person usually becomes unaware of her surroundings and may appear to go into a trance.

- In a mild case the person may simply stop and appear to stare into the distance.

- In a *grand mal* convulsion, the person goes rigid and stiff, loses consciousness and may have trouble breathing. Her limbs jerk and she may bubble saliva, bite her tongue and lose bladder and bowel control.

- The movements gradually stop and the person may fall asleep. On waking she may be confused and irritable.

First-aid guidelines

You cannot do anything to prevent or stop a seizure and you should not attempt to do so. You may, however, be able to prevent the child from being hurt.

1 If the child is likely to fall over, hold her gently and if possible lower her carefully to the nearest soft ground available. Put something soft under her head and as soon as possible, usually after any convulsions have ceased, place her in the recovery position to reduce the danger of swallowing any vomit.

If a child has had a seizure, she may fall asleep once the convulsions are over. Place her in the recovery position and stay with her until she wakes.

2 If the child is carrying something, she may drop it, especially at the end of the seizure when the muscles start to relax. You may not be able to remove anything from a tight grip during the seizure, but you should hold the object until it can be gently taken away from her.

3 If the seizure occurs in a dangerous situation – for example, one involving road traffic – try to reduce the danger, or gently guide the child away.

4 Stay calm and remain with the child until she regains awareness. Be reassuring and try to prevent others from crowding round.

5 Do not put anything in her mouth. Loosen clothing around the neck, if possible.

6 Check to see if she has a card or ID jewellery that indicates that she suffers from epilepsy and how long the seizures normally last.

When to call for help

You should telephone for an ambulance or doctor when:

- A child collapses for any reason and epilepsy has not yet been diagnosed.
- The seizure lasts for longer than usual or, if this information is not available, for more than five minutes.
- A second seizure immediately follows the first.
- The child injures herself.

Diagnosis and treatment

Epilepsy will not be diagnosed until a number of seizures have occurred. Drugs to control epilepsy are not started until epilepsy has been diagnosed by a specialist.

- To help the doctor make a diagnosis of a child, try to make a note of how many seizures he has had, how long they lasted, how the child felt beforehand, what happened just before and during the seizures and any other factors, such as family history or previous injuries, that may be relevant.

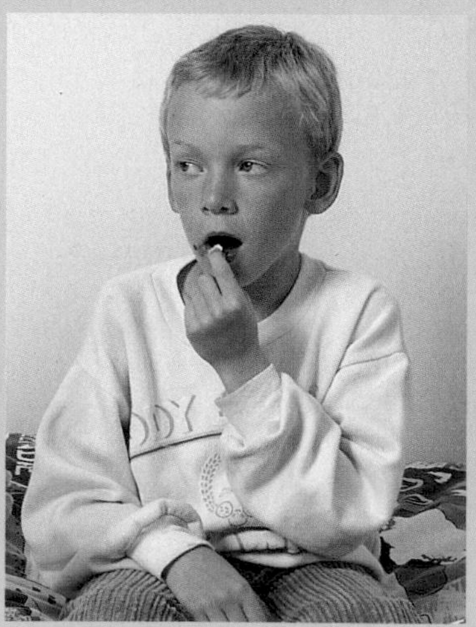

- Sleepiness can be a short-term side-effect. This usually passes as the body adjusts to the drug.
- Some people are allergic to certain drugs and develop skin rashes or other symptoms. In such cases, the doctor will prescribe another drug.
- Some drugs used to treat epilepsy produce long-term effects such as poor memory and concentration, irritability and overactivity in children, swollen gums, acne and weight gain. If any such symptoms are noted, a doctor should be consulted.

There are a number of drugs that are used to control epilepsy. Parents may find that it takes several attempts to find the right one for their child.

Outlook

Many people are able to stop taking drugs after a period without seizures.

- No one should stop taking anti-epileptic drugs suddenly. If the doctor considers it appropriate, the treatment will be reduced gradually.
- For most children with straightforward epilepsy the outlook is good. They have the same range of intelligence and abilities as other children and are able to enjoy a normal, active life as long as a few sensible safety precautions are taken.
- Some children have physical or mental problems as well as seizures. These may be linked to the brain damage or disease that has caused the epilepsy.

Useful address

NCYPE (The National Centre for Young People with Epilepsy)
St Piers Lane,
Lingfield
Surrey RH7 6PW

Tel: 01342 832243
www.nycpe.org.uk

EYE INFECTIONS

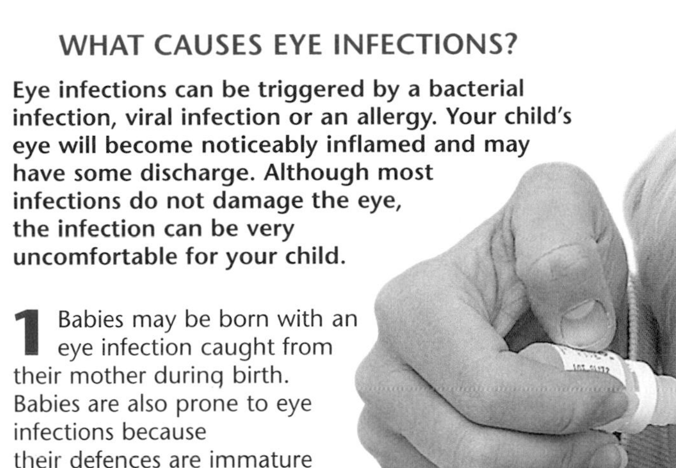

WHAT CAUSES EYE INFECTIONS?

Eye infections can be triggered by a bacterial infection, viral infection or an allergy. Your child's eye will become noticeably inflamed and may have some discharge. Although most infections do not damage the eye, the infection can be very uncomfortable for your child.

1 Babies may be born with an eye infection caught from their mother during birth. Babies are also prone to eye infections because their defences are immature when they are first born.

2 Children often have eye infections, especially when they start to go to nursery or school. Infection spreads easily between children because they are not very good at keeping their hands away from their eyes when they are infected.

Your doctor may prescribe drops to clear the eye infection. Putting these drops into the eye will be easier if you hold your child steady on your lap. Looking into a mirror will help you guide the drops in.

When to call the doctor

You should always take an eye infection seriously. Consult your GP if:

- The whites of his eyes are red.
- There is green or yellow pus in your child's eye.
- The eyelids are swollen and red.

What your doctor will do

- If your baby is less than one month old, your GP will take swabs for common bacterial infections, such as staphylococcus, and less common ones, such as gonorrhoea or chlamydia. Your baby may be referred to an ophthalmogist for treatment.
- In babies over one month, your GP may take a swab from your baby's eye and treat with antibiotic drops.

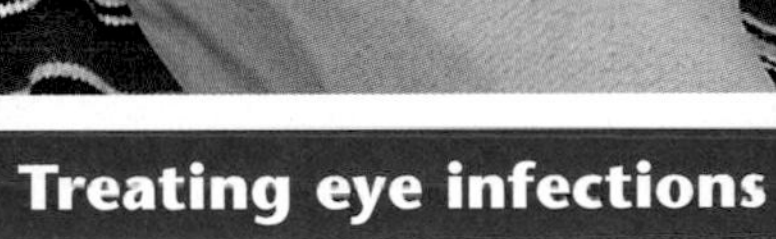

Treating eye infections

Washing the eyes

This is a useful technique in all babies at bathtime and any child with crusty eyes from a stye or conjunctivitis.

1 Take one cotton wool ball and soak it in cooled, boiled water.
2 Draw the cotton ball across the eye from the inner to the outer corner. Throw it away.
3 Use the next cotton wool ball to do the same thing with the other eye, drawing it from the nose outwards.

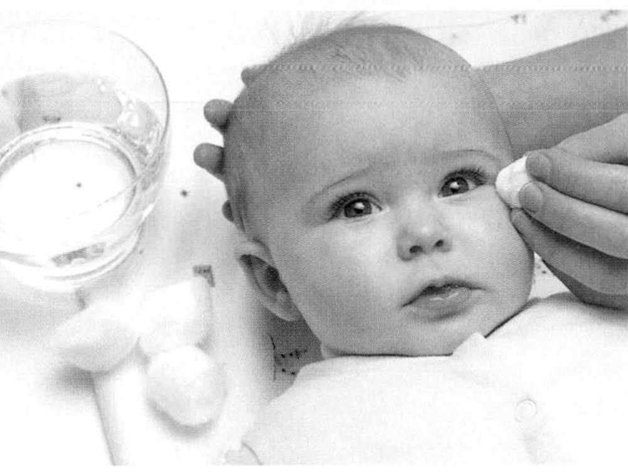

To prevent infection spreading from eye to eye, use a clean piece of cotton wool for each eye. Wipe the eye outwards from the inner corner.

Putting drops into the eye

The best time to put drops in a baby's eye is when he is asleep. If you are having problems applying drops or ointment to your child's eye, try squeezing the liquid gently into the corner of the eye.

1 Sit your child on your lap with his back against your chest.
2 Put one of your arms across his arms and chest and hold him fairly tightly. Place the other hand across his forehead.
3 Gently pull down the skin below the lower eyelid and squeeze the antibiotic into the lid – you may find it easier to have somebody else to help you to do this. The antibiotic will melt into the eye as he closes it.

Eye infections in babies and children are quite common and, in most cases, can be treated by prescribed antibiotics at home. Here are the four main eye conditions that your baby or child may contract.

Sticky eyes

This is a very common problem in babies and is not usually due to infection, although parents often worry that it is. It happens because the tear duct is not fully formed in babies.

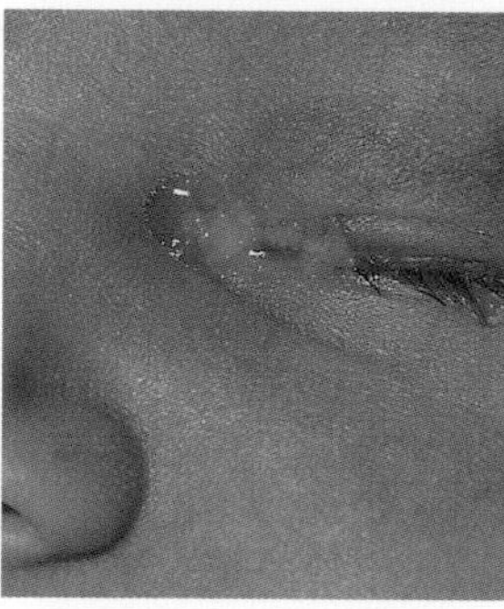

Sticky eyes affects newborns as their tear ducts are undeveloped. A discharge of yellow pus can stick the eye shut.

Symptoms:
- Pooling fluid in one or both eyes.
- Overflow of tears.
- Crusting around eyelids.

Treatment:
- Massage the eyes twice a day with a clean finger.
- Clean with cooled, boiled water.
- See the GP for antibiotics if there is a lot of discharge. If it is still a problem after one year the baby may need a small operation to probe the tear duct.

Styes

This is an infection of the eyelash follicle, usually with staphylococcus bacteria.

Symptoms:
- Small tender, red lump on the eyelid margins.
- Discharges pus.
- Develops rapidly.

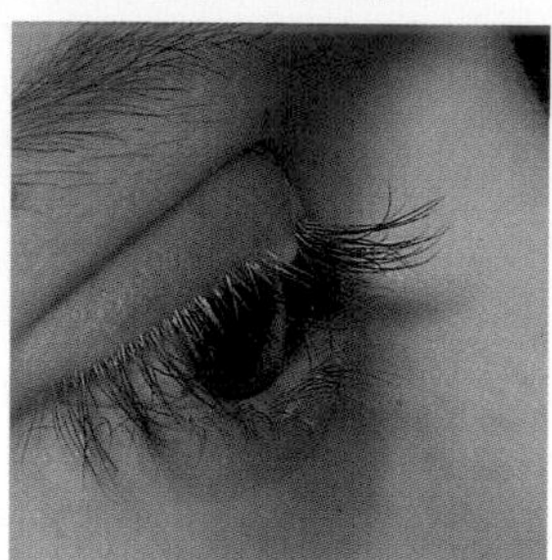

A stye may develop on your child's eyelid when the gland at the base of a eyelash becomes inflamed. Remove the eyelash to allow the pus to drain out then bathe the stye in warm water.

Treatment:
- Hot compresses applied to the stye will relieve the pain and draw out the pus.
- Pulling out the eyelash from the stye will allow the pus to drain out.
- Styes usually resolve within two to three days, especially if the pus is allowed to drain out. Remember, if there's pus about, let it out.
- If the stye does not seem to be settling down or the redness is spreading to the eyelids, antibiotics may be needed. These will be in the form of oral antibiotics because drops will not be as effective.
- Sometimes a stye needs surgical incision and drainage.

Conjunctivitis

Inflammation of the conjunctiva, the white part of the eye, is the commonest reason for children to complain of uncomfortable, bloodshot eyes.

Bacterial symptoms:
- There is often a lot of yellow pus pouring from the eye.
- The eyes are often stuck together in the mornings when the child wakes up.
- Both eyes invariably will be affected.
- Vision is unaffected.

Treatment:
- Antibiotic eye drops. Your GP will always advise you to use the antibiotics in both eyes regardless of whether the infection has reached the other eye.

Viral symptoms:
- The child will often also have a cough or cold as well as the conjunctivitis.
- The eyes feel gritty, like there is sand in them.
- The discharge is watery.
- Lasts longer than a bacterial conjunctivitis.

Treatment:
- The infection will settle with no treatment but sometimes needs steroid drops if intractable. These must be prescribed by a specialist.

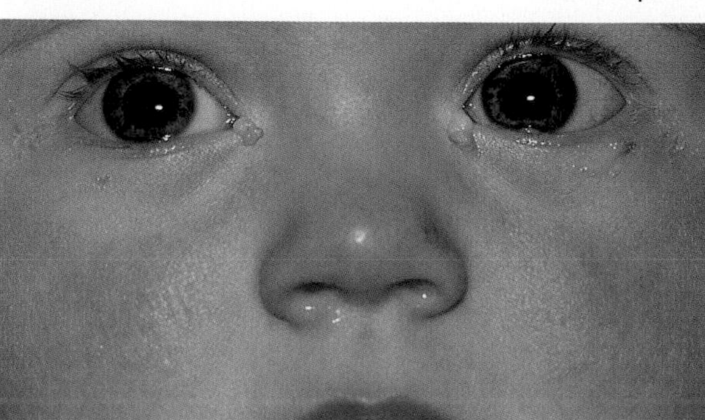

With conjunctivitis, the eyes may first become bloodshot and watery, followed by a build-up of discharge in the corner of the eyes. However, your child's vision should not be impaired by this condition.

Blepharitis

Blepharitis can be triggered by lice, a bacterial virus, dandruff or poor hygiene.

Symptoms:
- Inflamed, watery eyes.
- Warts on the eyelids.

Treatment:
- Antibiotic ointment will clear a bacterial virus, and daily cleansing with a moistened cotton wool bud will get rid of scales and crusts.
- Warts can interfere with vision, so your child may be referred to a specialist for removal.
- Emollients such as E45 will soften the eyelid skin.

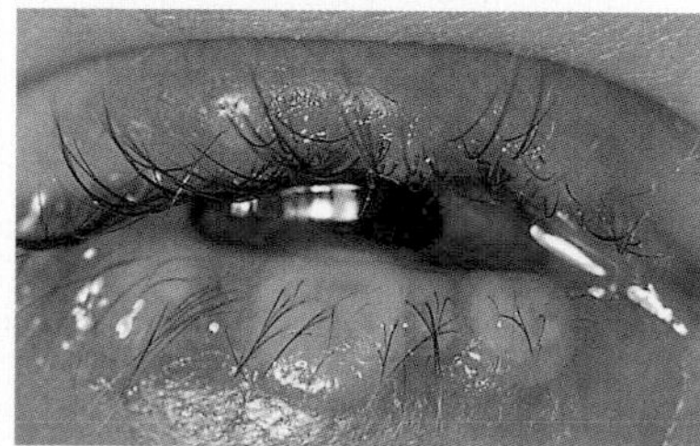

Blepharitis makes the eyes red, inflamed and watery. Although condition can affect both eyelids, it is not contagious.

EYESIGHT

HOW EYESIGHT DEVELOPS

Sight informs us about our environment and plays a major role in communication. Good vision aids your baby's development from the early stages of infancy.

- The development of the visual system is not complete when your baby is born and requires clear stimulation to develop fully.

- At birth, all babies have very poor visual acuity, which is the measure of how well a person can see detail. The acuity improves rapidly during the first year of life, but does not reach the adult level until a child is three to five years old.

- Many other aspects of seeing, such as the control of eye movements, are not fully developed at birth and mature alongside the visual acuity.

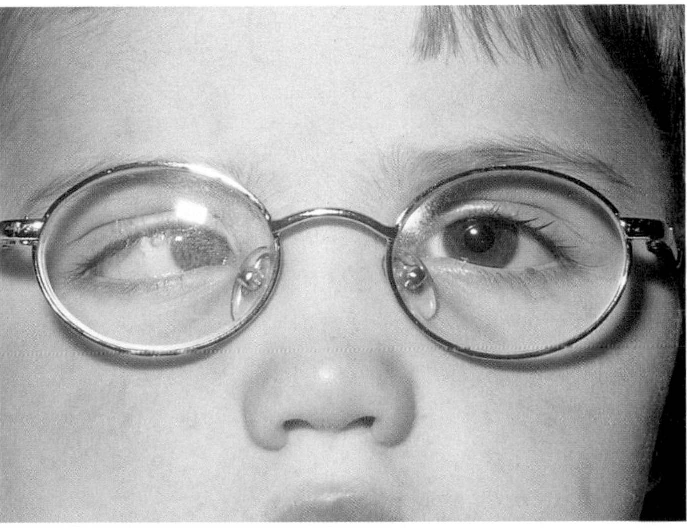

If your child has a squint (strabismus), which is when an eye turns in or out, a lazy eye or high astigmatism, glasses will be prescribed. The glasses must be worn constantly to correct vision.

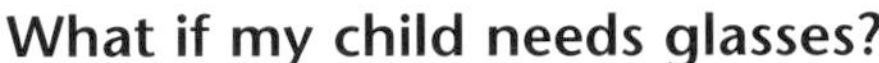

What if my child needs glasses?

Most babies are born with long-sightedness and astigmatism, but this decreases over the first year of life. If you or your partner have worn glasses since you were very young or have a lazy eye, there is a much higher chance of your child having eye problems. In these situations, your child should be examined regularly from a young age.

Usually, children's eyes should be examined at yearly intervals, but the optician (optometrist) will advise on this if more regular checks are needed.

Lazy eye

If one of your child's eyes has a retractive error, it will become lazy. He will therefore depend on his good eye.

- The 'lazy' eye needs to be corrected while your child is very young, otherwise the sight in the eye will always be poor.

- An optometrist may recommend that a patch is worn over your child's good eye for part of the day. This should encourage the lazy eye to work.

Identifying eye problems

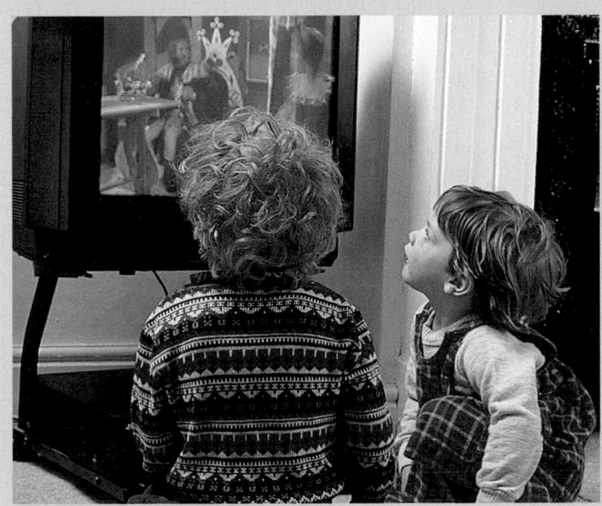

Sitting too close to the television can be a sign that your child's vision is impaired. She may also screw up her eyes when trying to focus on an object.

Very young children with poor sight accept this as normal because they have never known anything else. All children should therefore be examined before starting school. Signs to watch out for include:

- **Screwing up the eyes, rubbing the eyes, or excessive blinking:** this could be associated with difficulty seeing, an eye that tends to wander or a dislike of bright light.

- **An eye that turns in or out:** below the age of three months, many babies will have an eye that occasionally turns in, but if it stays in or out or turns after three months, help should be sought.

- **A family history:** if you, your partner, or a member of your family has a squint, lazy eye or strong glasses.

- **Sitting too close to the television:** your child may require glasses, although it could also be just a habit.

- **Difficulty distinguishing colours:** one in 10 males and fewer females have 'colour blindness'. Often this runs in families.

The eye examination

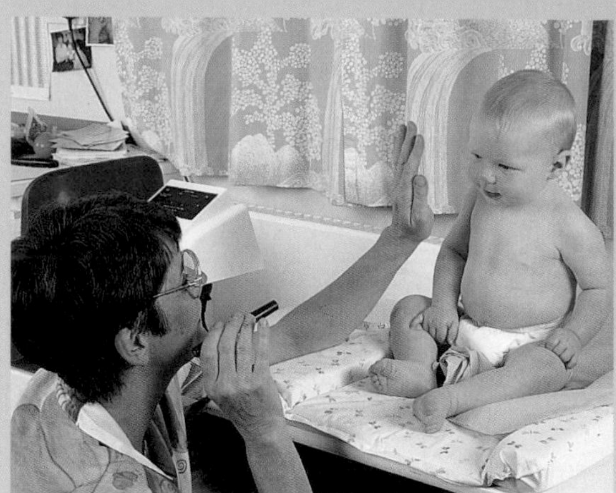

This baby is being tested for a suppressed squint, which causes blurred vision and may lead to loss of sight. A squint can be corrected with glasses, a patch over the normal eye or surgery.

Your baby's eyes can be examined from birth onwards, but the examination will differ in many ways from the examination of an adult. The optometrist will rely on what are called 'objective tests'.

- An optometrist may shine a light into your baby's eyes to check that there are no cataracts. The light reflections of each eye are compared to check that there is no squint.

- To test your baby's vision, the optometrist will show your baby special cards and note the direction of her gaze. Toddlers may need to match letters or pictures. Your child can practise this matching technique at home before the test.

- Other sight tests will be carried out to check that your child's eyes are working together. The optometrist will look into your child's eyes using a special instrument, called an ophthalmoscope, to ensure that they are healthy.

- Drops may be used to make your child's eye muscles relax and give the optometrist a better idea whether glasses are necessary or not.

Fitting the right glasses

A child with impaired vision will need to be fitted with glasses. A special range of children's frames give a good and comfortable fit.

- Young children should have plastic lenses in their glasses, so that damage to the eye is less likely in an accident.

- Expect glasses to break regularly and take this into account when considering the cost.

- Only in very exceptional circumstances would contact lenses be appropriate for a pre-school child. In these cases, the lenses would be fitted at hospital.

- Children should not have refractive errors corrected by laser because the eyes are still developing.

- Children's sight tests are available through the National Health Service at no charge and a voucher is also provided towards the cost of glasses, if these are necessary.

Long sight, short sight and astigmatism

In normal sight, the image of an object is focused on to the back of the eye (retina). If this doesn't happen, the person is said to have a refractive error or ametropia and cannot see without glasses. There are three main types of refractive error:

1. **Long-sight or hyperopia:** this is an inability to focus on objects close up. It usually occurs when the eyeball is too short, making the light focus beyond the retina.

2. **Short-sight or myopia:** this is the inability to focus on a distant object. It usually occurs when the eyeball is too long, which means that the sharpest image forms in front of the retina.

3. **Astigmatism:** where the light comes to a focus at two points, rather than one.

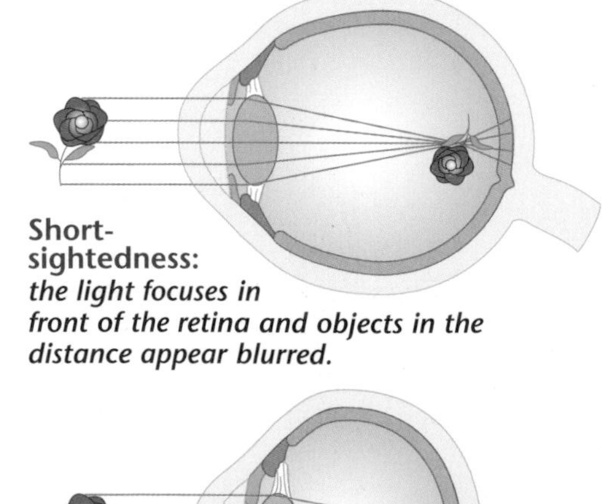

Short-sightedness: *the light focuses in front of the retina and objects in the distance appear blurred.*

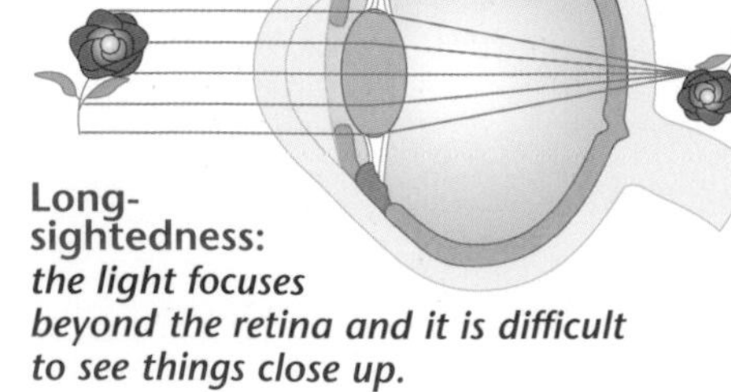

Long-sightedness: *the light focuses beyond the retina and it is difficult to see things close up.*

Eyesight professionals

Screening checks are carried out at various stages of your baby's development, but you can take her to have her eyes tested by an optometrist at any time.

- Optometrists are often known as opticians, although this is a general term to cover anyone who is involved with the provision of glasses.

- Optometrists are professionally qualified to examine eyes to check the sight, establish whether glasses are necessary or whether there is any eye disease. They often work with dispensing opticians, who help with frames and lenses.

FEVER

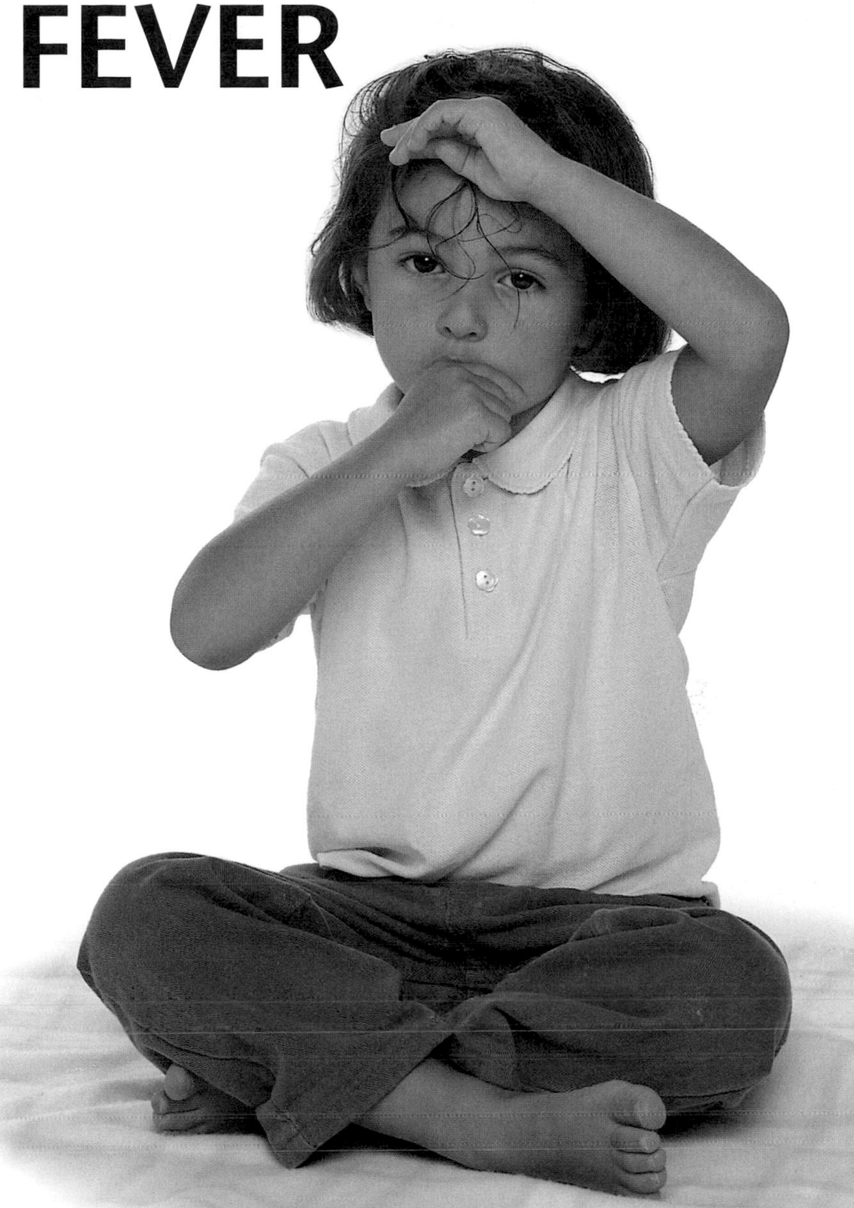

STAYING CALM

Finding that your child has a raised temperature can be a very frightening experience. Parents worry that a high temperature may cause brain damage, convulsions or even death, and fear that the temperature will continue to rise inexorably unless something is done to stop it.

In fact, a raised temperature usually means that your child is fighting infection. The fever activates the body's immune system and most fevers are caused by viral infections, which do not respond to antibiotics.

A high temperature is not the only indicator that a child is ill – children, especially babies, can be very poorly and not have a fever at all. On the other hand, a healthy child can get a raised temperature in hot weather, from doing exercise, wearing clothes that are too warm or heavy, having a hot bath, or even a hot drink. What counts is how ill your child seems to you.

If you suspect your child has a fever, take her temperature and then again half an hour later when she's rested. If it is still raised, check for other signs of illness. Try to get her to drink as much fluid as possible – little and often is the key to prevent her vomiting it back up.

Symptoms

Temperatures above the following are considered to be fevers:

Method	°C	°F
Under arm	**37.2**	**99**
Oral	**37.5**	**100**
Rectal	**38.0**	**100.4**

Symptoms include:
raised temperature, sore throat, vomiting, diarrhoea, runny nose, earache, achiness, shivering, rash, tummy pain.

When to call the doctor

It is not always easy to decide when to seek medical advice. Always trust your instincts – it may be that your baby or child just doesn't appear 'right' to you. Ring your GP immediately if any of the following symptoms are apparent:

- Your baby is less than three months old and has a low-grade fever, 37.2°C (99°F), unless the fever follows immunisations.
- Your baby is not feeding.
- High fever is 39°C (102°F) or more.
- Your child cannot be comforted.
- She will not wake up, or is drowsy or floppy.
- She cries if you touch her.
- Her neck is stiff.
- She is vomiting.
- She has a rash – if not typical of chickenpox or other common viral illnesses – and particularly if they have purple spots that do not fade when pressed.
- Your baby/child has trouble breathing even after you have cleared her nose of mucus.
- Your baby/child cannot swallow anything and is drooling saliva.

Within 24 hours if:

- It hurts when she passes urine or she is going more often.
- Fever is still high even if symptoms are not apparent.
- She has a history of febrile convulsions.

Treating fever at home

A normal temperature for your child is 37°C (98.4°F) – higher than this may indicate a fever. Try to keep your child calm and follow the guidelines below for treating her effectively and making her comfortable while she is feeling unwell.

1 If you suspect your child has a fever, ask her where she has a pain. Call the doctor immediately if she shows any of the symptoms requiring urgent medical help.

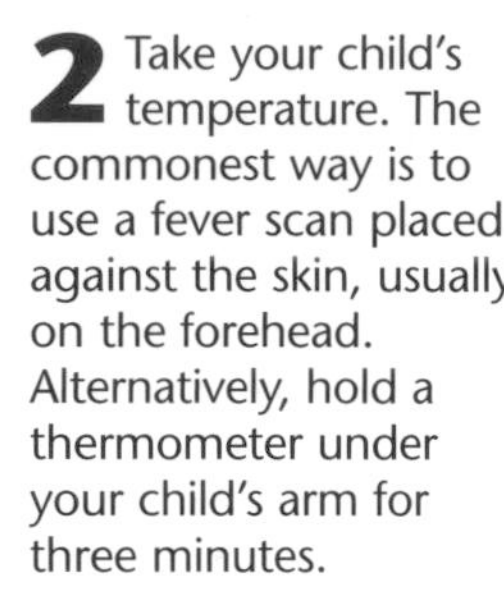

2 Take your child's temperature. The commonest way is to use a fever scan placed against the skin, usually on the forehead. Alternatively, hold a thermometer under your child's arm for three minutes.

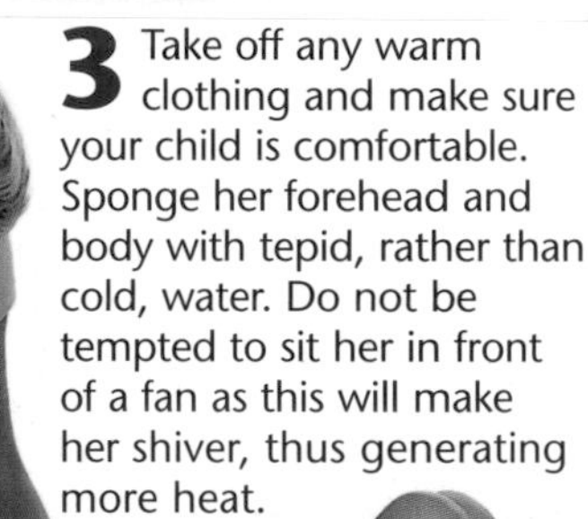

3 Take off any warm clothing and make sure your child is comfortable. Sponge her forehead and body with tepid, rather than cold, water. Do not be tempted to sit her in front of a fan as this will make her shiver, thus generating more heat.

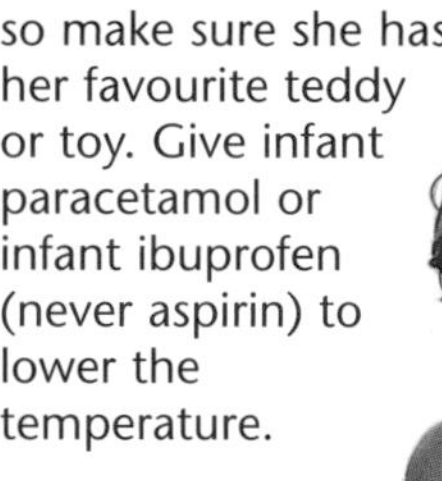

4 She'll be more clingy than usual and need to feel secure, so make sure she has her favourite teddy or toy. Give infant paracetamol or infant ibuprofen (never aspirin) to lower the temperature.

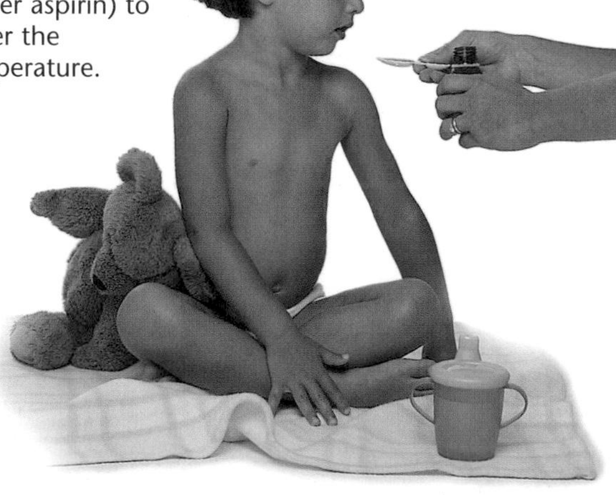

Fever fits

Febrile convulsions are the reason we worry about a child having a temperature. They often happen as the temperature is rising for the first time, before the parent is even aware that their child has a fever. These fits are very common, affecting mainly children between the ages of six months and three years. The characteristic stiffness followed by jerking or twitching movements usually lasts less than five minutes.

- Try not to panic. A short fit does not damage your child. Febrile convulsions are not epilepsy. She will grow out of them usually after the age of three.
- Try to lie your child on her side to stop her injuring herself.
- Don't put anything in her mouth but pull her jaw gently forward to stop her choking on her tongue.
- Seek medical help once the fit has stopped or if she is still fitting after five minutes.

Treating babies with fever

If your baby is under six months, he should not be given paracetamol syrup, unless advised to do so by your doctor. Undress your baby to his nappy and sponge him lightly with tepid water. Try to keep him calm. You should call the doctor immediately if his temperature is 39°C (102°F) or more – and he is under a year old – and you can't bring it down.

FOOD ALLERGIES

WHAT ARE FOOD ALLERGIES?

Food allergies and food intolerance are controversial issues. One fifth of people believe that they have a bad reaction to certain foods, while surveys show that only about two in every 100 have an adverse reaction that is measurable.

Young children are more likely than adults to be affected, however, and some allergies, such as peanut allergy, are on the increase. The good news is that most children grow out of their food allergy by the age of five.

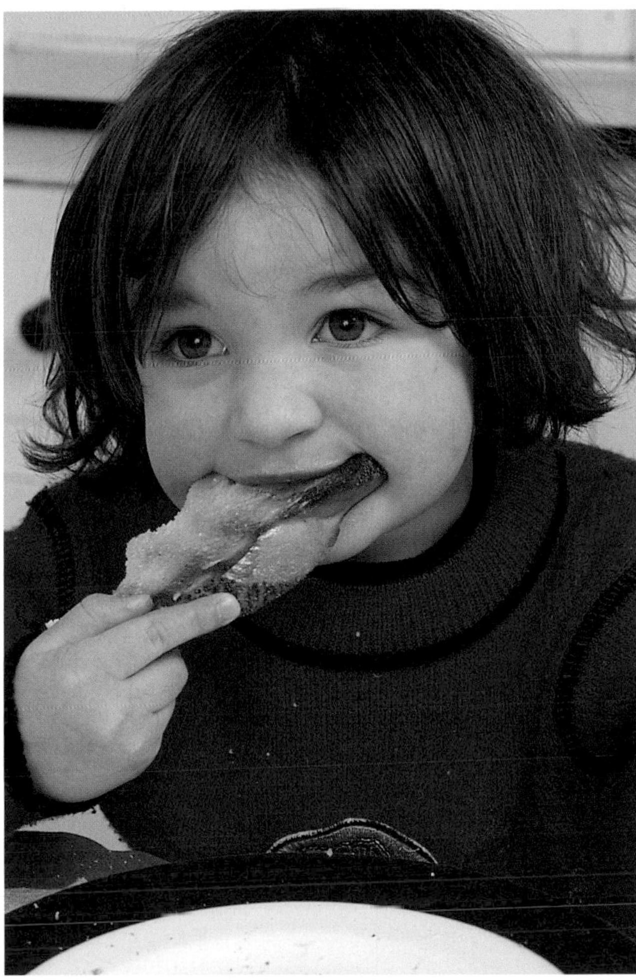

A child suffering from an allergy should take 'safe' food with her to a party. Chain restaurants offer standardised dishes that can be relied upon not to vary.

Symptoms

If your child has a food allergy, her immune system sees a certain food as a foreign invader (allergen), and, as with an infection, produces antibodies. The next time your child eats the food, a war breaks out between the allergen and the antibodies. The symptoms this causes include:

- Diarrhoea
- Vomiting
- Abdominal pain
- Wheezing
- Runny nose, sneezing
- Rash
- Burn-like rash around the anus
- Facial swelling
- Sinus headaches
- Glue ear
- Bloodshot eyes
- Your child may also seem irritable and have difficulty sleeping, due to the effects of the allergic reaction

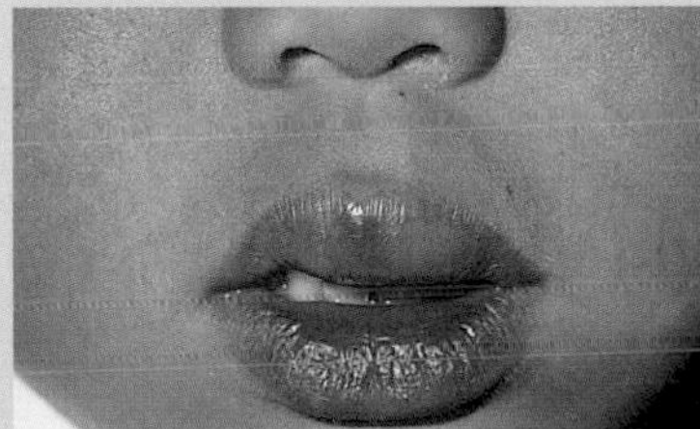

LEFT: A close-up of the swollen upper lip of a six-year-old, caused by peanut allergy – an increasingly common problem among children.

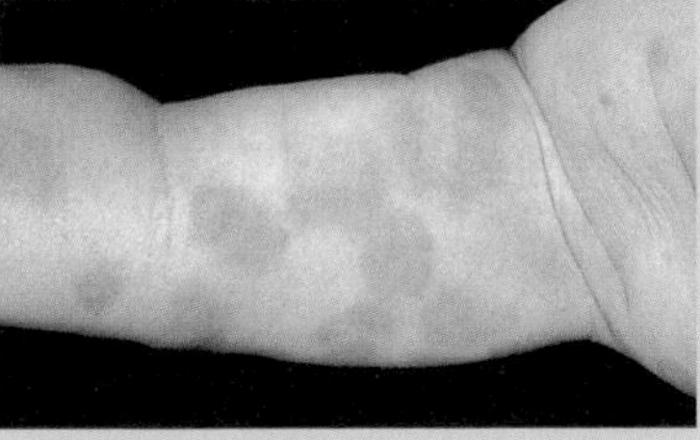

RIGHT: The arm of this four-month-old baby is marked by a red rash, triggered by an unknown food. Treatment includes antihistamines.

Food allergy or food intolerance?

Food allergy can produce the same symptoms as food intolerance. An allergy involves the immune system, intolerance is linked to an inability to digest food.

Food allergy: these are of special concern to parents because in their most severe form they can cause life-threatening reactions. A food allergy triggers an abnormal reaction in the immune system.

Food intolerance: this is an adverse reaction that doesn't involve the immune system; it may be related to an enzyme deficiency. If a child is lacking in the enzyme lactose, it may lead to an intolerance of milk.

WHO IS SUSCEPTIBLE?

Some children may be more sensitive to general allergic reactions than others and this condition is known as atopy. It means your child is more likely to suffer from eczema, asthma and hayfever.

Atopy runs in families – if both parents suffer from allergies, a child has a 60 per cent chance of developing them, too.

Some argue that the increase in peanut allergy reflects the general increase in atopy over 20 years. Others think that it is due to mothers eating peanut butter when breast-feeding, and recommend that foods known to cause allergies should not be given in allergy-prone families until the immune system has a chance to mature, usually between the ages of two and three.

Difficulties with diagnosis

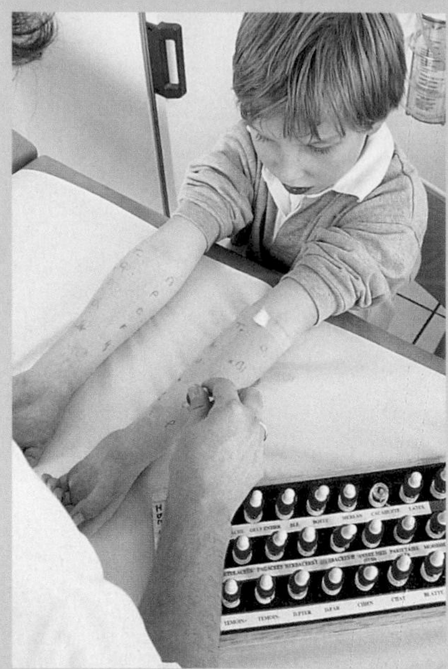

A boy undergoes an allergy test. His arms are pricked and soluble allergens are applied; a reaction shows a possible allergy.

In a wide-ranging diet, it is not always easy to pinpoint the cause of an allergy – some children are sensitive to more than one food or to other allergens as well, for example, pollen or cat fur.

- If you suspect a particular food, keep a diary of what your child has eaten, where he's been and what he's been doing, then talk to your GP. You may be referred to an allergy clinic where specialists will take a detailed history and carry out tests to diagnose the problem food.

- There are two main types of test. In the skin prick test, a small amount of an allergen is placed in a solution on the forearm or back and then the skin is pricked with a lancet through the drop. A weal and raised red area after 15 minutes generally show an allergic reaction.

- The RAST test is a blood test that checks for the presence of specific antibodies produced to defend against typical allergens.

- Neither of the tests are always accurate, particularly with young children, as it takes time for their antibody response to build up. Sometimes a skin prick test may produce a false negative result if antihistamines have been taken previously. The skin type and the quality of testing can all affect accuracy, too.

- Occasionally, if these tests fail to identify the allergy, an elimination diet may be suggested, which means cutting out the foods that commonly cause allergic reactions and then re-introducing them gradually.

- A food challenge test introduces your child to a likely allergen, in the presence of a doctor, to diagnose the problem of food intolerance.

Peanut allergy

An estimated one in 200 UK children are allergic to peanuts, which can trigger a potentially fatal reaction, anaphylaxis. Symptoms include abdominal pain, facial swelling, breathing problems and asthma. It requires immediate treatment with an adrenaline injection.

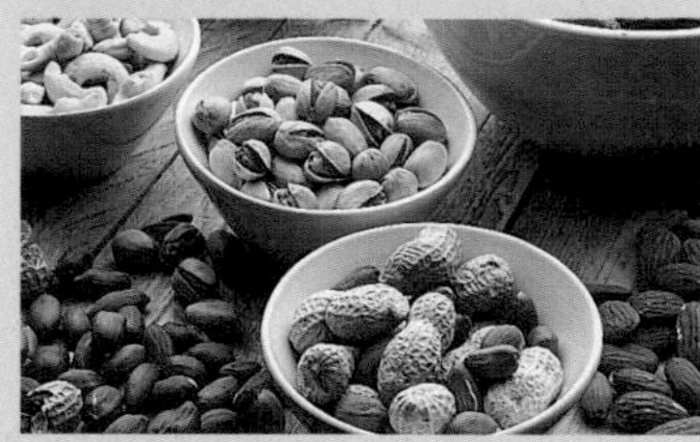

Useful addresses

British Allergy Foundation
Deepdene House, 30 Bellegrove Road, Welling, Kent DA16 3PY
Tel: 020 8303 8525

Helpline: 020 8303 8583
(Mon–Fri, 9 a.m.–5 p.m.)
www.allergyfoundation.com

Anaphylaxis Campaign
PO Box 275, Farnborough, Hants GU14 6SX
Tel: 01252 373793
www.anaphylaxis.org.uk

Prevention better than cure

Once a problem food is diagnosed, the basic treatment is excluding it from your child's diet. This should always be done with the help of a dietitian to ensure that the child's diet remains balanced.

There are substitutes for most allergenic foods, for example, with a cow's milk allergy a soya milk substitute is suggested.

But foods appear under unexpected names – milk may be listed as casein, whey, lactalbumin and lactose; eggs as albumen and egg lecithin; wheat flour as durum semolina and farina; peanuts as groundnuts.

A family with a history of allergies should cut out trigger foods during pregnancy and breast-feeding, delay weaning until six months and avoid eggs and nuts for two years.

Common food allergens

Four of the most common food allergens are:

- Dairy products
- Wheat
- Egg whites
- Peanuts

These are responsible for nearly 90 per cent of allergies. Other allergenic foods are tree nuts (walnuts, almonds, brazils, hazelnuts, cashews), sesame seeds, citrus fruits, soya, fish and shellfish. Some children react to additives, e.g. tartrazine (E 102), antioxidants and preservatives.

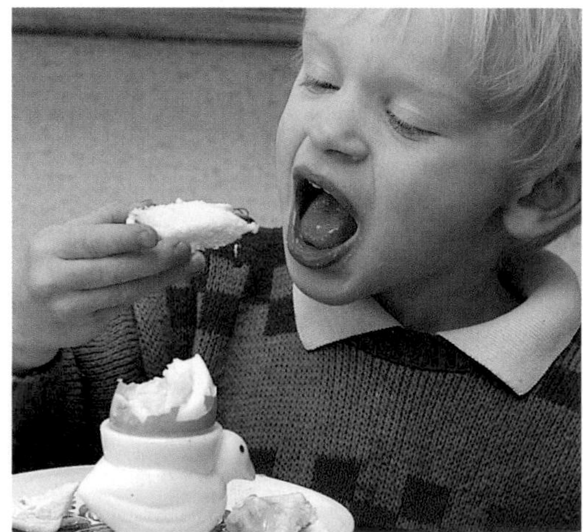

Most food allergies in children fade by the age of five, but you should teach your child to ask if foods contain the substance he's allergic to, and inform his friends and carers.

GASTROENTERITIS

WHAT IS GASTROENTERITIS?

Gastroenteritis is an inflammation of the stomach and intestine, and typically causes vomiting and diarrhoea. It is a common condition in young children.

- In developed countries, this infection is usually mild and curable, but in developing countries, especially where clean water is in short supply, gastroenteritis kills millions of young children each year.

- Some of the symptoms of gastroenteritis are vomiting, diarrhoea, nausea, stomach cramps, fever and headache.

- Sometimes symptoms can occur within hours of taking in germs, but they usually take longer than this to manifest.

- Since most infections are viral, antibiotics are rarely prescribed. Drugs that stop diarrhoea are also avoided because they tend to prolong the time the bug stays in the gut.

- This illness usually lasts between three to five days, during which time the child should be closely monitored and given plenty of fluids.

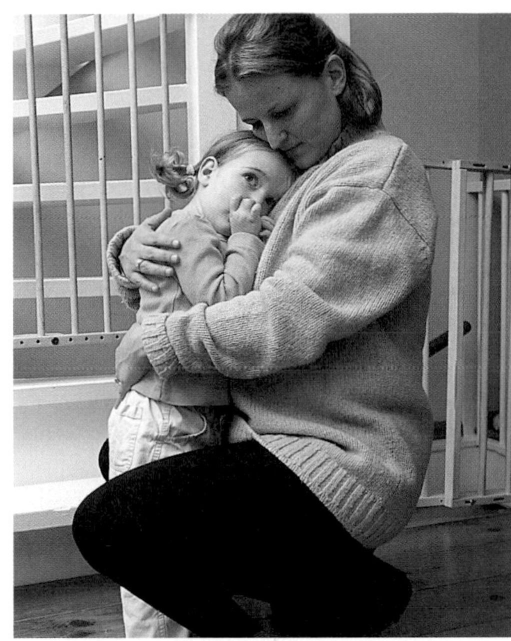

Your child will feel unwell, and weak due to her inability to store fluids. It is important to give her lots of love, understanding and attention.

Causes

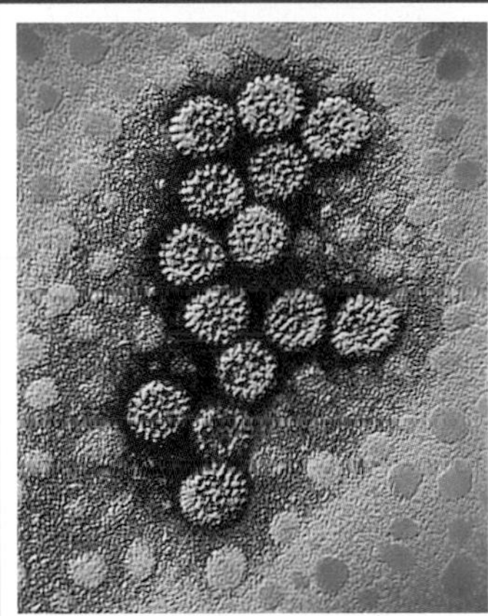

If the membrane of the stomach and intestine become inflamed, your child cannot absorb nutrients and water from the food as it passes through. Gastroenteritis is caused by a 'bug' – a virus, bacteria or parasite – and caught by eating infected food, or from contact with an infected person.

- **Viruses:** 60 per cent of all cases of gastroenteritis in the developed world are caused by the rotavirus, an organism that is especially virulent in the winter months.

The rotavirus is the main cause of gastroenteritis. Rotavirus infections may be contagious and can be passed on through human contact.

- **Bacteria:** the bacteria campylobacter jejunii is found in uncooked meat and can cause gastroenteritis if food is not cooked thoroughly. Salmonella, found in eggs, dairy products and undercooked poultry, can also be responsible for the infection.

- **Parasites:** these bugs, for example giardia, can cause gastroenteritis and are often picked up when travelling abroad.

Symptoms

The symptoms of gastroenteritis are persistent vomiting and diarrhoea, but vary depending on the type of infection.

- Diarrhoea is often watery, to the extent that it may be difficult to distinguish it from urine. In some types of gastroenteritis, the stools may contain blood and mucus.

- Some children with gastroenteritis have a high temperature, which can cause a febrile convulsion (fit) in children under five. These convulsions are usually short-lived and are easily avoided by taking steps to bring the temperature down.

- Bacterial and viral infections can also cause abdominal (tummy) cramps and tenderness.

When to call the doctor

Call the doctor if your child has been vomiting for more than 12 hours and is not getting better, or if your child won't drink and is dehydrated.

- Current medical advice is that you should continue to breast-feed or bottle-feed even though your child may be less hungry.

- Your doctor can prescribe oral rehydration solutions to replace the lost fluid, and advise how often to give them.

- If your baby has severe dehydration, or if he is unable to drink for a prolonged period, he will be admitted to hospital for treatment with nasogastric or intravenous fluids.

Dehydration

A potentially serious effect of gastroenteritis is dehydration. It is important to be aware of the signs:

- Dehydration can happen very quickly in babies and toddlers because they have a large surface area of skin in relation to their body weight. This means that they lose fluid through their skin quickly.

- Depending on the extent of dehydration, a baby will lose weight noticeably. The amount of urine he passes will decrease.

- The skin becomes dry, as do the mouth and lips, and you may notice that your baby's eyes and his fontanelle (the soft area on the top of his head) appear sunken.

- Children with dehydration may feel hot to the touch. If the dehydration is quite severe, your child will become drowsy and floppy.

Dealing with dehydration

If your child has any of the symptoms of dehydration, it is important to seek medical advice. In most cases, the dehydration will be mild and you can start to resolve the problem by encouraging your child to drink.

- Frequent small sips (i.e. every five minutes) of any fluids will help to avoid serious complications. You may have to persevere – a child who feels nauseated and unwell may not be willing to drink.

- There are oral rehydration solutions that can be bought at your chemist or prescribed by a GP. Read the packet carefully to check whether they are suitable for your child. These solutions contain glucose and various salts – exactly the substances that are lost in diarrhoea.

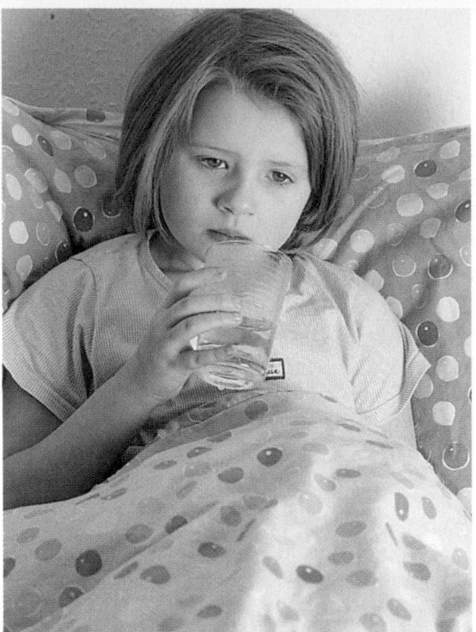

Constant diarrhoea and vomiting can cause dehydration, so it is essential to keep up your child's fluid intake, even if she is nauseous and reluctant to drink.

Stomach ache and sickness

There are several ways that you can make your child comfortable when he is suffering from gastroenteritis:

- The first priority is to keep up the fluid intake, preferably with plain water, rehydration salts or very dilute fruit juice.

- Remember that your child will be feeling very unwell so comfort and cuddle him.

- If his temperature starts to rise, remove heavy bed clothes, make sure the room is well ventilated and use a fan if you have one. If he is not being sick, you could give him a dose of junior paracetamol to help keep the fever down.

- Constant diarrhoea may cause your child's bottom to be sore. Gently wash the area with warm water and apply barrier cream.

- Do not worry if your child refuses to eat for several days, it will not harm him as long as he is drinking – it's essential that he stays hydrated.

- Your child may continue to have diarrhoea for several days after the fever and the vomiting have improved.

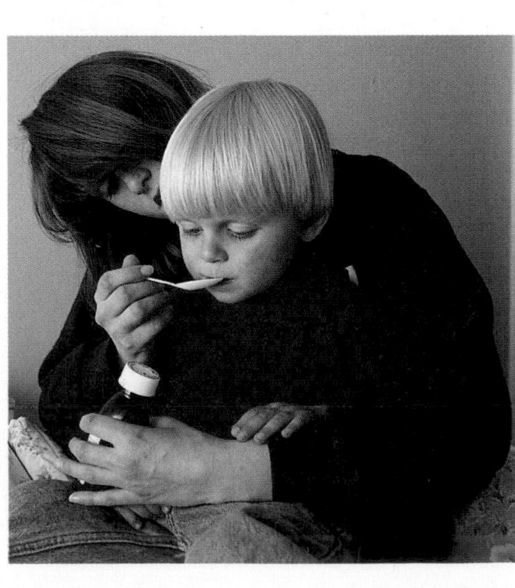

If your child is feverish and has a high temperature but is not vomiting, giving him a dose of junior paracetamol may help to reduce his fever.

Preventing gastroenteritis

It may not be clear how your child has contracted gastroenteritis, but bear in mind the following:

- Always thoroughly cook food, especially meat and make sure that you wash vegetables thoroughly, even if they are organic.

- When travelling with small children, always drink bottled water and eat at 'tourist restaurants'. Try to avoid eating from market stalls and street vendors.

- Try to make sure that your child does not come into contact with anyone who has gastroenteritis.

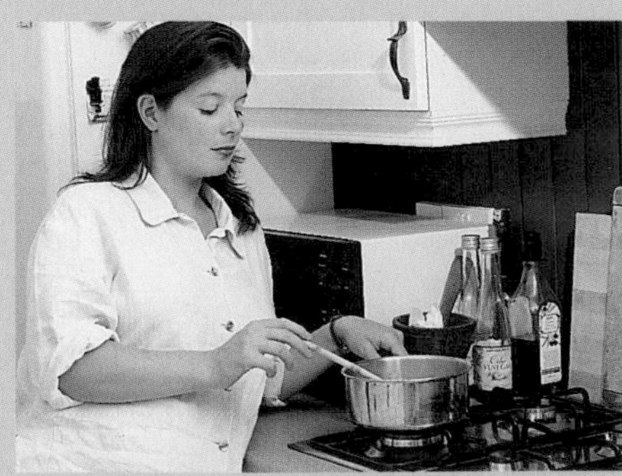

To help prevent gastroenteritis, prepare and cook all food hygienically and thoroughly to limit bacteria.

GLUE EAR

WHAT IS GLUE EAR?

Glue ear is a condition seen mainly in children where a sticky, thick, glue-like material collects behind the eardrum. It is most common in two- to five-year-olds, where some 20 per cent of children will have glue ear at any one time.

- The main danger with glue ear is that it can affect both ears, causing deafness. In this age group, at the stage when a child is learning to talk, even temporary deafness can have harmful effects on learning and development.
- Children with glue ear may be noisy and naughty because they cannot hear what is going on around them. They are too young to pinpoint the problem for themselves and it is common for the condition to go unrecognised.
- The child's inability to hear properly can lead to misunderstandings between parents, teachers and children and cause a great deal of unhappiness and potentially delayed development.

Glue ear is a common childhood condition that can cause temporary deafness. It occurs when the swollen or blocked eustachian tube cannot clear any of the mucus into the back of the throat.

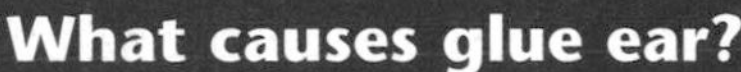

What causes glue ear?

Children are prone to develop glue ear when they have a cold or flu, as the build-up of mucus can't be drained by the eustachian tube.

- Children have large tonsils and adenoids (lymphoid tissue at the back of the throat) that block the eustachian tubes.
- A baby's eustachian tube runs fairly horizontally. It becomes more vertical as the baby gets older, improving drainage.
- If your child spends time with other children, she is more likely to get a cold and therefore glue ear.
- It occurs more often in winter and spring.
- Children whose parents smoke are at more risk of developing glue ear.

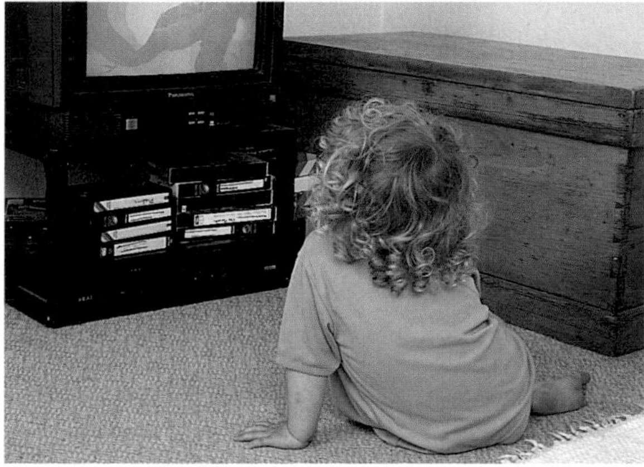

Symptoms

Glue ear can be difficult for a parent to diagnose. However, if your child experiences any or all of the following symptoms, it may be an indication that she has the condition:

Hearing loss: your child may have the television volume turned up very loud, sit close to the television, or shout all the time. You may also find it difficult to get her attention.
Change in behaviour: deafness is a very isolating condition, especially if it goes unrecognised. A previously sociable and friendly child may become introverted and shy.
Earache: glue ear in itself does not often cause pain in the ear, but it can lead to painful ear infections, which in turn make the condition worse.
Delayed speech: if your child is affected at around the time she is learning to talk, glue ear may be identified by a speech therapist as a cause of her speech problems.

If your child sits too close to the television it may be a sign that she has glue ear. She may not be able to hear clearly because of the blockage in the middle ear.

How is glue ear diagnosed?

If glue ear is suspected, the GP will examine your child's ears. The ear drum may be shrivelled and there may be a build-up of fluid.

If your GP suspects that your child is suffering from glue ear, he may carry out the following tests:

1 Auroscope: the GP may be able to diagnose glue ear by using an auroscope to look at the appearance of the ear drum. If it's healthy it should look opaque, pale pink, smooth and shiny. If there is glue ear, the ear drum may look dull and shrivelled. Sometimes a fluid level can be seen on the other side of the ear drum, or bubbles within the fluid. Some specialists use an auroscope with a pump attached to puff air on to the ear drum. If the ear drum is healthy it will move; if there is glue ear, the fluid behind the ear drum may stop it moving.

2 Hearing tests: glue ear causes a significant hearing loss in each or one of the ears. A test, which can be done by the health visitor, involves whispering about three feet from behind the child's ear. If she cannot hear the sound, she will need more formal hearing testing. This may reveal hearing losses of up to 50 decibels and the child may only hear normal speech as a whisper.

3 Tympanometry: this machine measures how well the ear drum moves. When there is glue behind the ear, the drum does not move.

Surgery to treat glue ear

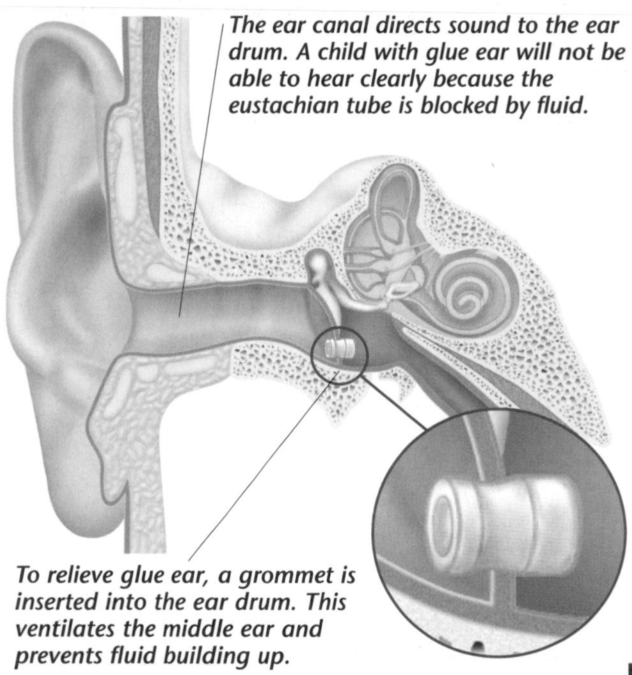

The ear canal directs sound to the ear drum. A child with glue ear will not be able to hear clearly because the eustachian tube is blocked by fluid.

To relieve glue ear, a grommet is inserted into the ear drum. This ventilates the middle ear and prevents fluid building up.

Most episodes of glue ear are short-lived, but children with continuing problems such as speech delay, deafness, or persistent ear infections will be offered surgery. A hearing loss of more than 20–30 decibels in both ears is sometimes used as a guide to justify surgery, which involves some or all of the following:

- **Myringotomy:** a small cut is made in the ear drum and the sticky glue is sucked out of the ear.
- **Grommet:** this is a tiny plastic tube that looks like a miniature empty cotton reel. It is placed through the slit ear drum keeping the ear drained. It slowly works its way out of the ear drum and comes out with the ear wax over several months.
- **Adenoidectomy:** the adenoids are lumps of lymphoid tissue. These may also be removed during the operation if they seem large and are blocking the eustachian tube.

If antibiotics do not relieve the condition, your child may need surgery. A doctor will make an incision into the middle ear and insert a grommet, which can be as small as 3mm (⅛in) long.

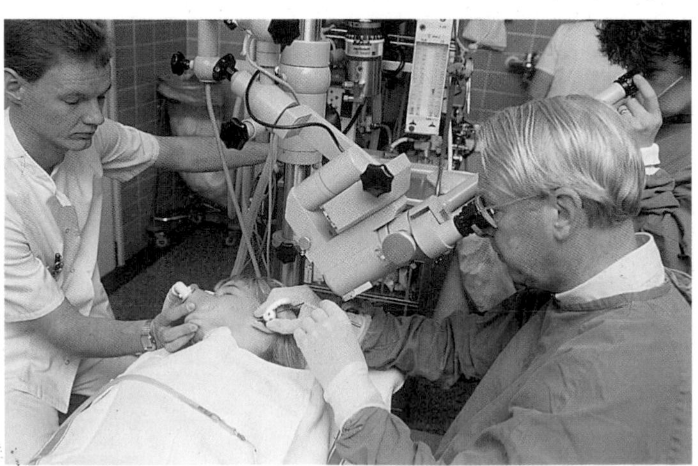

Risks from surgery

Glue ear surgery is a safe operation that usually lasts for 10–15 minutes. However, there are three minor drawbacks:

- **Perforation:** there may be a slight risk of the ear drum remaining open long term, with a chronic perforation.
- **Infection:** there may be discharge and frequent infections.
- **Durability:** the effects of surgery are not long-lasting. Grommets fall out after about six months. If glue ear is still present a second operation may be necessary.

GROWTH RETARDATION

WHAT IS GROWTH RETARDATION?

Growth retardation is a slower rate of growth than expected for a child's age. It is a term generally applied to children over a year old.

- Many healthy children are small for their age, but eventually catch up and become normal-sized adults.

- Often there is a familial tendency to being a 'late developer', so you need to compare your child's height with your own at a similar age – your parents may be able to help you.

- As a rough guide, birth length doubles by approximately four years of age and trebles by approximately 13 years.

- Your health visitor will have plotted your child's weight, length and head circumference in her early years, on a standard growth chart (found in your child's health record book). The chart shows printed growth curves, known as centiles. In normal growth, a child's height is plotted between the first and last centile. There is cause for concern if the rate of growth does not follow the curve of the chart.

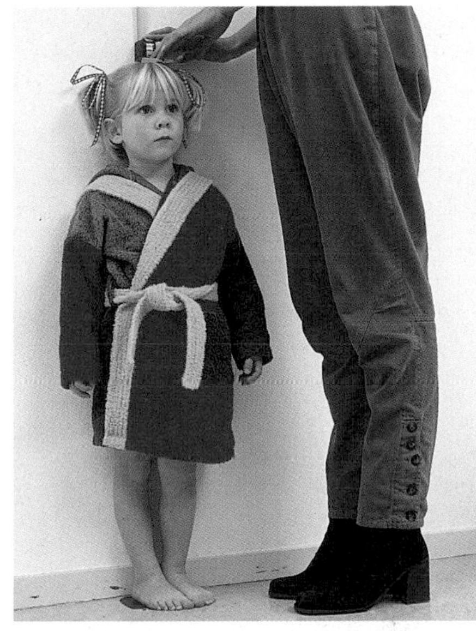

Growth retardation refers to a slow rate of growth compared to the normal rate for the child's age.

Causes of growth retardation

There are many different possible causes of growth retardation. They include:

1 Genetic: your child may have inherited slow growth, eventually achieving a normal, average adult height; or she may have inherited a family tendency to short stature, and will have a short final adult height. Genetic disorders include achondroplasia, one of the commonest forms of dwarfism. Another is precocious (early) puberty, which can result in short stature because puberty is closely associated with the maturation of the long bones and the cessation of growth.

2 Chromosomal disorders: these include Down's syndrome and Turner's syndrome.

3 Endocrine (hormonal) disorders: these include growth hormone and thyroid hormone deficiencies. Growth hormone deficiency is more common in boys than girls. Congenital thyroid hormone deficiency is tested a week after the birth. If detected, this can be treated successfully.

4 Chronic medical disorders: particularly disorders affecting the bowel and therefore absorption of nutrients, e.g. coeliac disease. Other chronic disorders adversely affecting growth include kidney and heart disorders, diabetes, thalassaemia and cystic fibrosis. A child who suffers repeated infectious illnesses, with loss of appetite, may also suffer growth retardation.

5 Social factors: poor nutrition with a consistently inadequate diet, or emotional neglect or abuse, will sometimes result in growth retardation.

Premature and small babies

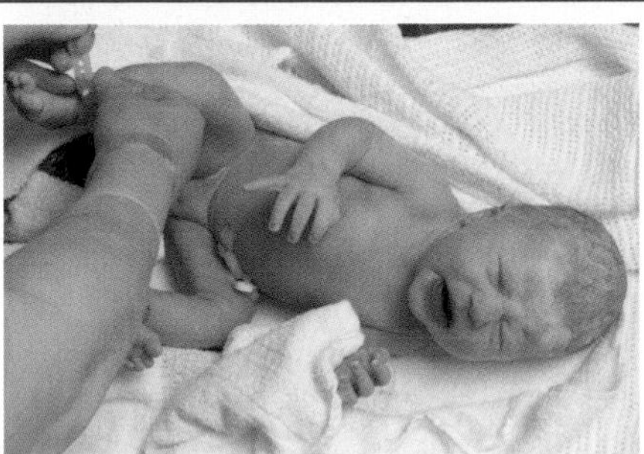

Premature babies won't necessarily suffer from long-term growth retardation – they usually make up any shortfall.

At birth the weight of some babies falls below the 10th centile on the standard growth charts.

- Babies can fall into this category whether born prematurely or at full term.

- Babies who are small may have suffered intrauterine growth retardation, which has many causes, making it difficult to assess expected growth outcome. Possible causes include placental insufficiency, poor maternal nutrition and chromosomal abnormalities.

- Premature babies are often an appropriate weight for their gestational age. Most premature babies catch up in growth by the age of two years, but some do not, and it is very difficult to predict which ones will.

- If your baby was premature, you must remember to correct his age according to his due date when assessing his growth.

Helping your child

Children who are small for their age are often taken to be younger than they are, and treated as such. As a parent, there are ways you can help.

- **Encourage self-confidence:** encouraging your child to develop self-confidence and to defend himself can help. After all, character and personality matter far more than height. This is particularly important at school, where bullying can be a problem. Any unkind comments or hint of bullying should be addressed immediately with your child's school.

- **Provide reassurance:** delayed onset of puberty is associated with growth retardation, and this can cause embarrassment to adolescents, especially boys. Reassure your child that he will catch up and that everyone develops at different rates.

- **Discuss your worries:** inherited slow growth or short stature do not make your child more likely to have delayed intellectual development, but if you feel your child is not attaining the developmental milestones, do discuss this with your doctor or health visitor.

- **Seek specialist help:** children with some chromosomal abnormalities, such as Down's syndrome, may need additional stimulation in the early years to encourage their development. In some areas special groups are set up for this purpose, which your doctor or health visitor should be able to arrange for you. These children may be able to attend a mainstream primary school in the early years, but may then need to transfer to a special needs unit.

- **Provide support:** remember that whatever the cause or extent of your child's growth retardation, your reassurance and support are vital.

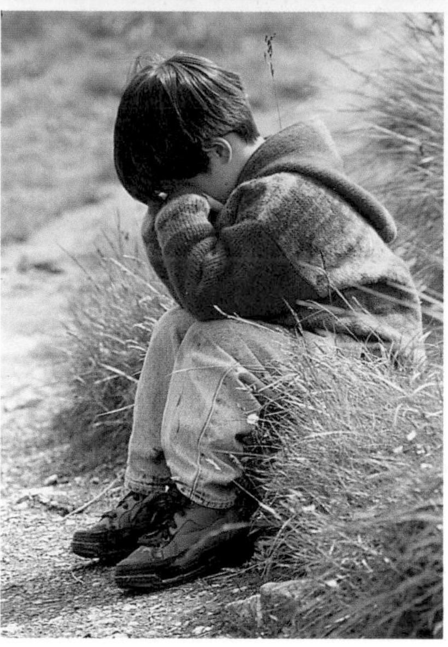

If your child is short for his age, he may be more susceptible to bullying. Your support and reassurance are vital for his self-esteem and wellbeing.

Possible treatments

If you are concerned about your child's height, you should consult your GP or health visitor. There is a series of tests and investigations that can be done to monitor any problems.

1 Your health visitor may take measurements over a period of 12 months. She will plot them on a special growth chart. Your child's health record book, which includes the original growth charts, should be taken into consideration, too.

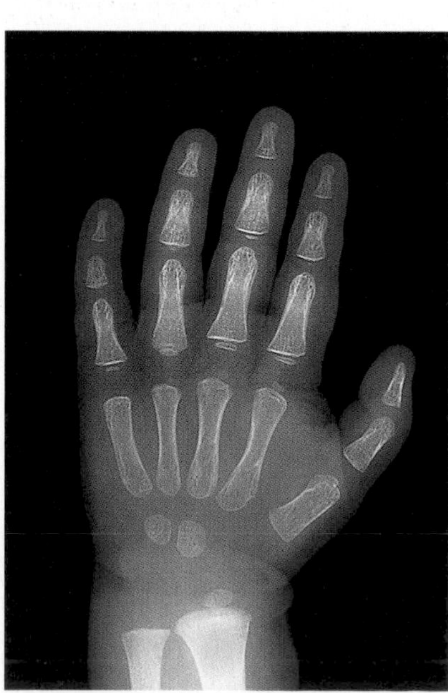

2 Plotting the measurements will show whether your child is below average or of normal height and weight for his age. If your child's rate of growth is normal, the plotted curve will follow the curve of one of the printed centile lines on the chart. If the plotted growth curve falls away from the printed curves, your child's rate of growth is slowing down. If it falls away across more than two centile lines, the cause usually needs investigating, and your child may be referred to a paediatrician or to a specialist growth clinic.

3 Investigations may include an X–ray of your child's hand and wrist (or feet and legs if your child is under 18 months) to assess his 'bone age' – an indication of the maturation of the bones.

4 If your child's bone age is significantly less than his chronological age, there is more growth potential in the bones and a possibility that he may eventually reach a normal adult height. However, if your child's bone age is very similar to his chronological age, he is more likely to remain short.

5 Blood tests may also be carried out to check for any deficiencies or abnormalities that may cause or contribute to growth retardation.

6 Growth hormone deficiency can be demonstrated using a series of blood tests and exercise tests. Either growth hormone itself, or growth hormone releasing factor, may be used to treat a deficiency, and with early recognition, the treatment can often be very successful. It does, however require daily injections up until adulthood.

7 If the underlying cause of growth retardation is nutritional, you will be given dietary advice and possibly special supplements to supply extra calories and nutrients.

If your child's rate of growth is slower than normal, he may be referred to have hand and wrist X-rays. These are used to assess bone maturation.

HAND, FOOT & MOUTH DISEASE

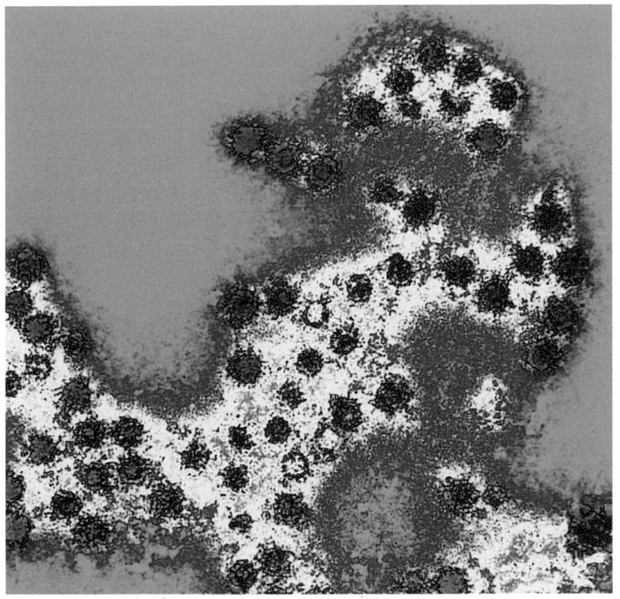

WHAT IS HAND, FOOT AND MOUTH DISEASE?

Hand, foot and mouth disease is a common, contagious viral infection that generally affects children under the age of four. The illness is seen most often during the summer months and in early autumn.

- Hand, foot and mouth disease (entirely different from the animal foot and mouth disease) is caused by a particular virus – the Coxsackie virus – and it usually takes about four days after infection for the child to start to feel unwell. At this stage a distinctive rash usually appears.

- Hand, foot and mouth is not a serious condition. Its effects last from only a few days, up to a maximum of a week. While it is advisable with any rash to consult your GP, many cases of hand, foot and mouth are so mild as to pass undetected.

The Coxsackie virus is responsible for a number of diseases, including hand, foot and mouth and, in a different variation, the common cold. It is highly contagious.

How the virus is spread

The virus that causes hand, foot and mouth disease is passed from child to child in tiny airborne droplets of mucus. Transmission can occur in different ways.

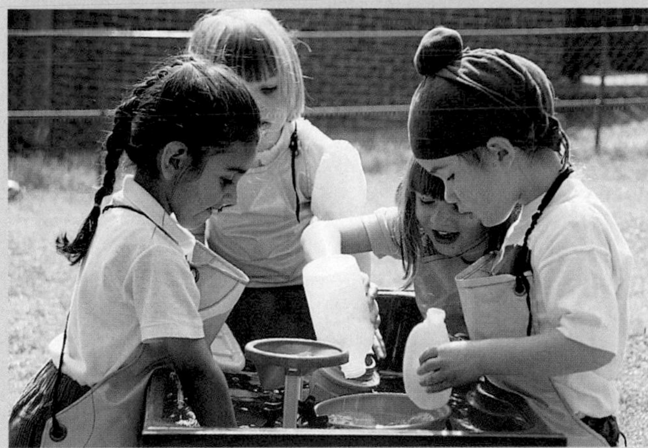

Children playing in close proximity can facilitate the spread of a virus such as hand, foot and mouth.

1 An infected child may cough or sneeze in close proximity to others, who then inhale the droplets.

2 Close personal contact, for example by kissing, can spread infection.

3 It is common for the brothers and sisters of toddlers infected with hand, foot and mouth to become infected as well. The virus is prevalent in children only, so adults in the family are usually immune.

Recognising the symptoms

As implied by its name, hand, foot and mouth disease affects those specific parts of the body. The symptoms include:

- A fever, poor appetite, sore throat.

- Small red spots that appear on the tongue, gums and inside the cheeks one or two days later. These turn into blisters, ending up as white ulcers about 3mm (⅛in) in diameter.

- Raised, red spots that become noticeable on the hands and feet, which sometimes turn into blisters that resemble those found in chickenpox.

- Sometimes a child may also have a rash on the buttocks.

Painful spots on the feet and hands are typical of the disease. They are not unlike the spots found in chickenpox infection.

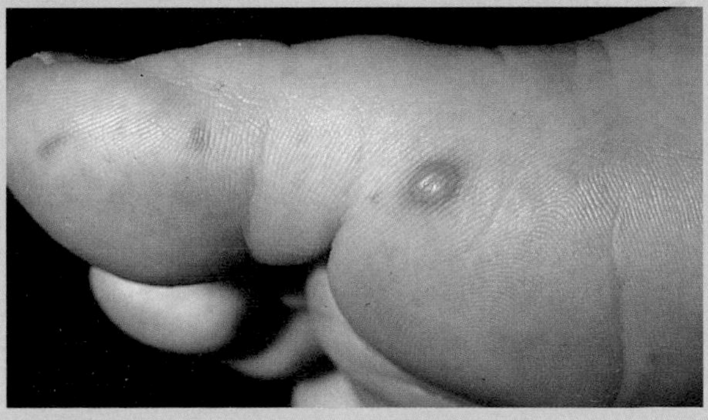

Home nursing

There is no specific treatment for hand, foot and mouth disease and viral infections do not respond to antibiotics. Once the condition has been diagnosed, the doctor will probably want to monitor the child's progress, but there is generally no cause for concern. There are, however, several steps that parents can take to ensure that their child is as comfortable as possible.

- If a fever is present, remove most of the child's clothing and cover her with a cotton sheet.

- Make sure that the room is well ventilated and use an electric fan if you have one.

- Liquid paracetamol is particularly effective at reducing a temperature, and it has the added advantage of helping to relieve any discomfort from the rash or mouth ulcers.

- If none of these measures seem to help, gentle sponging of the skin with tepid water (never ice-cold) can be effective in reducing the child's temperature.

- Making sure that a child drinks plenty of fluids is important in any infection. Mouth and throat ulcers may be painful; ensuring that liquids are not too hot or ice-cold, and are as bland as possible, may help. A child may eat very little during the acute stage of the illness but it is more important to maintain a high level of fluid intake than trying to 'force' food down her. A short period of time without food will do no harm.

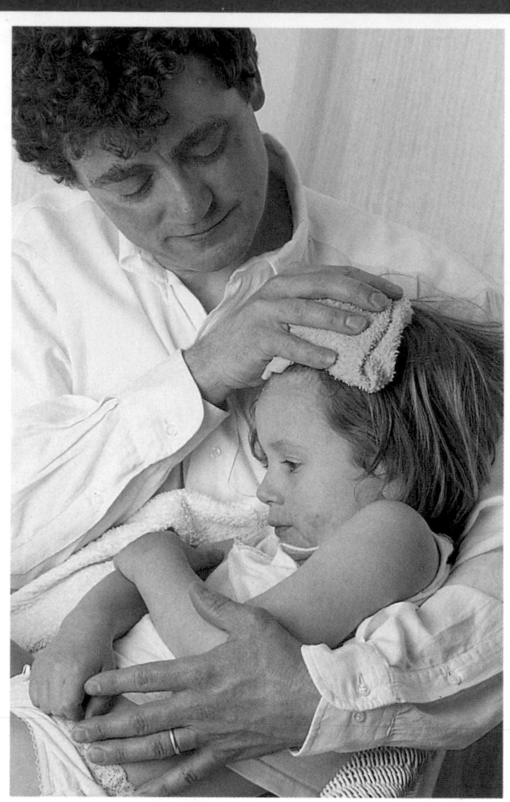

Although the symptoms of hand, foot and mouth may be mild and of short duration, it is important to take steps to lower the temperature of a feverish child as quickly as possible.

How to treat the rash

The mouth ulcers and skin rash usually disappear within a week, but during this time a child may complain of discomfort (especially in the mouth) and itching. Mouth ulcers, if severe, can be particularly worrying for a parent as they can make a child reluctant to eat or drink.

- Several over-the-counter products can help soothe inflammation inside the mouth. Gels containing local anaesthetic can be effective but it is important to check that the product is suitable for a young child. Some medicated mouthwashes claim to help heal ulcers, and, if they are antiseptic, may prevent a secondary infection developing.

- The itchiness of the skin rash may be relieved by calamine lotion, which is also available over the counter.

- Hot baths will make the rash on the skin feel even more uncomfortable. Ensure that the child's bath is run with warm water only, and avoid the use of bubble baths.

- Use lightweight cotton rather than man-made fabrics for your child's bedding to reduce skin irritation.

Lesions on the tongue and around the mouth can be extremely sore and distressing to a pre-school child. Consult your GP for advice if the symptoms worsen.

Nutrition

If a child is suffering from the painful mouth ulcers that are symptomatic of hand, foot and mouth, it may be necessary to adapt her diet for a few days.

- Serve food that is soft and relatively bland, taking special care to avoid salty or spicy flavours. Salt should never be added to children's food either during cooking or serving.

- Offer frequent drinks, but take care to avoid acidic fruit juices. Water and milk are the best options; citrus flavours may irritate the mouth ulcers.

- Feverishness diminishes the appetite, so allow your child to eat at her own pace. Her appetite will revert to normal.

HAYFEVER

WHAT IS HAYFEVER?

Hayfever, also known as allergic rhinitis, is an allergic reaction to particles that enter the nose and throat.

- Hayfever is the most common of all allergies, affecting 10–15 per cent of the population. Its incidence is rising, though the reasons for this are unclear.

- Hayfever is more common in boys than girls. Children from well-off families and single and first-born children are more susceptible. Many doctors believe that this may be because such children are not exposed to enough infections and foreign substances during the first few years of life.

- There are two types of hayfever: the first is seasonal (mainly spring and summer) allergic rhinitis; the second is perennial (all year round) allergic rhinitis.

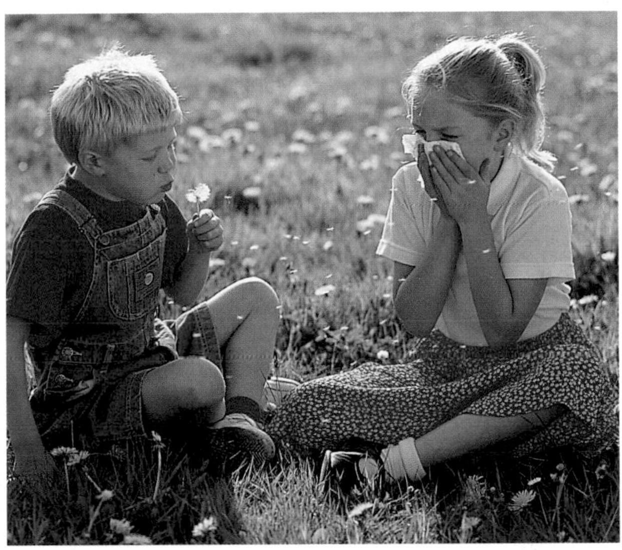

Seasonal hayfever attacks are usually intermittent throughout the spring and summer months.

What triggers hayfever?

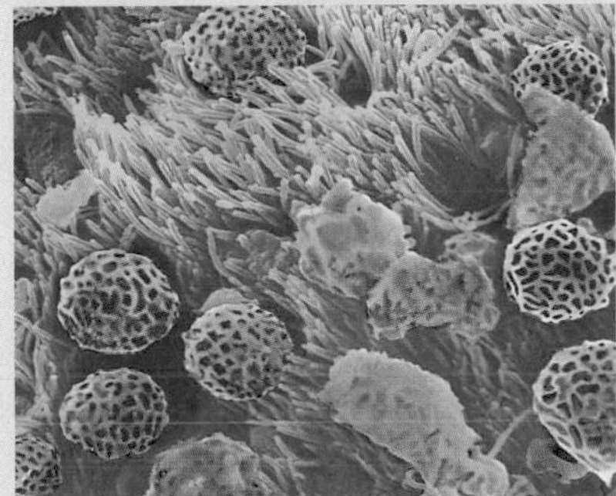

The trachea or windpipe covered in allergens – pollen (orange) and dust (brown).

Hayfever is an allergy that can be triggered by many different proteins entering the body. The triggers can vary from person to person.

- Hayfever occurs when the body reacts with unusual sensitivity to a substance (known as an allergen). When the substance is next present, the body's antibodies mark it and attract defensive cells, some of which are called mast cells. These release chemicals such as histamine.

- Histamine is a substance that causes an inflammatory response and produces allergy symptoms.

- Hayfever allergens include tree pollens in the spring, grass pollen in the summer and mugwort and hybrid flowers, such as chrysanthemums, in the autumn. Other allergens include dried cat saliva and skin from pets. Perennial hayfever can be caused by the droppings of house dust mites and the spores from fungal moulds.

- Nasal hypersensitivity to tobacco smoke and dust, for example, can exacerbate symptoms.

What happens during an attack?

The symptoms of hayfever vary according to how the body reacts to specific allergens and the amount of histamine that is produced.

- **Allergic reaction:** histamine contracts smooth muscles, such as those of the airways, and widens small arteries and blood vessels, which become more permeable, allowing fluid to escape into the tissues. This causes the membranes to become swollen and inflamed.

- **Symptoms:** the result of an attack can be frequent sneezing, with either a runny or congested nose, coughing, watery, itchy, puffy eyes and sometimes wheezing and a burning sensation in the throat.

- **Duration:** symptoms may subside, only to reappear two to12 hours later when more histamine is released from slower-reacting mast cells.

NOTE: sufferers from perennial allergic rhinitis may have low-grade symptoms throughout the year, often worse in the morning and evening, with occasional severe attacks.

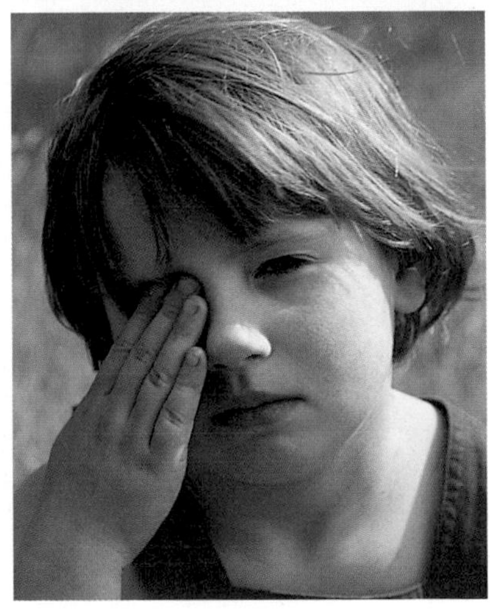

The symptoms of hayfever can be very irritating for the sufferer. The eyes often become itchy and appear puffy during an attack.

Wet combing step-by-step

Although you can buy chemical treatments for head lice, these are costly, potentially toxic, unsafe to use on toddlers and do not always work. The wet combing method is safe and reliable, if you follow the instructions below.

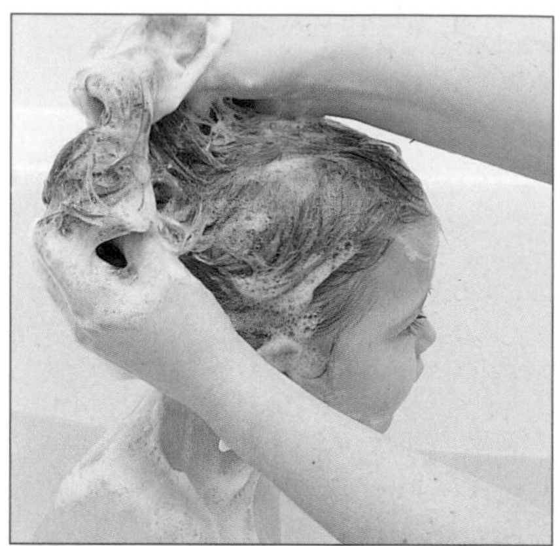

1 Wet your child's hair then shampoo as usual. Next, apply a very liberal amount of conditioner all over the head. (This should be around twice or three times the amount you might use for a normal hairwash.) Smooth the hair down carefully.

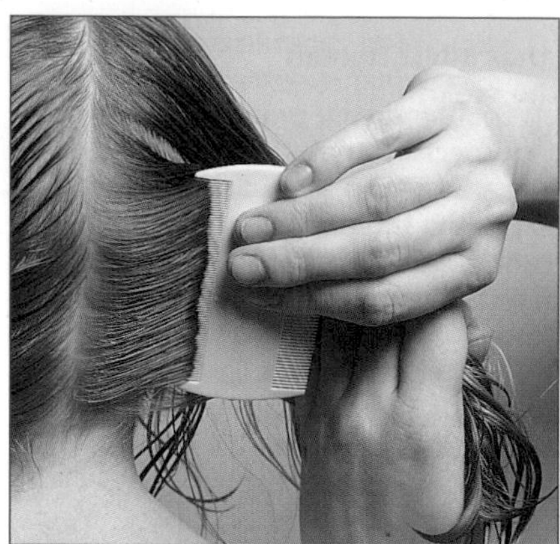

2 Without rinsing off the conditioner, start combing the hair into sections, using a special nit comb. Work from the roots upwards, lifting the hair as you comb. Pay particular attention to the area behind the ears and at the nape of the neck.

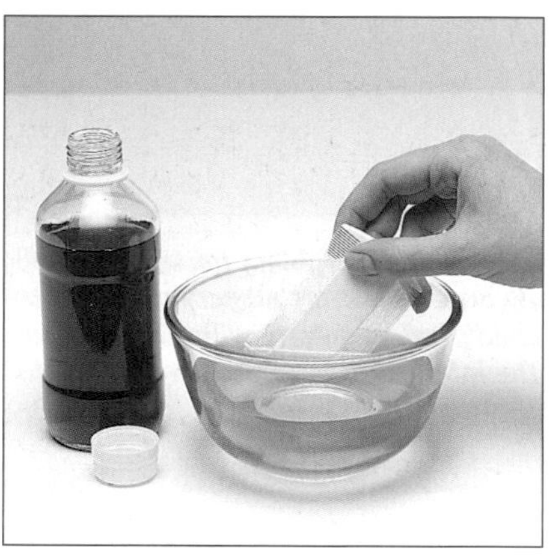

3 Check for lice on the comb after each stroke, and rinse them away, preferably by dipping the comb into a bowl of hot water mixed with a drop of vinegar. Continue working until you have combed all of the hair.

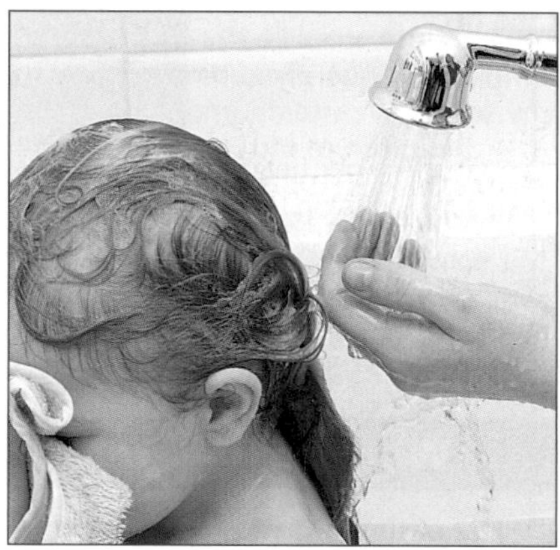

4 Rinse the conditioner off and dry the hair as usual. Repeat the process every two to three days for at least two weeks. Check the rest of the family, including yourself, for infestation, and treat if necessary.

Treatment

If you choose to use a chemical treatment to get rid of lice, make sure you ask your pharmacist's advice first. Avoid an alcohol-based treatment if your child is asthmatic.

- It can take up to two weeks to eliminate an infestation of head lice. Affected family members should be treated, but there is no benefit in treating non-infested members.
- There is a range of chemical preparations available over the counter from your local pharmacist, or on prescription from your GP. Treatment is usually in the form of a shampoo or lotion.
- All chemical head lice treatments are potentially toxic if misused, so it is vitally important to carefully follow the instructions.
- Chemical treatments usually need to be repeated and don't always work: head lice are becoming more and more immune – this is why infestations are increasingly common.

Caution!

Children under the age of two, pregnant women and asthmatics should not be treated with chemical preparations for killing head lice. Ask at your health food shop about natural remedies, or try the wet combing method, as described. This is laborious, but can be just as effective as any special preparation – and there are no side-effects.

Getting help

Generally, there is no need to consult your doctor if your child has head lice, but it is best to bear the following in mind:

- If your child's scalp looks inflamed, it is worth seeking medical advice, as some of the sore spots may have become infected.
- It's usually possible to self-treat head lice as described above.
- Remember to avoid chemical preparations for children under the age of two. Wet combing is the safest way to deal with the problem, and is also the cheapest.

Your home and family pets

Although an infestation of head lice is unpleasant for the whole family, there is no need to panic if you detect lice in your child's hair.

- Head lice need warmth as well as human blood to survive, which is why eggs are laid close to the scalp. Any lice that crawl off on to pillows, furniture, carpets or clothing will not survive, so there is no need to take any action around the home.
- As the Latin name suggests, the common head louse lives on human scalps only, so family pets will not be affected. If your dog or cat suddenly starts scratching, it's probably a case of fleas. Ask your vet for advice.

HEART DISORDERS IN NEWBORN BABIES

WHAT IS A HEART DISORDER?

Nearly one in 100 babies has a heart disorder at birth. These disorders are usually caused either by a fault in the 'plumbing' – those parts of the heart blood moves through – or in the 'electrics' – the pacing of nerve messages which tell the heart when to beat and how fast.

Typical 'plumbing' faults could be a narrowing or a hole in the heart, while pacing faults cause arrhythmia, when the heart beats too fast, slowly or is irregular.

There are many kinds of disorders of the heart – most are minor and need no treatment, some may need medicines or medical procedures to cure them and, in a few cases, a baby will need heart surgery.

Babies often have a heart murmur when they are born. It usually disappears within a few days.

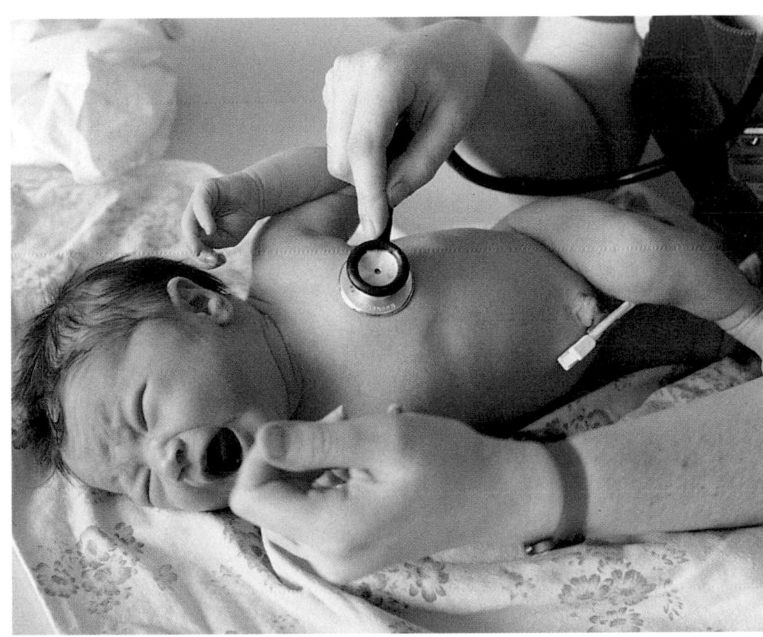

Symptoms

Almost all babies with heart disorders look normal and behave normally. However, symptoms may include:

- More frequent chest infections
- Looking pale
- Difficulties feeding because the baby tends to tire quickly
- Blueness or breathlessness

Heart murmurs

A 'murmur' describes extra sounds that blood makes as it passes through the valves and blood vessels of the heart. Newborn babies often have murmurs because parts of the system they used before birth are closing.

- An unusual murmur in a newborn, or one picked up at the routine eight-week check, could mean there is a heart disorder – the sound could be made by blood crossing through a hole, or a valve that is too narrow.
- If your baby has an unusual murmur your GP will refer her to a paediatrician. If he is not satisfied that the murmur is normal, your baby will be referred to a cardiologist.
- The Children's Heart Federation (freephone 0808 808 5000) offers information on heart disorders.

Tests for heart disorders

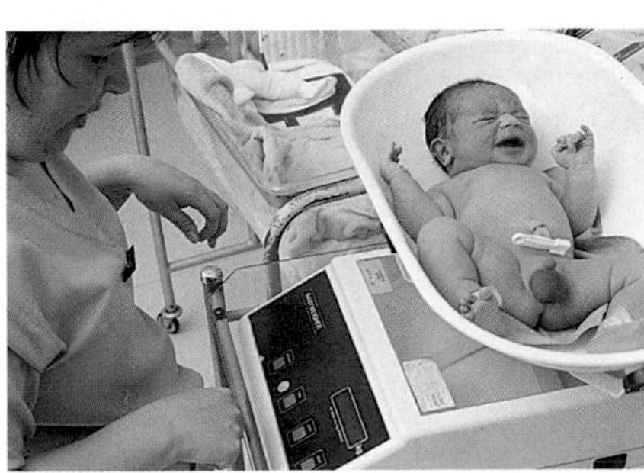

The heart specialist will want to know how much your baby weighed at birth. A baby with a heart condition may be slow to gain weight after birth.

Tests to determine the nature of the problem may include:

1 Health check: the cardiologist will look at your baby to see if he is showing any signs of heart disorder, such as blueness or breathlessness. He will also want to know your baby's birthweight (in kilos) and may ask about your baby's feeding and sleeping habits.

2 Chest X-ray: this is sometimes needed to look at the position of the organs in the chest.

3 ECHO (echocardiogram): this is similar to the ultrasound you may have had in pregnancy, but looking at the baby's heart this time.

4 ECG (electrocardiogram): leads are placed over your baby's chest and a reading is taken of the electrical activity of the heart.

5 Pulse oximetry test: this test checks the amount of oxygen in your baby's blood by using a clip on the finger, ear or toe.

Common types of heart disorder

Congenital: when a baby is born with the problem. Some congenital conditions are inherited from the baby's parents, others occur in the womb while the baby is developing.

Patent, or Persistent, Ductus Arteriosus (PDA): patent means open. Persistent means that it remains after the birth. When the baby is in the womb, blood bypasses the lungs through the ductus arteriosus. If it doesn't shut after birth, too much blood will be pumped through the lungs.

Ventricular Septal Defect (VSD): when a hole appears between the two ventricles, red blood is pumped from the left ventricle to the right, instead of round the body.

Atrial Septal Defect (ASD): this means that there is a hole between the two atrial chambers: red blood will mix with blue blood and be pumped to the lungs.

Pulmonary Stenosis: the pulmonary valve is narrowed. This means that there is a reduction in the amount of blue blood that can get to the lungs.

Aortic Stenosis: the aortic valve is narrowed. This means that there is a reduction in the amount of red blood that can get to the body.

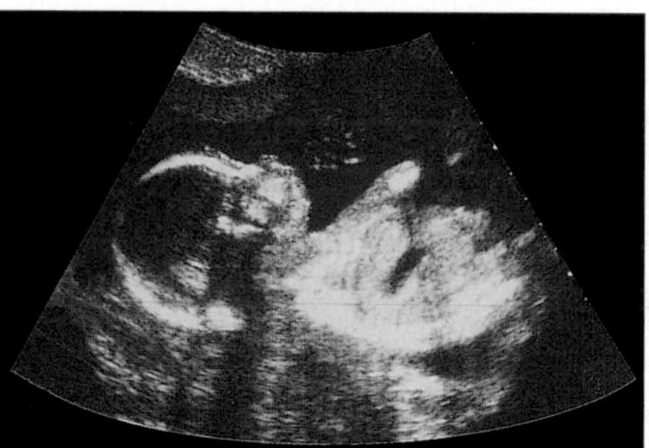

A heart defect in an unborn baby may be detected by an ultrasound scan when the baby is still in the womb.

What is the treatment?

Medicines: used to regulate a very fast heartbeat, or to get rid of a build-up of excess fluid in the heart.

Catheter intervention: used to close an ASD or PDA by putting a device on the end of a fine tube and feeding this through a vein into the ductus or hole.

Open-heart surgery: sometimes needed for larger VSDs and ASDs, although many VSDs will close spontaneously as the child gets bigger.

Monitoring: your child will be monitored before and after treatment.

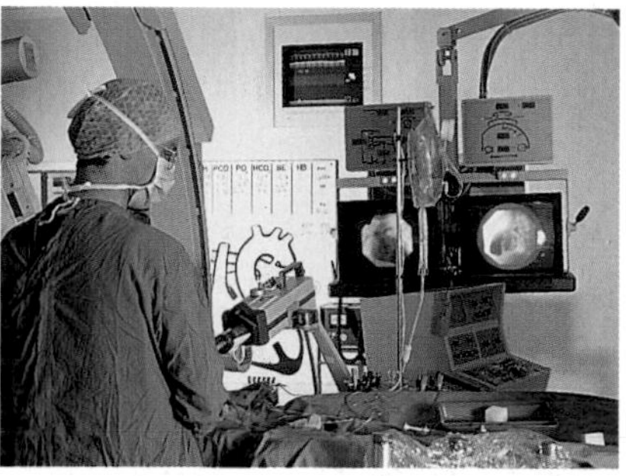

Surgeons will need to assess the blood flow to the heart before any surgery. A catheter is inserted into the artery and guided by X-ray to the heart.

How the heart works

The right side of the heart collects blue blood (de-oxygenated), which returns from the body, into the right atrium. The left atrium collects red blood, which has picked up oxygen from the lungs. Both atria contract, pumping blood through the valves into the left and right ventricles. As the right ventricle contracts, it pumps blue blood through the pulmonary valve, into the pulmonary arteries and so to the lungs. The left ventricle pumps at much higher pressure through the aortic valve into the aorta and so round the body.

NORMAL HEART

Aorta
Pulmonary artery
Right atrium
Left atrium
Mitral valve
Tricuspid valve
Left ventricle
Right ventricle

VENTRICULAR SEPTAL DEFECT

Aorta
Pulmonary artery
Right atrium
Left atrium
Mitral valve
Tricuspid valve
Ventricular septal defect
Right ventricle
Left ventricle

Parts of the heart

Aorta: the artery through which red blood is pumped to take oxygen to the body.

Aortic valve: the valve that lets blood into the aorta and stops it from leaking back into the heart.

Atrial chambers: the two chambers of the heart in which blood collects.

Mitral valve: the valve that lets blood into the left ventricle, and stops it from leaking back.

Pulmonary artery: the artery through which blue blood is pumped to the lungs to pick up oxygen.

Pulmonary valve: the valve that lets blood into the pulmonary artery, and stops it from leaking back.

Septum: the wall between the right and left sides of the heart.

Tricuspid valve: the valve that lets blood into the right atrium and stops it from leaking back.

Ventricles: the two pumping chambers of the heart.

HERNIAS IN BABIES

TYPES OF HERNIA

Your baby may be born with a weakness or gap in the muscles at the base of the umbilical cord. This causes the abdominal contents to bulge under the skin, which forms a soft lump. This is an umbilical hernia.

Another type of hernia is an inguinal hernia, when part of the bowel protrudes through the groin. Other variations are diaphragmatic hernias, which are life-threatening, and strangulated hernias, which are much rarer.

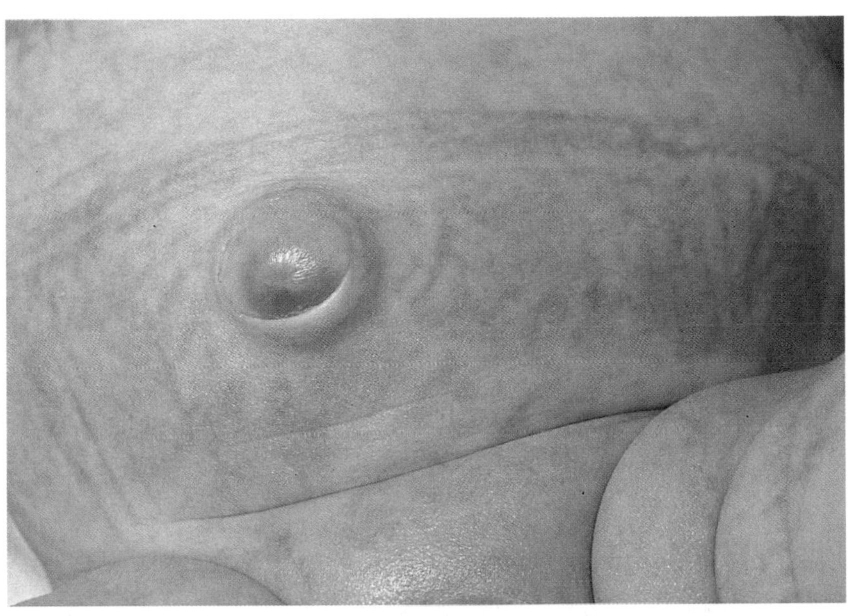

An umbilical hernia occurs when the abdominal organs protrude through the abdominal wall. If it occurs, it is usually present at birth but should not cause the baby any pain or discomfort.

Umbilical hernias

Umbilical hernias affect one in five babies and are more common in low birthweight or premature babies and those with Down's syndrome. If you suspect that your baby has an umbilical hernia, consult your GP.

- Your baby may have an umbilical hernia if you notice a slight lump under his skin around the navel. The lump is caused by part of his intestines bulging through the hernia.
- An umbilical hernia varies in size from that of a pea to a small plum – your GP can determine the size by feeling the lump under your baby's skin.
- The hernia may be present at birth or appear a day or so afterwards.
- The hernia is most visible when your baby cries, strains or coughs, as pressure pushes his abdominal contents through the hole.
- The lump can be pushed back by simply pressing on it gently with your finger.
- Although an umbilical hernia is rarely dangerous, it can be confused with other, more serious conditions.
- Sometimes, the lump is a sign of exomphalos, a rare defect causing the intestines to protrude through the umbilical cord. It may leak fluid whereas umbilical hernias do not. Exomphalos requires surgery.

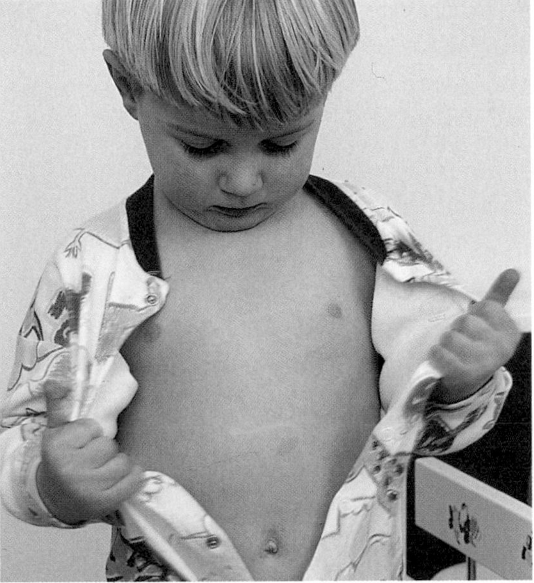

Treating an umbilical hernia

An umbilical hernia does not usually require medical treatment. Instead, the parent needs to keep a watchful eye on the swelling, which should get smaller as the baby grows.

- If your baby has an umbilical hernia, check it regularly, especially at bathtime, to make sure it's not growing or hardening and that it goes back in when gently pushed.

An umbilical hernia usually disappears without any need for medical attention. Your child's belly button should return to its normal size and appearance by the time he is four or five years old.

- Don't compress your baby's hernia with a bandage, tape or plasters, as this can increase the risk of an infection and skin irritation.
- Surgery is rarely necessary in young babies, although some parents request it for cosmetic reasons. Older children may have surgery if an umbilical hernia shows no sign of closing by about three or four years, or if the gap gets larger.

Inguinal hernias

An inguinal hernia occurs when part of the bowel protrudes into the groin (inguinal ring). This type of hernia affects 3 to 5 per cent of healthy full-term babies, but is more likely to occur in boys. In 10 per cent of cases there is a family history of the condition.

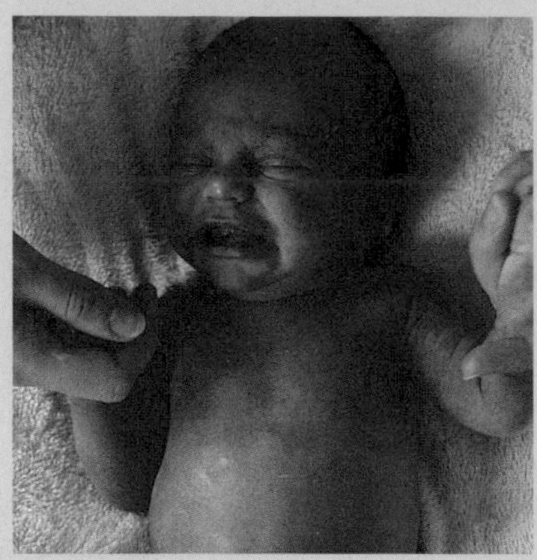

- In about the seventh month of pregnancy, a baby's testes descend into his scrotum. They pass through his abdominal wall via the 'inguinal canal', which should then close. However, sometimes the canal remains open and part of the baby's intestines escape from his abdominal cavity down into his groin, forming an inguinal hernia.

Occasionally, an inguinal hernia is noticeable when the baby cries, passes a motion or coughs. The condition is more common in premature babies.

- Your baby may have an inguinal hernia if there is a swelling or puffy area in his groin. The bulge may be visible all the time or it may appear only when your baby cries, coughs or has a bowel movement. It should be soft and can be gently pushed back into place.
- The hernia usually appears in one groin. Occasionally, the hernia is accompanied by a hydrocele, which is an accumulation of fluid around your baby's testicles, or an undescended testicle.

Repairing inguinal hernias

An inguinal hernia is repaired surgically. The hernia is not a direct threat to your baby's health, but there is a risk that it will become twisted (strangulated), when it will need to be corrected immediately. If the hernia is not strangulated, surgery may be delayed until your baby is five months old, when he will be stronger.

1 Surgery: the operation to repair an inguinal hernia is a simple day-case procedure performed under general anaesthetic. Your baby's lower abdomen and scrotal region are washed with antiseptic. Then the surgeon makes a small cut in your baby's groin, pushes his intestines back into place and sews up the opening. The hole in your baby's abdominal muscles usually closes by itself as he grows.

2 Aftercare: once your baby wakes up after surgery, you can resume his feeding routine and you may be able to return home within a few hours. The medical staff will show you how to change the dressings and will recommend you give your baby suitable painkillers over the next day or two. After a few days, you can give him a bath and he can move around normally. You don't need to return to the hospital to have the stitches removed – they should be self-dissolving. As there is a slight risk of infection after surgery, you need to keep an eye on the cut as it heals.

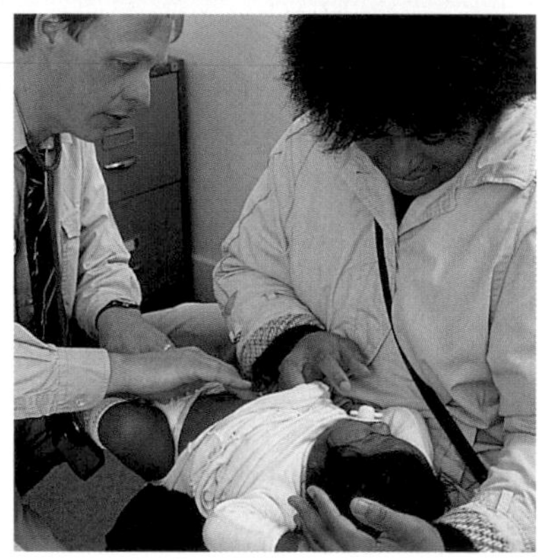

Check your baby's scar daily to make sure it is healing well. If it appears red, hot or your baby seems in pain, see your GP.

Strangulated hernias

A strangulated hernia occurs when part of the intestines becomes trapped. As a result, the hernia can't be pushed back in and becomes red and painful.

A strangulated hernia cuts off the blood supply to the intestines, which may burst. This can lead to gangrene within five to six hours.

If your baby has an inguinal hernia and you are waiting for surgery, you need to watch for hernia strangulation. If you see any of the following symptoms, call an ambulance straightaway:

- A hard tender swelling in the groin that won't disappear.
- The hernia is growing or changing colour.
- A swollen testicle or scrotum that won't subside.
- Abdominal pain, nausea and vomiting.

Diaphragmatic hernias

A diaphragmatic hernia may occur if a baby's diaphragm (the muscular wall separating his chest and abdomen) fails to develop normally before birth, leaving a hole. As a result, some of his abdominal organs enter his chest.

- In severe cases, this compresses the baby's heart and lungs, stopping them from developing properly.
- When a baby with a diaphragmatic hernia is born, he will have breathing difficulties and may be blue with a sunken or hollowed abdomen, vomiting and severe colicky pain.
- A diaphragmatic hernia can be fatal and needs immediate surgery. The procedure is complicated and the survival rate depends on the state of the baby's lungs.
- Following surgery, the baby may need help with breathing for several days or months before his lungs can work on their own.

IMMUNISATIONS

WHY ARE BABIES IMMUNISED?

Immunising babies helps to protect them from serious infectious diseases. Although born with some natural immunity from their mother's antibodies, which can be boosted by breast-feeding, this immunity gradually wanes over the first few months. Premature babies are particularly vulnerable to infection and should not have their immunisations delayed.

Now that children are routinely immunised against diphtheria, whooping cough, tetanus, polio, Hib, meningitis C, measles, mumps and rubella, these diseases are fortunately rare.

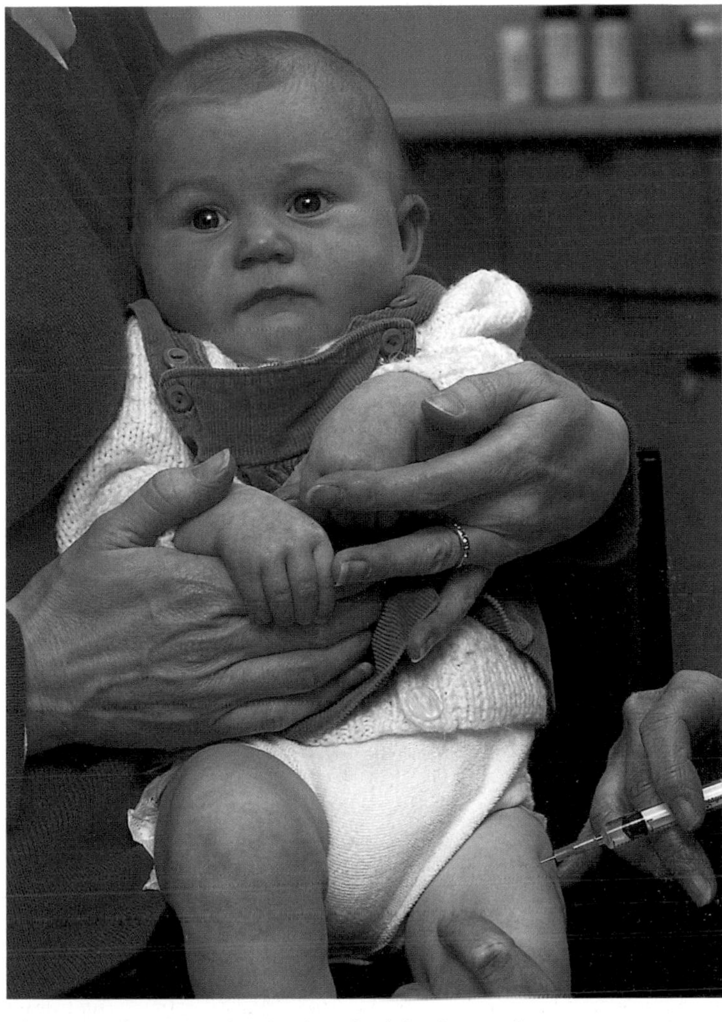

The DTP-Hib vaccination is given by injection to the upper arm or thigh, usually at the age of two months. This protects against whooping cough, tetanus, diphtheria and Haemophilus influenza B. Meningitis C is given by injection to the other side.

Starting vaccinations

Vaccinations generally start when a baby is two months old with a combined diphtheria, tetanus, whooping cough and Haemophilus influenza B injection (called DTP-Hib), a second injection (meningitis C) and a polio vaccine by mouth. Three doses of DTP-Hib, meningitis C and polio are given at four-weekly intervals and will protect the child until the pre-school booster injection is given at age four. Most vaccines are given at the GP's surgery, often by the practice nurse, but in some areas immunisations are given at the child health clinic. Parents will be given an appointment for the first injection. If the baby has a fever on that day, the injection should be postponed. It is quite safe to vaccinate a baby who has a mild cold or is taking antibiotics, but the doctor needs to know if your child is taking medication, such as steroids, for a chronic illness.

If you haven't been notified of a vaccination by the time of your baby's six-week examination, check with the GP's surgery or health visitor.

First-year immunisations

Age given	Name of immunisation	Diseases protected against	Form
From birth* ** given at birth in some areas only*	BCG – the acronym stands for bacille Calmette-Guérin. (Calmette and Guérin were the French bacteriologists who developed it). BCG does not cause tuberculosis, but retains its ability to produce immunity	tuberculosis (TB)	1 injection
At 2, 3 and 4 months	DTP-Hib (The P in DTP stands for pertussis, the bacterium that causes whooping cough)	diphtheria, whooping cough tetanus, and Hib meningitis	1 injection
	meningitis	meningococcal C meningitis	1 injection
	polio	polio	by mouth

How they work

Vaccines contain a very small amount of the particular virus or bacteria, which is carefully treated so that it does not actually cause the disease. The vaccine stimulates the blood to make antibodies that would fight the disease if a child is ever exposed to it in the future. Booster doses of certain vaccines, such as tetanus and MMR (measles, mumps and rubella), are needed to prevent immunity wearing off.

Your baby will also be offered the meningitis C vaccine, which protects against one of the three strains of meningococcal meningitis – the C strain.

Reactions

After the first injections, many babies have no reaction at all, but it is quite common for a baby to cry and be irritable or get a slight temperature. If this happens, a dose of Calpol will relieve the pain and help lower the temperature.

At the site of the injection, some babies develop redness up to the size of a 10p piece or a lump that may last several weeks. The correct treatment is simply Calpol. If the area of redness is more than about 10cm (3in) it should be reported to the doctor or nurse, but it is rarely necessary for antibiotics to be given.

The risks

Parents often worry about the long-term risks or complications of vaccinations. In fact, the possible risks of vaccines are now known to be far smaller than the real risks of the diseases themselves.

- In the 1970s there was a scare about the whooping cough vaccine, which was linked with a few cases of children suffering from brain damage, but this link has not been confirmed in more recent studies. As a consequence, many mothers did not vaccinate their children and the number of unnecessary cases of whooping cough, a distressing and serious illness, soared.

- For those thinking of alternative medicine, homeopathic vaccines have now been found definitely not to work and even the governing body for homeopathic doctors recommends that babies have the routine immunisations. The decision to withhold any immunisations from a child should not be taken lightly.

- If in doubt, ask to be referred to the local specialist immunisation clinic for up-to-date information. Your baby's eight-month developmental check-up is a good opportunity to discuss the next immunisation, the MMR, which is due between 12 and 15 months.

Polio

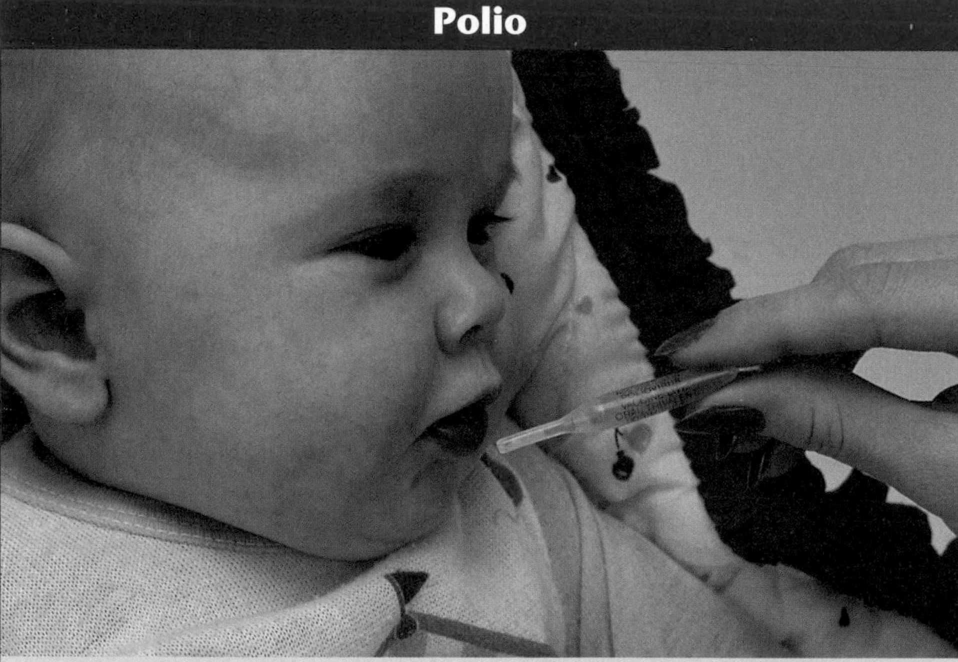

The polio vaccination is usually given by three drops on to the tongue. Polio is an infectious disease that can damage the nervous system.

At the surgery, the person giving the vaccine will explain about any possible side-effects and may give some written information to remind parents.

Your baby will be given three drops of polio vaccine on the tongue. This tastes rather bitter, so your baby's chin will be gently pressed to stop him spitting out the vaccine. If he is sick within one hour, the dose should be repeated. If in doubt, it is perfectly safe to give an extra dose. After your baby has had the polio drops, the vaccine is excreted in the faeces for up to six weeks.

It is important to make sure that anybody changing your baby's nappy has been previously immunised against polio and thorough handwashing is needed. If uncertain, check with the doctor, as the carer may need a polio booster.

Occasionally, if a family member is immunosuppressed, a 'killed' polio vaccine is used instead to prevent the theoretical risk of transmission.

BCG

In some inner-city areas where tuberculosis is re-emerging, newborn babies are being offered a BCG injection by the community paediatrician. This involves a small scratch on your baby's upper left arm, which usually develops as a small lump in the weeks following and may discharge pus. Generally, this will not require any treatment. The timing of the BCG injection does not affect the timing of your baby's other vaccinations, but the same arm must not be used for an injection for at least three months.

In areas where TB is less of a risk, BCG is offered to children aged 10-14 years. A skin prick test is performed first in all children over three months to ensure that they have not been exposed to tuberculosis as BCG would then not be given.

Useful address

Immunisation programme:
Department of Health
Room 602A, Skipton House
80 London Road
London SE1 6LH

www.immunisation.nhs.co.uk

IMPETIGO

WHAT IS IMPETIGO?

Impetigo is a common and extremely contagious skin infection caused by staphylococcus (staph) or streptococcus (strep) bacteria. The condition can affect anyone, although it is more common in children as they are in closer contact with one another.

How is it contracted?

Usually, although not always, staph or strep bacteria have to pass through the barrier of the skin to cause impetigo.

- Bacteria are always present on the skin, although their numbers are reduced by regular washing and good hygiene. Sometimes, impetigo can develop on what seems to be perfectly normal, healthy skin. In this case, the first sign is a small area of inflammation, resembling eczema.
- More often, impetigo develops when staph or strep bacteria gets into a minor break in the skin – a small cut or an insect bite, for example. Children with eczema or other skin conditions are particularly at risk, since they have many skin breaks.
- When the blisters that impetigo causes are scratched, bacteria-rich fluid seeps out of them. These can contaminate other breaks in the skin or be transferred to other people. This can happen either by physical contact or by contact with shared items, such as towels and face-cloths.

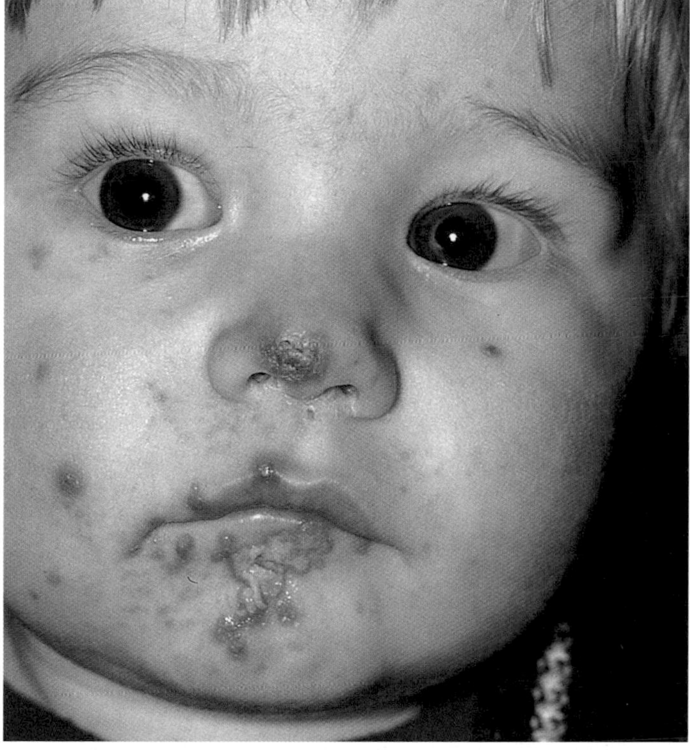

Impetigo is a highly contagious skin infection, normally affecting the face. The condition is usually contracted when bacteria enter a break in the skin. If left untreated, impetigo can spread to other parts of the body.

Good hygiene is essential to reduce the risk of impetigo spreading. If your child has the condition, make sure that she uses a separate towel and face cloth.

Symptoms

Impetigo is unsightly and irritating, but it is rarely a serious condition. The symptoms include:

- A small red, inflamed lesion on the skin, usually on the face, upper chest and arms, but sometimes on the legs or buttocks.
- A cluster of tiny blisters that are filled with a yellowish, honey-coloured fluid.
- The blisters itch and eventually ooze – especially when scratched – and a thick crust forms over them.
- If the blister bursts, a raw, reddish area is left behind.
- A rash may form in the area of the blisters as the condition is spread by scratching. Other areas may become infected.
- Lymph glands may be enlarged in the area of the infection.
- On rare occasions, when strep bacteria are involved, impetigo may lead to a potentially serious kidney infection called post-streptococcal glomerulonephritis. Very rarely, impetigo may cause ulceration of the skin and scarring.

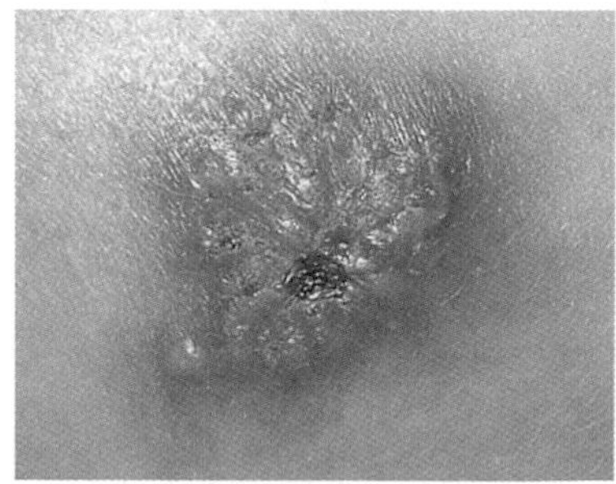

Impetigo appears as a small red lesion on the skin with yellow blisters. These blisters will burst forming a yellow crust.

Treatment for impetigo

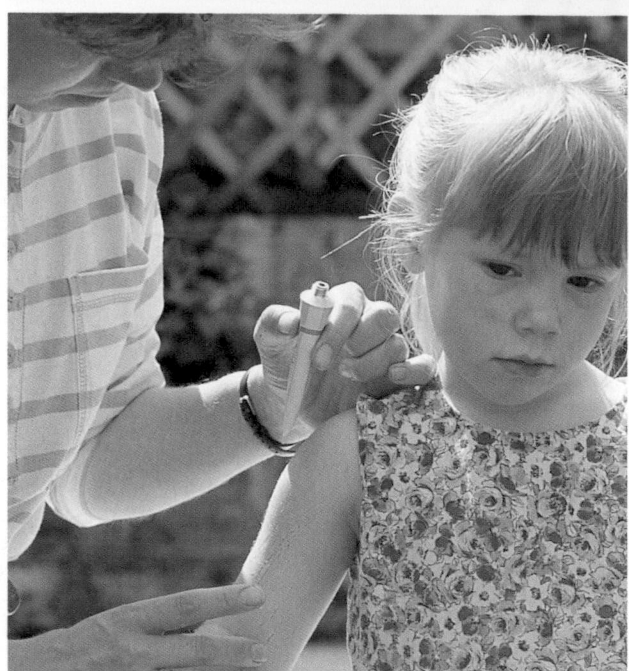

If your child has a mild case of impetigo, your GP may prescribe antibiotic cream. Tell your child not to touch the infected area, as this can make it worse.

Impetigo can be treated by your GP. The level of treatment depends on the severity of the outbreak.

- In mild outbreaks of impetigo, anti-bacterial ointment is applied to the blisters and scabs. The affected area should be washed regularly and left uncovered to dry out. Mild antiseptic, such as povidone-iodine, may be applied to the crusts under which the bacteria live, to soften them.

  The ointment is usually applied to the infected skin three times a day for seven days, or for a maximum of 10 days. If there is no improvement to the condition after using the ointment for two days, the GP is likely to recommend giving your child antibiotics by mouth.

- In more severe outbreaks, a course of antibiotics by mouth may be recommended from the outset.

- On rare occasions, impetigo may prove resistant to antibiotics. In this situation, swabs will be taken to examine the infection more closely. It is possible that repeat courses of antibiotics may be given.

- Strict hygiene measures are essential. These will help to ensure that the condition does not become worse, especially that it doesn't spread to other parts of your child's body.

Preventing impetigo from spreading

If no precautions are taken, impetigo will spread to other areas of your child's body, as well as to other members of the family – including you!

- Stress to your child that she must not touch the blisters and scabs.

- Explain that a special effort is needed with hygiene. Make sure that your child has her own face-cloth and towel and that she washes her hands regularly.

- Remember to wash your own hands immediately after touching your child's blisters or scabs.

- Cut your child's fingernails short, and make sure that there is no nose-picking, nail-biting or finger-sucking.

- Children with eczema are particularly susceptible to impetigo, and if they contract the condition the presence of other breaks in the skin make it much more likely to spread. In such cases, a strict hygiene regime is necessary and a course of antibiotic tablets is likely to be prescribed.

- If your child has repeated bouts of impetigo, as may be the case with children who have eczema, your GP may advise that she washes with a gel that contains benzoyl peroxide.

- Ask your GP for advice regarding the application of any ointment, but remember to make sure that any cream you apply to your child's face does not come into contact with her eyes or mouth.

Keeping your child off school

Even if your child's impetigo is being treated, it is important to prevent her from passing on the condition to other children.

- Keep a pre-school child away from a nursery or playgroup until the scabs or blisters have disappeared. Impetigo is spread by contamination with the fluid within the blisters and the tissue of the scabs. Unfortunately, young children cannot be trusted not to scratch itchy scabs and blisters, which is why the incubation period is longer.

- Older children should also be kept from school at the start of an attack of impetigo. As long as they do not touch or scratch any blisters or scabs, they may return to school after treatment has been under way for a week. They must be scrupulous about personal hygiene and avoid sharing items such as clothes, towels, flannels and brushes.

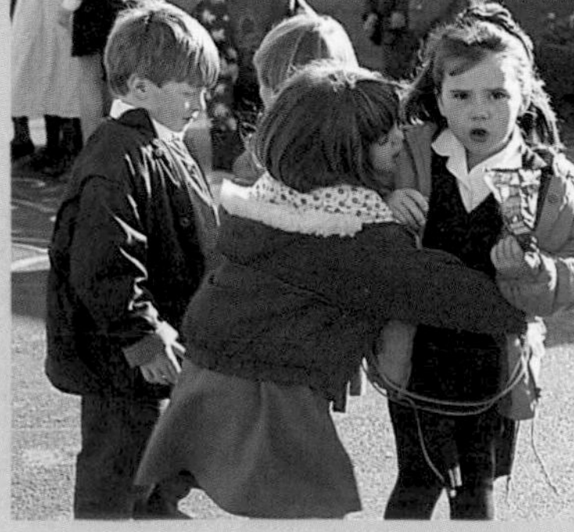

As impetigo is highly contagious and can be passed on by physical contact, it is advisable that your child doesn't go to school until the infection has cleared. She should also be kept away from young babies.

JAUNDICE

WHAT IS JAUNDICE?

Jaundice is a condition in which the skin and whites of the eyes turn yellow. Jaundice is not a disease in itself. Like a rash or a high temperature, it can be a sign of underlying disease. There are two distinct times when jaundice occurs: at and just after birth and later in childhood. Many newborn babies suffer from physiological jaundice, which indicates an immature liver. Haemolytic jaundice affecting newborns and jaundice in children is rare.

What causes it?

The yellow colouring is the result of a build-up of a bile pigment called bilirubin, which is produced by the breakdown of red blood cells. The bilirubin attaches to a protein in the blood called albumin. This moves to the liver where it is metabolised. It is then excreted into the gut. Broken down, bilirubin is what makes stools a dark brown colour. However, if, for whatever reason, the bilirubin is not being disposed of by the liver, its accumulation in the blood will affect skin colour.

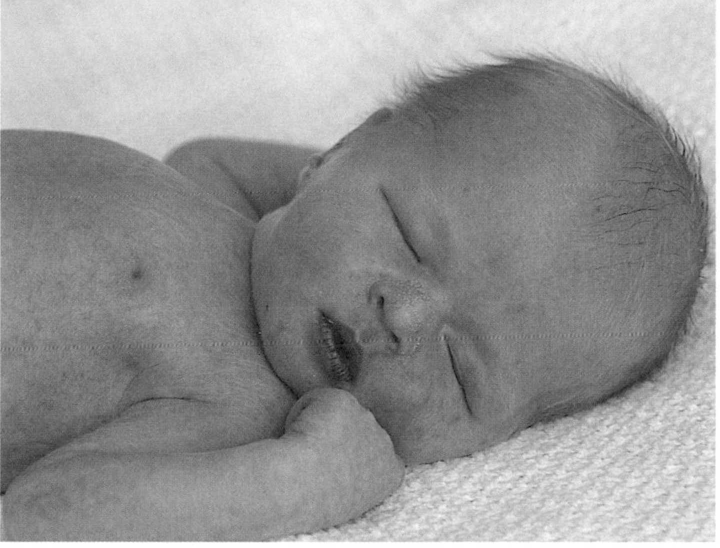

When a baby is first born, his immature liver may not be able to remove all the bilirubin from his blood. The bilirubin then builds up and causes a yellow colouring of the skin.

Physiological jaundice

Around 60 per cent of normal, healthy, full-term babies develop what is known as physiological jaundice.

- Suddenly the baby's liver has to struggle to get rid of the bilirubin, a job previously taken care of by the mother's placenta.

- Newborns have to deal with a lot of red blood cells as they swap their foetal haemoglobin for adult haemoglobin.
In addition, any bruising as a result of the birth will have to be broken down to bilirubin too.

- Because of the immaturity of the liver, there is usually a small delay before its enzymes kick into action. Premature babies are particularly slow at getting rid of the bilirubin and so are more prone to physiological jaundice.

- Physiological jaundice only ever appears on day two after birth; never within the first 24 hours. It peaks on day four and usually clears by the end of the first or second week.

Haemolytic jaundice

A baby may develop haemolytic jaundice if his blood group is incompatible with his mother's, particularly if the mother is rhesus negative.

- The difference between the mother and baby's blood is often not a problem in a first pregnancy. However, if the first pregnancy involves a rhesus positive baby this may sensitise the mother's blood to her baby's blood.

- If the rhesus negative mother is not given a special injection at the time of the first birth, miscarriage or termination, the blood of the next rhesus positive baby she carries will be attacked by her immune system.

- Such extreme situations are usually avoided as antenatal tests during a first pregnancy reveal whether the woman has a rhesus negative blood group – if she does, the required injection will be given.

- If, for some reason, a rhesus negative woman has not been treated in this way, a blood test will check whether she might have blood cells that will attack her baby. If so, both mother and baby will be monitored closely.

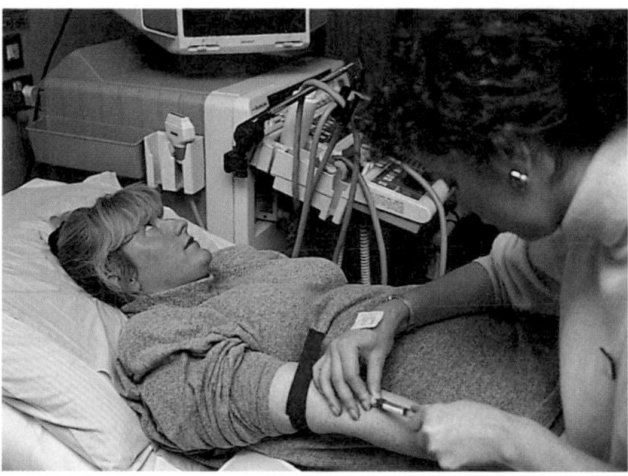

If the mother is found to have a rhesus negative blood type, it is likely to be incompatible with her baby's, which can result in the baby developing haemolytic jaundice before or after birth. Close monitoring during pregnancy is required as this type of jaundice can cause damage to the baby's brain and circulation.

Treatment

Treatment depends on the severity of the condition and how early it is picked up. A simple blood test can be taken to ascertain the bilirubin level.

1 Sunshine: for mildly jaundiced babies, a short spell each day in the sun is usually all that is needed, as light breaks down bilirubin.

2 Fluids: the baby needs plenty of fluids, by drip if he is not feeding.

3 Phototherapy: the baby will be put under a light and assessed every 24 hours.

4 Exchange transfusion: only used when the bilirubin level is rising fast and/or other measures have failed. The baby's blood is slowly removed and 'new', healthy blood – free of bilirubin – replaces it. This may be done repeatedly to ensure that the baby is out of danger from long-term injury.

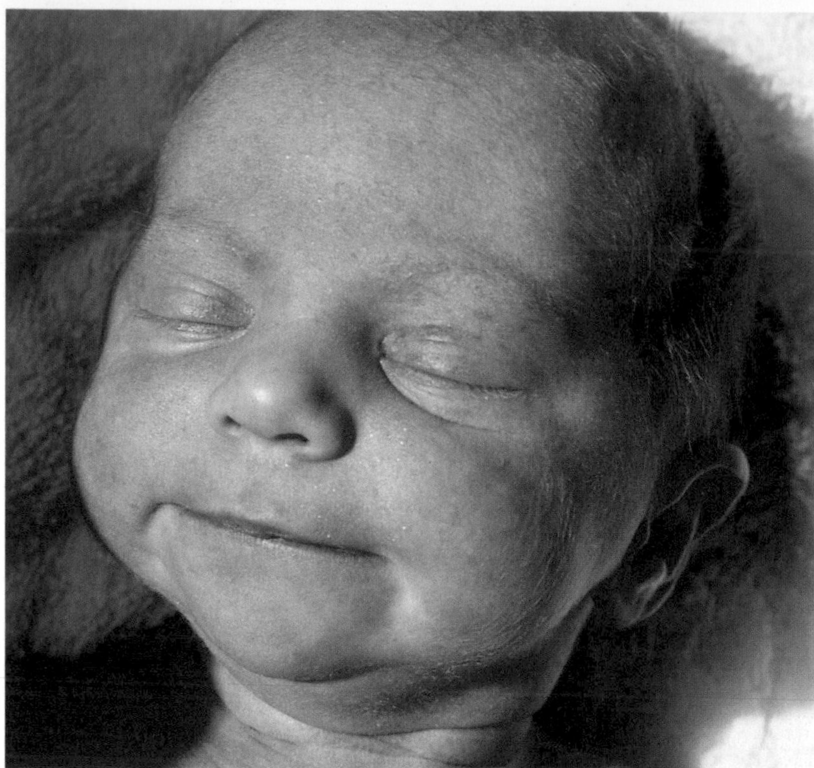

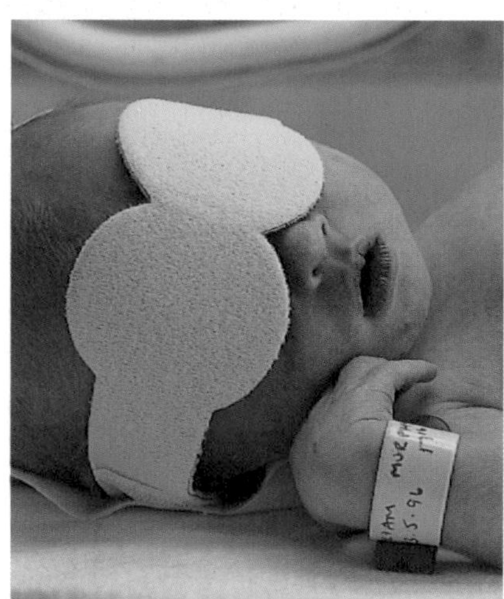

LEFT: A newborn with jaundice may be treated by phototherapy – a type of fluorescent light that breaks down bilirubin. His eyes are protected from the glare with eye patches or masks.

ABOVE: Half of all newborn babies develop jaundice two or three days after birth. Doctors recommend a few hours each day in the sunlight and it usually disappears within a week.

Complications

If the bilirubin level is very high, it can lead to a life-threatening condition called Kernicterus. If a baby recovers, he may be left with cerebral palsy and deafness.

Symptoms include:

- Abnormal behaviour
- Poor feeding
- Fitting
- Opisthotonus – a condition whereby a baby throws back his head and arches his back

Jaundice persisting over one week

As jaundice is a symptom of an underlying illness, any discolouration lasting for more than a week needs to be investigated, especially if it is associated with dark wine or pale stools. It is important that the baby is checked for liver disease or other conditions.

Breast-milk jaundice: this may result from infrequent feedings, starvation and dehydration, rather than from the breast milk itself. The bilirubin level does not usually rise very high and, with treatment and giving up breast-feeding for 72 hours, the jaundice soon clears up.

Biliary atresia: a rare condition in which bile fails to drain from the gall bladder in the liver into the bowels. Urgent surgery is needed before irreversible liver and brain damage occur.

Urine or other infections or hypothydroidism (underactive thyroid gland): these may cause jaundice and may be checked for by a doctor at this stage.

Hepatitis: type A is spread by eating or drinking food infected with hepatitis A, often while abroad. Children usually have a mild illness and recover well. Types B and C are spread via blood products (such as HIV) or the virus is given to the baby by the mother's placenta, and may cause serious long-term damage to the liver.

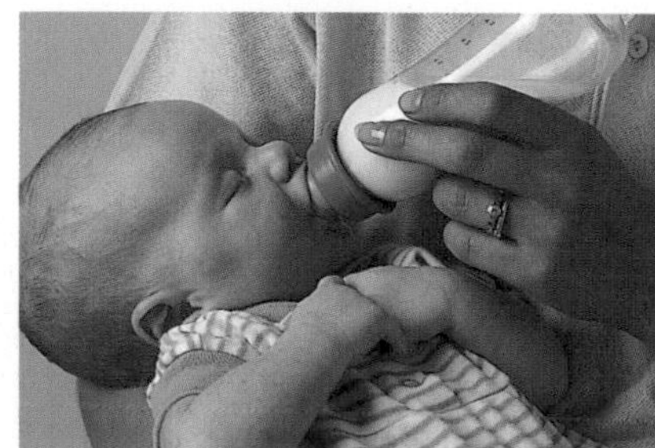

A baby suffering from breast milk jaundice may need to be fed formula milk until the jaundice clears.

KAWASAKI DISEASE

WHAT IS KAWASAKI DISEASE?

Kawasaki disease, or mucocutaneous lymph node syndrome as it is also known, is a rather unusual illness that mainly affects pre-school children.

- Kawasaki disease was first identified in Japan in 1967. This rare condition causes inflammation of the blood vessels, which can lead to a wide range of symptoms.

- Although most children recover from Kawasaki disease, there may be long-term problems because of damage to the heart.

- No one knows what causes Kawasaki disease. Many doctors think it must be due to a virus, or another type of infectious microbe, because the disease can occur in outbreaks and it only affects children who have not had time to become immune to it.

- However, there seem to be other factors at work; Japanese children are much more likely to get Kawasaki disease, and it rarely seems to spread from person to person.

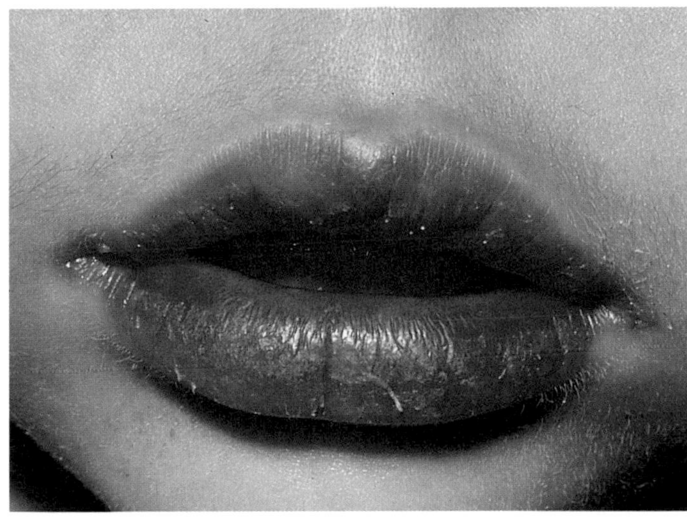

A swollen tongue and cracked lips are symptoms of Kawasaki disease, as well as a rash, conjunctivitis and fever. A child must have five or more specific symptoms to be diagnosed.

Who is affected?

Kawasaki disease is fairly uncommon. In the UK, out of every 100,000 children under five, about four will be diagnosed with Kawasaki disease every year. However, it is likely that more children do get the disease but are never diagnosed.

- Kawasaki disease is an illness that usually affects pre-school children, although older children do sometimes suffer from it.

- Four out of five cases of Kawasaki disease occur in children who are less than five years old.

- Toddlers, from one to two years, are the most likely to be affected.

- Kawasaki disease is harder to diagnose in very young children and they are, unfortunately, more likely to have complications involving the heart.

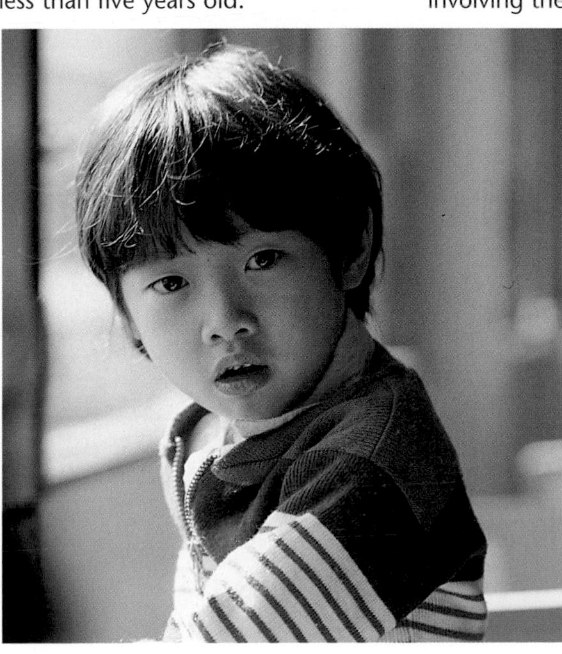

- Boys are more commonly affected than girls. The reason for this is unknown.

- Although children from all racial groups may get Kawasaki disease, it is up to ten times more common in Japanese children (one in every 1000).

Kawasaki disease occurs most commonly in children under five and affects more boys than girls. It is most prevalent in Japanese children.

How Kawasaki disease is diagnosed

The illness must be diagnosed on the basis of the child's symptoms. He must have five of the following symptoms:

1. A fever that persists for five days or more.
2. Conjunctivitis – both eyes may be red and sore.
3. Swelling, redness and then peeling of the hands and feet.
4. A skin rash appearing anywhere on the body.
5. A swollen red strawberry tongue and cracked lips.
6. Enlarged lymph nodes in the neck.

NOTE: other symptoms may mimic measles, or include distress, painful joints, diarrhoea, vomiting and abdominal pain.

Effects on the heart

Kawasaki disease is the most common cause of heart disease acquired by children in developed countries today. If Kawasaki disease is suspected, a special investigation of the heart – called an echocardiogram – will be performed to check for damage.

- Although most children who get Kawasaki disease recover fully, about one in five may have further problems due to damage to the heart or its blood vessels.

- These effects may occur during the first, acute, illness or may happen some time afterwards.

- The heart muscle or membrane around the heart may become acutely inflamed, causing breathlessness and swelling due to heart failure.

- There may be damage to the coronary arteries, the blood vessels that supply the heart. These vessels may become wider due to weakening of the walls, and areas of ballooning known as aneurysms may form. In a few cases, this leads to a blood clot being formed, which may cause a fatal heart attack.

- There is a small risk that months or even years after the acute illness, the coronary arteries will become narrowed. This reduces the amount of blood (and therefore oxygen) that can reach the heart muscle, leading to angina and possible heart attack.

- Death, when it occurs, usually does so suddenly between the 10th and 28th day of illness. It seldom occurs in children over two years of age.

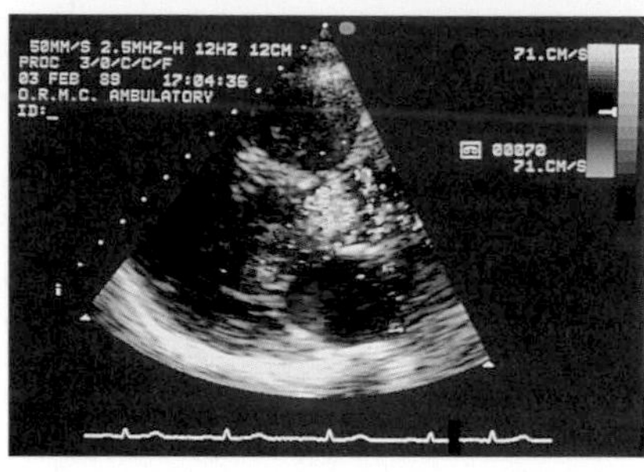

If a child has Kawasaki disease, an echocardiogram will be performed to check for heart damage.

What treatment is available

Even though doctors do not know what causes Kawasaki disease, there are some medicines that can help.

- Treatment for Kawasaki disease is aimed mainly at trying to prevent damage to the heart and coronary arteries.

- Intravenous gamma globulin may be given through a vein. This medicine contains proteins from human blood that help with immunity. If given within 10 days of the start of the illness, it can help to reduce the risk of heart damage.

- Although we think of aspirin as a painkiller, it has many useful actions. In Kawasaki disease it helps to reduce fever and inflammation, but also helps to thin the blood in order to prevent clotting. If there is damage to the coronary arteries, low-dose aspirin may be continued for a long time.

- Aspirin is not normally used in children under 12 years, but in the case of Kawasaki disease its use is felt to be justified.

- A specialist in child heart conditions, a paediatric cardiologist, will ascertain if the heart has been damaged.

- New studies are being made all the time to see if better ways can be found to treat this potentially serious disease. One recent study showed that taking a combination of heparin, a blood thinning medicine, and regular exercise, may help the damaged blood vessels to repair themselves.

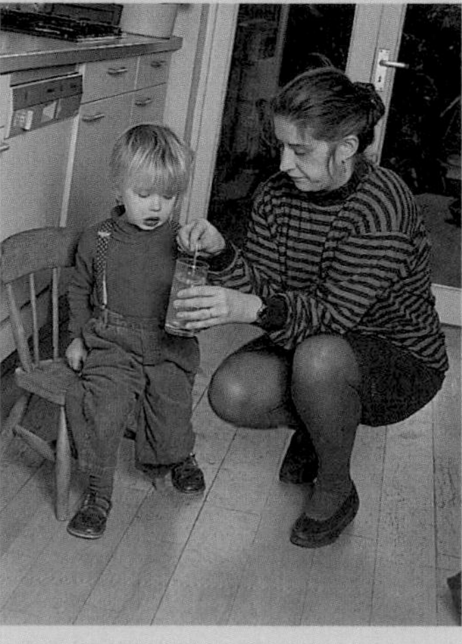

Although aspirin is not usually given to young children, it is used to treat Kawasaki disease because it helps to thin the blood, preventing clotting.

Difficulty in diagnosis

As Kawasaki disease is so unusual, many GPs have never seen a case before. This can make it much harder to diagnose than the more common viral illnesses that Kawasaki disease resembles.

- Diagnosis is particularly difficult in the case of children who may not have distinctive symptoms. Some children, particularly very young ones, have what is called an atypical illness, where only a few of the symptoms of Kawasaki disease are present. In these cases the doctor may not recognise the disease.

- The Kawasaki support groups, together with the medical experts, are trying to raise awareness of this disease among family doctors and parents so that affected children will be diagnosed sooner. Earlier diagnosis will lead to earlier treatment, which in turn should reduce the risk of heart damage in these children.

Useful addresses

The following organisations can provide information, advice and support:

- **Kawasaki Support Group**
13 Norwood Grove, Potters Green, CV2 2FR
Tel: 024 7661 2178

- **Kawasaki Disease Foundation**
www.kdfoundation.org

- **Kawasaki Families' Network**
http://ourworld.compuserve.com/homepages/kawasaki/

LEUKAEMIA

WHAT IS LEUKAEMIA?

Leukaemia is a form of cancer in which the number of white cells in the body are permanently increased.

- There are four main types of leukaemia, of which two are acute (of sudden onset) and two are chronic (slow and progressive).

- The chronic types are rarely seen in a person aged under 20, but the acute types affect children and adults.

- Acute lymphoblastic leukaemia (ALL), is responsible for around 85 per cent of childhood leukaemia, while acute myeloid leukaemia (AML), also known as acute non-lymphocytic leukaemia (ANLL), accounts for the vast majority of other cases.

The most common form of childhood leukaemia is acute lymphoblastic leukaemia (ALL). This condition is usually contracted in children between the ages of two and five years.

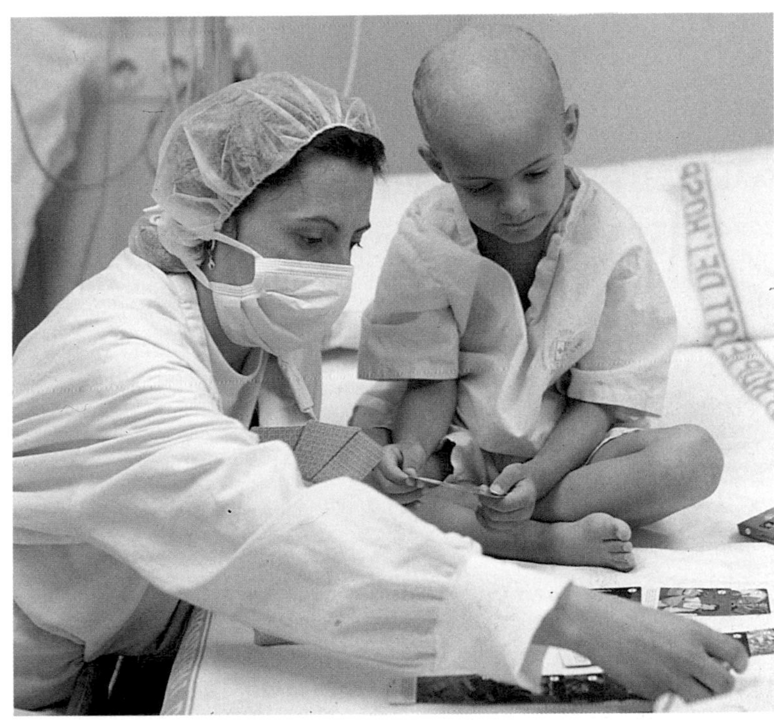

What causes leukaemia?

Although the causes of leukaemia are still unclear, there are several theories.

- Possible causes include a reaction to an infectious agent, exposure to radiation, chemicals or electromagnetic fields, such as power lines, and genetic factors.
- 'Clusters' of leukaemia cases have occurred in Britain and are being investigated. So far, little is known, other than that radiation may only account for less than 10 per cent of cases.

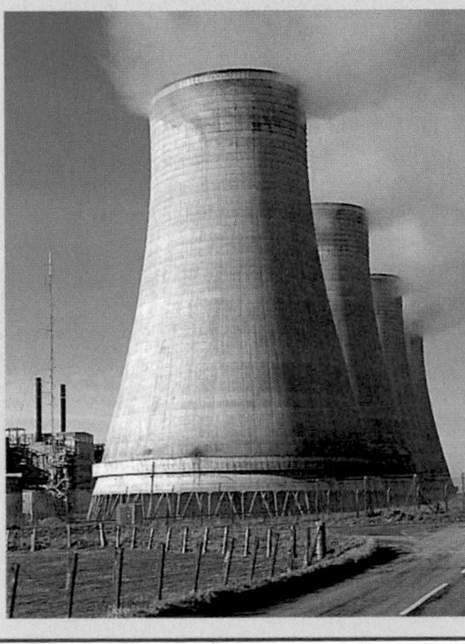

- These 'clusters' seem to occur in areas in which one population, often urban, has moved into a rural setting. One theory, which has considerable support, is that the presence of urban incomers affects the susceptibility of the local people.
- Certain viruses are known to cause leukaemia in domestic and laboratory animals. It is thought that a virus or viruses may be responsible for leukaemia in children who have a genetic susceptibility.
- In the early 1990s, it was reported that vitamin K injections, given to most babies at birth, caused an increased risk of leukaemia. However, in 1997, after a series of further studies, the Department of Health decided that there was no increased risk.

The incidence of childhood leukaemia has increased over the last 20–30 years. Factors thought to be responsible include exposure to chemicals and radiation.

Symptoms

Without treatment, leukaemia is fatal, and the earlier treatment starts the better the chances of remission or a cure. Symptoms include:

- Excessive and persistent tiredness
- Breathlessness
- Pain in the bones and arm and leg joints
- Recurrent and persistent infections
- Unusually severe bruising
- Abdominal swelling
- Bleeding gums or blood in the faeces

IMPORTANT: consult your GP immediately if your child has any of these symptoms or a fever that lasts longer than a few days.

Diagnosing leukaemia

If leukaemia is suspected, your child will need to have hospital tests.

- A blood test is taken to determine the levels of red and white cells and platelets, and to detect any abnormal cells.

- The diagnosis is confirmed by a bone marrow biopsy. The precise type of leukaemia involved is identified by examination of the leukaemic cells' chromosomes and by tests to establish which type of antibodies they would normally produce.

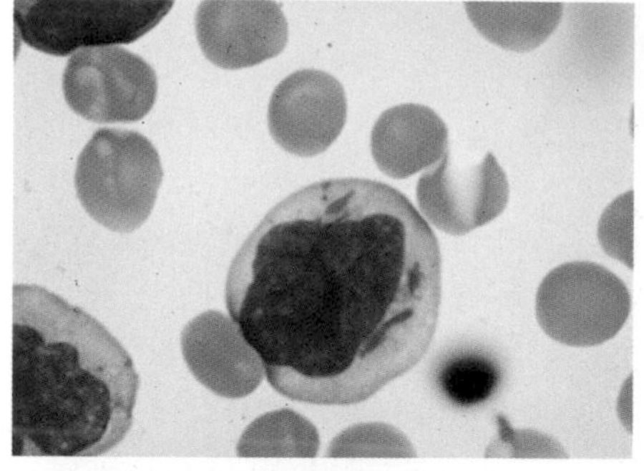

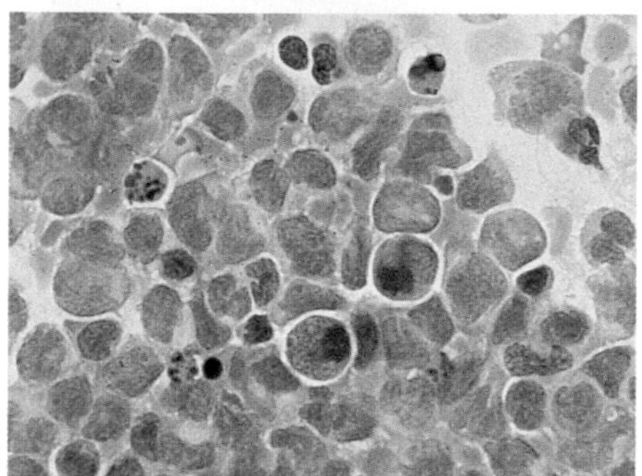

How does leukaemia develop?

ALL and AML both drastically increase the number of white blood cells, but each condition affects different types of white cells. The picture is complicated by the fact that there are different subtypes of both conditions.

- ALL increases the number of white cells called lymphocytes, produced in the lymph tissues and glands. Between 30 and 60 times more of them may be found in the blood than is usual.

TOP LEFT: Leukaemia develops when the bone marrow produces a large amount of white blood cells. Acute myeloid leukaemia (pictured) affects the cells in the myeloid tissue.

LEFT: Cells of a child with acute lymphoblastic leukaemia (ALL). This type of leukaemia affects the white blood cells in the lymph tissue and glands.

- AML increases the number of white cells called granulocytes, produced in the myeloid tissue of bone marrow.

- Normally, white blood cells cannot reproduce. However, in both types of leukaemia, they do reproduce, further increasing their number, but they do not mature sufficiently to fulfil their vital role – the immune response that defends the body against infection.

- In both cases, the numbers of red blood cells and platelets are much reduced. The result is tiredness and a tendency to bruising and bleeding.

Treating leukaemia

The object of treatment is to bring about remission and then to maintain it. Different techniques are used depending on the type of leukaemia involved.

- Most anti-leukaemia drugs work by killing cells that are dividing. Unfortunately, they may also kill beneficial cells that are dividing, such as red blood cells.

- A child with ALL is treated with a combination of drugs. Once the child is in remission, there will be a period of consolidation therapy, to suppress the production of the abnormal cells. Later, drugs will be given for a two-year period to maintain the remission (maintenance therapy).

- Children with AML are treated more intensively than those with ALL. Consolidation therapy is more intensive, too, but maintenance therapy may not be given.

- After treatment, normal life can be resumed, although with some follow-up care and testing.

- The drugs used to treat leukaemia have a number of side-effects. Depending on the drug, these may include pins and needles, tiredness, susceptibility to infection, constipation, weight gain, bone weakening, high blood pressure, diabetes, hair loss, nausea and vomiting.

- Whether a leukaemia sufferer relapses or comes out of remission depends to a certain extent on the individual child. However, those whose white blood cell counts were very high at the time of diagnosis and who had AML are more likely to relapse. In such cases, a bone marrow transplant may be given, depending on the availability of donor tissue that is immunologically matched to that of the child.

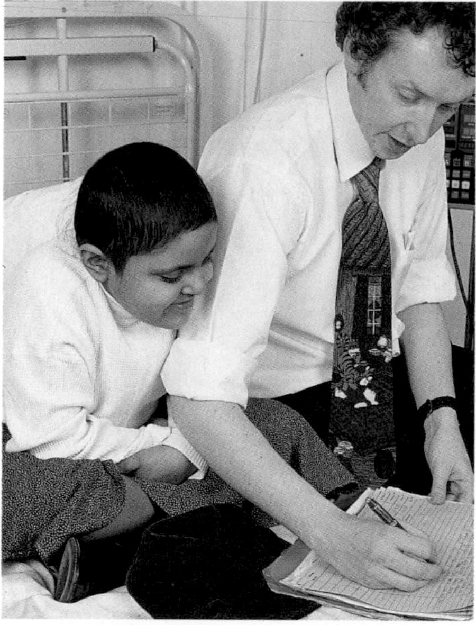

Most children with ALL can be treated effectively and around 75 per cent are cured. Drugs used to send childhood leukaemia into remission can cause side-effects, such as hair loss and weight gain.

Useful addresses

The side-effects of leukaemia treatment are often the worst part. The drugs can make a child feel as sick as the illness itself. It helps if you are honest with your child and prepare him for the investigations and treatment. Support and advice are available from the trained hospital staff, as well as specialist organisations.

The Anthony Nolan Bone Marrow Trust
Hotline: 0901 882 2234
www.anthonynolan.org.uk

The Leukaemia Care Society
Helpline: 01902 330 003
www.leukaemiacare.org

The Leukaemia Research Fund
Tel: 020 7405 0101
www.lrf.org.uk

MEASLES

WHAT IS MEASLES?

Measles is caused by a highly infectious virus found throughout the world. Although it was once a common childhood disease, measles is now rare due to a more effective immunisation programme.

- The incubation period (the time since the first contact with the disease to the appearance of any symptoms) is about 10–14 days, and the rash often appears on the 14th day after exposure.
- Measles is infectious from four days before to four days after the appearance of the rash.

Who is at risk?

Anyone not vaccinated or immune against the disease is vulnerable.

- Measles is a very contagious disease and is spread by droplets of fluid. You can catch the disease from someone sneezing or even talking. If you enter a room an hour after a person with measles has left it, you can still catch measles from them because the droplets will be in the air.
- Unless you have a disease affecting the immune system, e.g. leukaemia or HIV, once you have had measles you cannot catch it again.
- Measles can cause a pregnant woman to miscarry or to give birth prematurely.

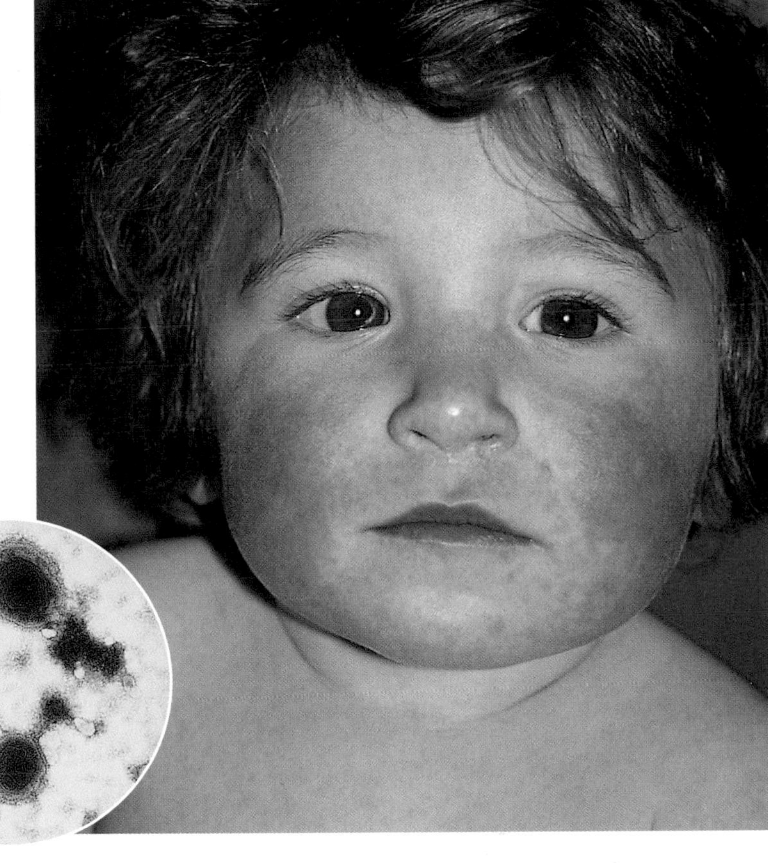

ABOVE LEFT: The measles virus is a highly contagious disease that can temporarily affect the immune system.

ABOVE: A child with measles may develop a high fever and flu-like symptoms. A red rash first appears on the face and ears, then spreads to the body.

Symptoms

- Your child will develop a fever of 39.5–40°C (103–104°F) – reaching its peak on day four or five.
- Your child will have a cough, runny nose, and red, sore eyes.
- Small, white spots appear inside the cheek called 'Koplik's spots', which are only ever seen in measles.
- The rash appears as red, flat spots which join up to form irregular patches.
- As the rash appears, your child's temperature rises rapidly and he becomes very ill. He may complain of earache, swollen glands in his neck, tummy ache and diarrhoea.

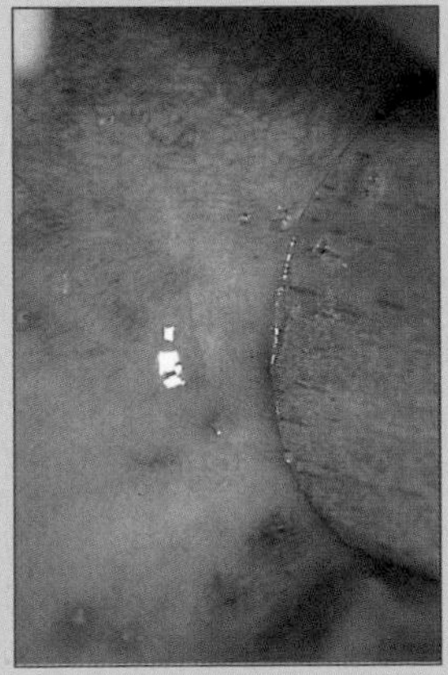

Koplik's spots are small, red spots with bluish-white centres. These appear in the child's mouth a few days before a measles rash is evident.

When to see the doctor

Some children with measles have relatively mild symptoms and suffer no complications. However, you should get medical assistance if you suspect your child is seriously ill.

Call your doctor immediately if:

- Breathing becomes laboured.
- Your child cannot be woken or becomes confused.
- He starts shaking or fitting.
- He develops a severe headache or neckache.
- Your child seems extremely ill.

Call your doctor within 24 hours if:

- Your child has a severe earache.
- His fever persists for more than four days after the appearance of the rash.
- He is unable to keep down fluids because of vomiting, or if he has severe diarrhoea.

Immunisation

Children can be immunised against measles as part of the MMR vaccination programme at about 12–15 months and three to five years of age. It is safe and effective, although your child may get a small swelling at the spot where the injection is given and he may have a fever which can last for seven to 10 days. He may also have a mild reaction to the vaccination, such as a slight rash, swollen glands or, rarely, a swelling of the joints.

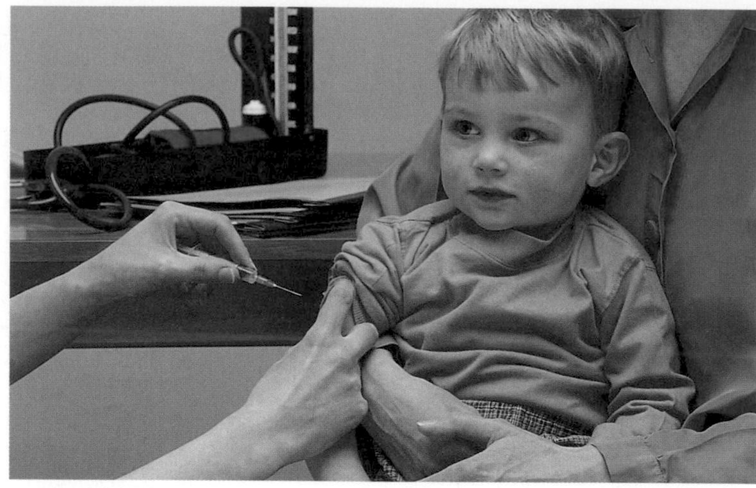

Immunising your child against measles – part of the MMR vaccination at around 12–15 months – offers the best defence against this potentially fatal disease.

What you can do at home

There is no specific treatment for measles. Unless you suspect any complications (in which case you should call the doctor) keep your child at home, especially in the early stages, when she is most infectious.

1 Keep your child well hydrated with regular drinks.

2 Ensure your child has plenty of rest, preferably in bed.

3 If your child has a cough, which is bad enough to hinder sleep, offer cough sweets or cough mixture.

4 Give infant paracetamol if your child's temperature is high and she feels miserable.

5 There was a belief that measles could cause children to go blind, but this is not true. However, if your child is disturbed by bright light, she may be more comfortable if you close the curtains.

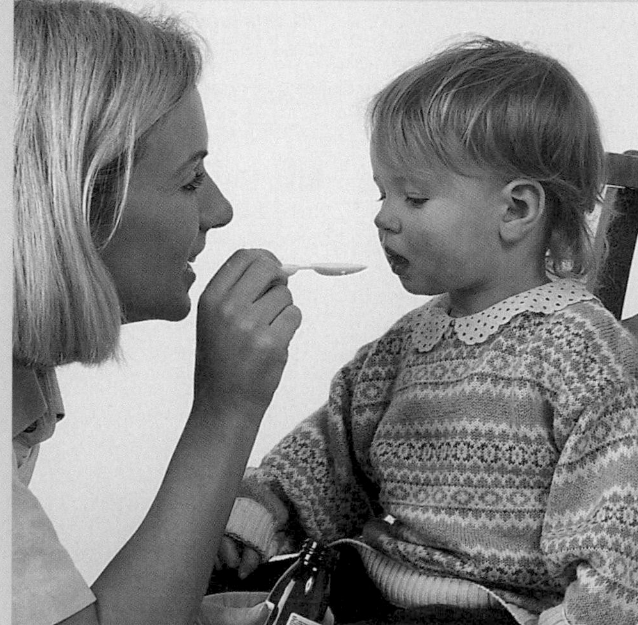

Although there is no specific cure for measles, you can make your child feel more comfortable by giving her infant paracetamol, plenty of drinks and lots of sympathy.

Complications

The rate of complications and death from measles in the UK has dropped dramatically this century, due to the vaccine and improved housing conditions, sanitation and nutrition of children. However, there are still several complications that make measles a very serious, even life-threatening disease.

- **Gastroenteritis and diarrhoea:** very common and can last for several weeks, especially in an undernourished child.
- **Encephalitis (brain inflammation):** rare and extremely dangerous, occurring seven to 10 days after the beginning of the illness, when the child develops a headache, neckache or even backache, feels drowsy and starts vomiting. In later stages, the child may even suffer fits.
- **Convulsions:** due to the fever caused by measles.
- **Pneumonia:** treated with antibiotics and/or hospital treatment.
- **Corneal ulcer:** the initial inflammation of the conjunctiva can lead to a more severe inflammation and breakdown of the front of the eye, which may cause blindness.
- **Thrombocytopenia:** measles may attack the child's immune system by causing a big drop in white blood cells. This may result in bleeding under the skin and bruising.
- **Subacute scelorising panencephalitis (SSPE):** a very rare, late complication of measles that occurs four to 10 years after the measles infection. It causes a slow deterioration of the child's nervous system, which is usually fatal.

Diseases with similar symptoms

Other illnesses, with similar symptoms to measles, can often be mistaken for the disease. These include:

- **Rubella (German measles):** a much milder illness, it produces a pale pink, bumpy rash and enlarged glands at the back of the neck.
- **Scarlet fever:** the symptoms are fever, vomiting and a scarlet rash that develops behind the ears and rapidly spreads to the face and chest. The tongue also becomes bright red (strawberry tongue).
- **Kawasaki disease:** an illness causing prolonged fever, rash, sore eyes, mouth, peeling hands and sometimes heart complications.

MEDICATION FOR BABIES & CHILDREN

FORMULATIONS FOR CHILDREN

Medicines are specially formulated for babies and children under five. Some have different ingredients from adult formulations, while others are diluted.

- Medication can be split into two types – prescription-only and over-the-counter medicines. Prescription-only medicines need a doctor's prescription, while you can buy most over-the-counter medicines from a local pharmacy or supermarket.

- Most children's medicines have added flavour and colour to make them more palatable.

Giving your child medication

When you are administering medication, always take care to follow the instructions.

1 When on a course of medication, your child should be given the correct dose as prescribed. Check with your GP or pharmacist if your child misses a dose.

2 Measure the dose accurately, using a measuring spoon or a syringe for liquid medication. By using an ordinary spoon, you could alter the dose.

3 Even if your child feels better, the treatment is not complete until the prescribed amount of medicine has been taken over the prescribed time. However, some medications, such as pain relievers, are prescribed as needed and can be stopped when the child is better.

4 Once your child is better, throw away any leftover 'as needed' medication. Don't give a medication prescribed for someone else, no matter how similar the symptoms or complaints.

5 Never give more than the prescribed dose. If your child is accidentally given the wrong dose, call the pharmacist or GP immediately and follow their instructions.

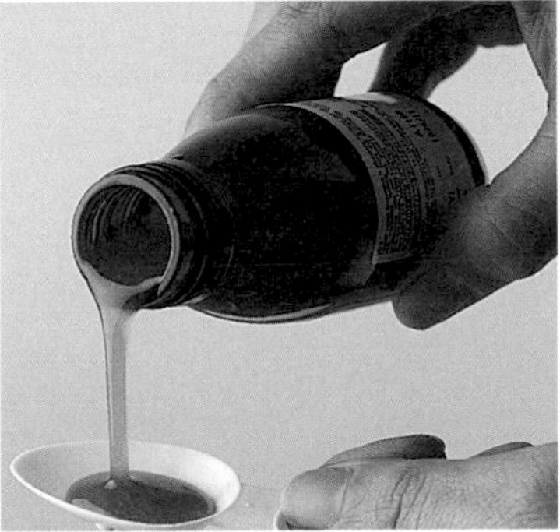

Always measure the dose of liquid medicine precisely with a measuring spoon or syringe. Do not keep the medicine once your child is well, as it will deteriorate over time.

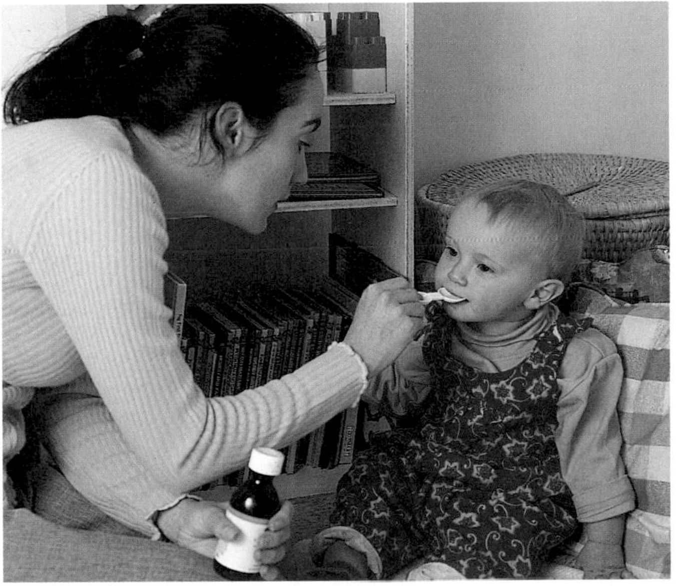

If your child is unwell, consult your GP or a pharmacist before giving her any medication. Never give your child medicine that has been prescribed for someone else.

Consulting your pharmacist

Pharmacists are qualified to provide valuable information about over-the-counter medication. When consulting the pharmacist, make sure you:

- Tell him your child's age and, if necessary, weight and height.
- Describe your child's symptoms.
- Ask about any side-effects.
- Tell him if your child has had any previous illness and is on any other medication.

NOTE: read the instructions on the medication before you leave the pharmacy. Ask the pharmacist if you are unsure about anything.

Age restrictions

Some medication suitable for adults cannot be given to babies or children. Always check the age guidance advice.

- **Paracetamol:** not suitable for children under 12 years old.
- **Bonjela (oral pain-relieving gel for treating teething or mouth ulcers):** not suitable for infants under four months old.
- **Liquid ibuprofen (for children):** not suitable for babies under six months.
- **Adult cold and cough remedies:** not suitable for children under 12.
- **Aspirin:** not suitable for children under 12.

Reactions to the medicine

Some medicines, such as painkillers, may cause side-effects such as drowsiness or sleepiness. Medicines can also cause allergic reactions.

- Allergic reactions to medications are rare, but do occur. Penicillin and other antibiotics are among the most common drugs to cause an allergic reaction.
- Adverse reactions include hives, itching, a rash or wheezing.
- Call your GP if any symptoms seem unrelated to your child's illness.

Storing medicines

- Always store medication according to the manufacturer's instructions.
- Before using a medicine, check the sell by date. Dispose of any medicine that has passed its expiry date. Most drugs lose their potency after one year.
- Do not keep medication in a bathroom cabinet, because of the steamy, moist environment.
- Always keep medication in its original packaging, so that you have the expiry date and instructions close at hand.
- Never put medicine into a different container or two different pills in the same container.
- If you have any questions or concerns about any medication, ask your GP or pharmacist.

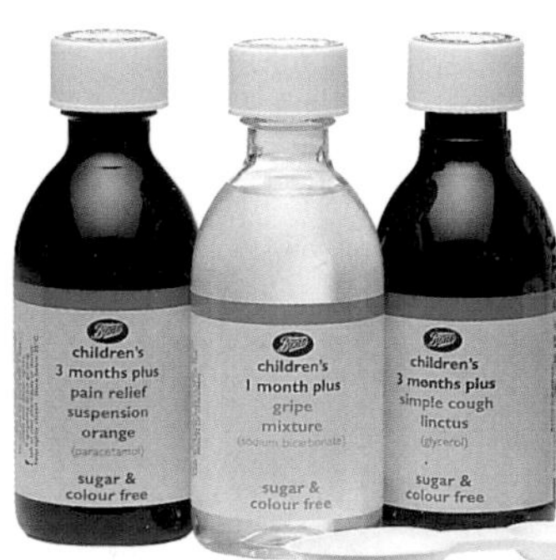

Keep all medicines safely in a locked cupboard. Left-over medicine should be returned to your local pharmacy.

Dos and don'ts

✔ Do comfort and cuddle your child, to make him feel a little better.

✔ Do consult your pharmacist, describing your child and his symptoms. Don't just buy a well-known over-the-counter medication.

✔ If you are concerned about your child's condition, do call your GP. Most doctors would prefer to be called rather than risk an illness becoming more serious.

✔ Do check your first-aid kit and stock of medication regularly, replacing missing items or those that are outdated.

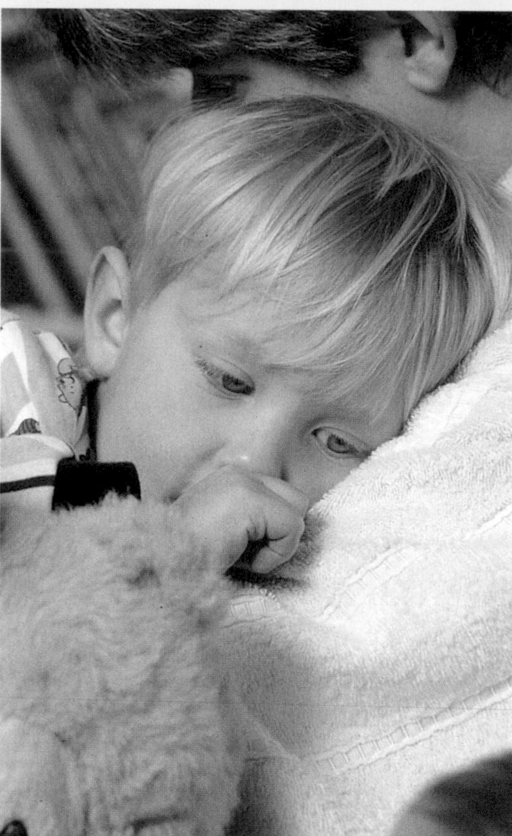

As well as the appropriate medicine, don't forget to give your child plenty of affection. Although it won't cure him, it should make him feel better.

✘ Don't be tempted to give your child adult medication or any medicine that you have used for his older siblings, no matter how similar the symptoms.

✘ Don't be disappointed if your child is not prescribed antibiotics, as they are not always the answer. Instead, your child's body should be allowed to fight the disease itself, by building up its own immunity.

✘ Don't give ibuprofen if your child has vomiting or diarrhoea as it could inflame his stomach.

✘ After the treatment has ended, do not save prescribed leftover medicine for next time.

✘ Do not exceed the dose of prescribed medication.

✘ Don't suffer in silence. Ask for help to nurse your sick child.

First-aid kit

A well-stocked first-aid kit, kept within easy reach of adults, is a necessity in every home.

- Preparing supplies ahead of time will help you handle an emergency at a moment's notice.
- Include an up-to-date list of emergency numbers, such as your GP and the casualty department.
- Ideally, you should keep one first-aid kit in your home and one in your car.
- Be sure to take a first-aid kit on family holidays, including enough prescribed medicines.

MENINGITIS & SEPTICAEMIA

WHAT IS MENINGITIS?

Meningitis is an inflammation of the layers of tissue that cover the brain and spinal cord – the meninges – and the fluid that circulates around the brain and spinal cord. There are two types of meningitis – viral and bacterial.

Viral meningitis is the most common, but least serious form. **Bacterial meningitis** is rare, but is the most dangerous. It can be caused by the meningococcus, pneumococcus, Hib and other bacteria. **Septicaemia (blood poisoning)** can be caused by the same bacteria as bacterial meningitis. It causes blood to leak out of the vessels into the skin, causing a characteristic non-blanching purple rash. It can be fatal.

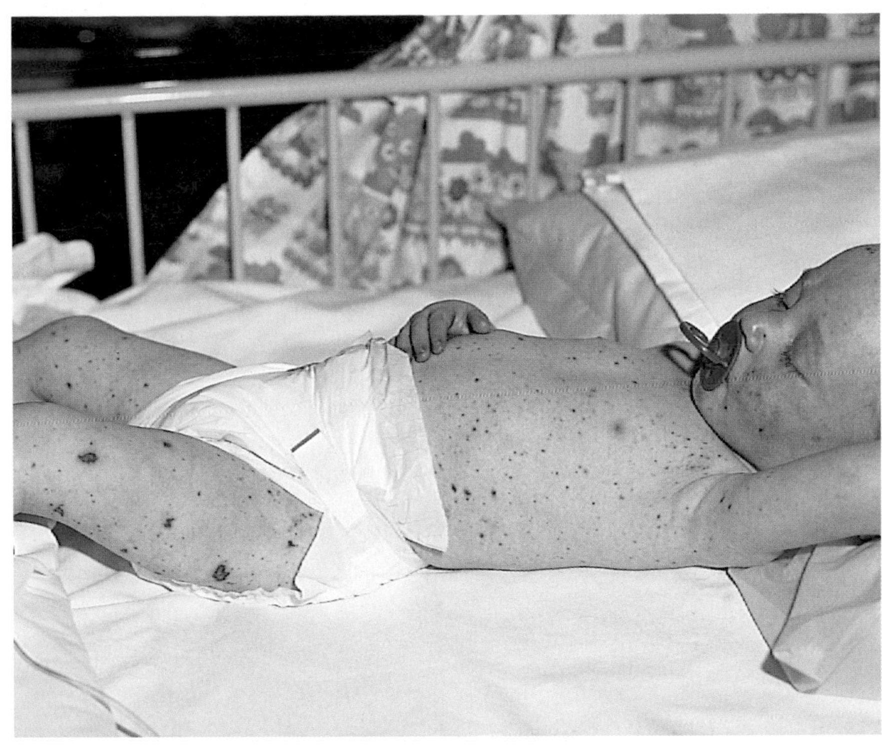

This child is recovering from meningococcal meningitis and septicaemia. The under-fives are particularly vulnerable.

Recognising the signs

Recognising meningitis and/or septicaemia early on, before the infection has taken hold on your child, is crucially important. Two or more of the following symptoms may indicate that your child is suffering from meningitis.

Newborn
- Floppy or unresponsive
- Poor feeding or off feeds altogether
- Weak cry and sucking poorly
- Vomiting
- Irritable behaviour
- Sleepy
- Jittery

Infants
- Drowsy
- High temperature or fever
- Off feeds/meals
- Staring
- Abnormal tone – increased/decreased
- Unusual breathing patterns
- Fast heart rate
- High-pitched cry, especially when being handled
- Vomiting and/or diarrhoea
- A purple-coloured rash (see the glass test)
- Neck stiffness* (often this symptom is absent in babies)
- Convulsion or loss of consciousness – often the first sign

Older child
- High temperature or fever
- Vomiting
- Irritable behaviour and lack of concentration
- Headache
- Stiff neck*
- Fit
- Dislike of bright lights, 'photophobia'

*** Neck stiffness is one sign of meningitis. Your child may be unable to touch his chest with his chin or flex his neck forward.**

When to call the doctor

A child infected with meningococcus bacterium can develop meningitis and/or septicaemia; fever and vomiting are common in both. If there is only meningitis there may be no rash, if there is only septicaemia there may be no headache but severe tummy ache or pain elsewhere. If you suspect that your child has meningitis or septicaemia, you should seek immediate medical attention.

All GPs are equipped to give an immediate first dose of injected antibiotic and you should go to them first. If your GP is not available, take your child straight to hospital.

The glass test

Hold a glass firmly against your child's skin. If the rash does not fade, you should suspect septicaemia. Seek urgent help. If it fades, but your child has become rapidly unwell, you should also seek urgent help.

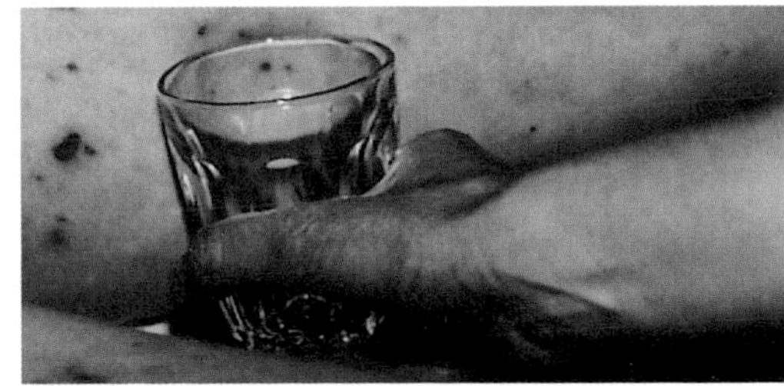

How meningitis is caught

Both viral and bacterial meningitis are caught by coughing, sneezing and kissing.

Around 10 per cent of the population will be carrying meningococcal bacteria in the back of their nose and throat and have absolutely no symptoms. The under fives, 16–25s and over 55s are more susceptible to meningitis than other age groups. This may be to do with a weakness of their immune system.

When a case of meningitis arises, a public health doctor is informed as a matter of law. This doctor ensures that all those who need antibiotics are contacted. These are usually limited to close household contacts and to any intimate kissing contact. The antibiotics kill the bacteria carried in the nose and throat. They do not get rid of the bacteria if they are multiplying and causing an infection, so all contacts should be especially vigilant for signs.

Complications

Bacteria that cause meningitis can also cause septicaemia, which is a type of blood poisoning. This may lead to a lack of adequate blood supply to parts of the body, and can cause loss of limbs or, if major organs such as the kidneys are affected, lead to death. In the long term, children will be affected differently depending on their age. They may fall back developmentally, have problems with balance and co-ordination, experience behavioural problems, or be left with deafness.

Vaccination

There is a vaccine available for one form of meningitis caused by Haemophilus influenza B (Hib). There is also a vaccine for one of the three strains of meningococcal meningitis called C strain. Currently, the three groups most at risk are first in line for the vaccine – all babies having their triple vaccines, toddlers having the MMR and teenagers. Unfortunately, the most common meningococcal strain seen in the UK is the B strain and there is no vaccine for this one. A natural source of protection for newborn infants is the acquisition of antibodies from the mother's blood – from the placenta before birth, and the mother's breast milk.

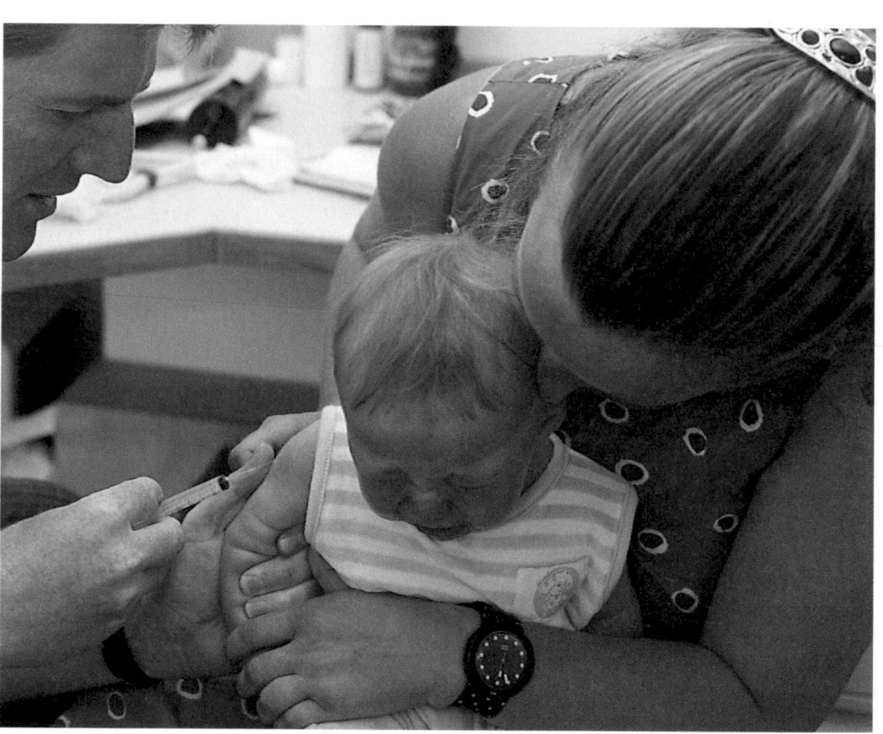

Vaccination against Hib and meningitis C will be given at two, three and four months of age.

Treatment

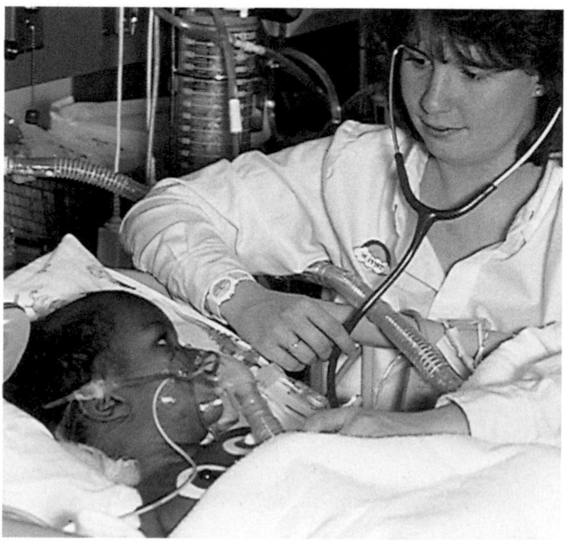

Bacterial meningitis

If antibiotics are given early, deaths from meningococcal and other bacteria causing meningitis are reduced. Benzylpenicillin given into a muscle or vein should be given as soon as meningitis is suspected. Chloramphenicol is the best alternative if there is an allergy to penicillin, but not in newborns. These antibiotics will be given intravenously for at least seven days.

Bacterial meningitis can be treated with antibiotics. Prompt diagnosis is essential.

Viral meningitis

Antibiotics are not effective against viruses, but most cases of viral meningitis run a short uneventful course and may never be seen by doctors. The mainstay of treatment in these cases will be rest, fluids and measures to control the fever and pain relief.

MMR VACCINATION

WHAT IS MMR?

MMR stands for measles, mumps and rubella (German measles). The MMR vaccine protects a child against these diseases. Until the MMR vaccine was introduced in 1988, these three diseases, although often mild, could lead to serious illness and complications.

What is the MMR vaccine and how does it work?

The MMR vaccine is made out of the measles, mumps and rubella viruses but they have been modified so that they do not cause serious illness in people. This is done by growing successive generations of the virus until eventually they grow a very mild strain. The vaccine works by stimulating a child's immune response so that when exposed to measles, mumps or rubella, his body can successfully fight them off. In 26 years, 250 million doses of MMR have been given in over 40 countries. No one has ever died from an MMR vaccine.

When is MMR given routinely?

The MMR vaccine is given routinely by injection at 12 to 15 months, with a second dose between three and five years as a pre-school booster. Before 12 months, babies still carry immunity from their mothers, and the vaccine would not work for them. The vaccine is given twice because not all children receive it as babies, and five to 10 per cent of children who had the first vaccine are still not immune to MMR. Among those children who do not respond to the first dose, 90 per cent have a good response to the second dose.

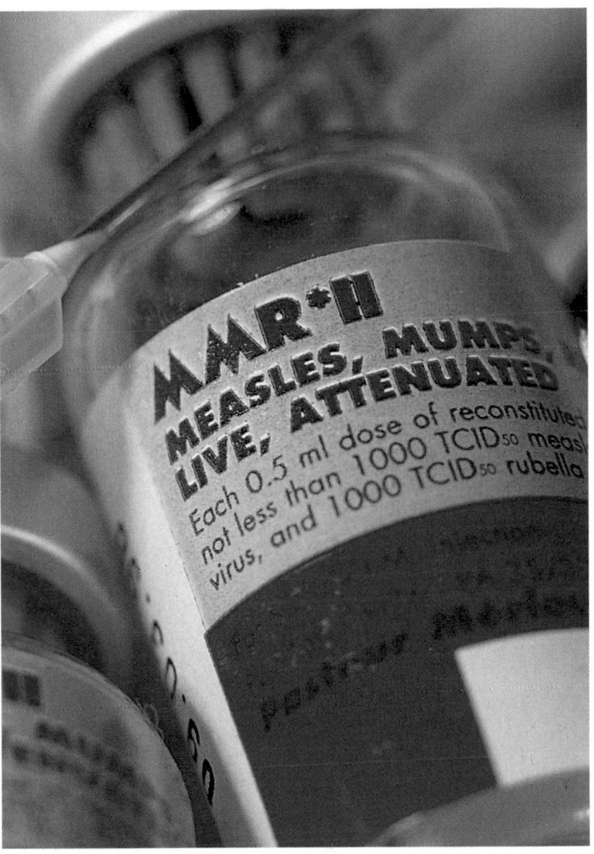

Vaccines against mumps, measles and rubella have helped to make these illnesses rare in the UK. If there was a drop in the number of vaccinations, the diseases would return. Between one and two million children still die worldwide each year from measles.

Complications of mumps, measles and rubella

- **Mumps vaccine** prevents mumps, which was the biggest cause of viral meningitis in children. Mumps can cause deafness in one in 25 cases, and in older males may cause painful, swollen testicles which can lead to infertility.

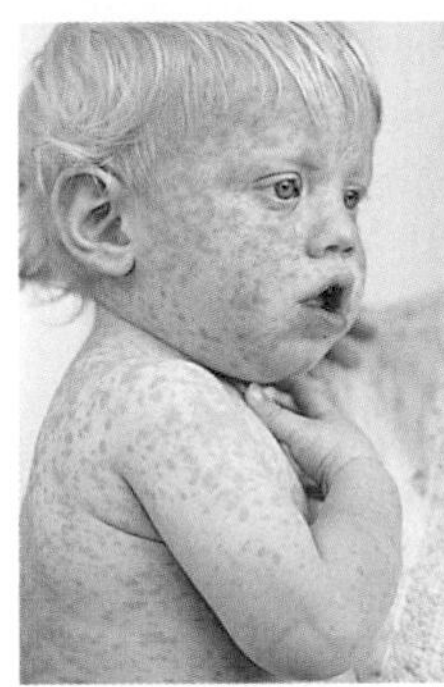

LEFT: This baby boy is covered with the measles rash. After symptoms of cold and fever, a blotchy rash appears behind the ears, and then on the face and rest of the body.

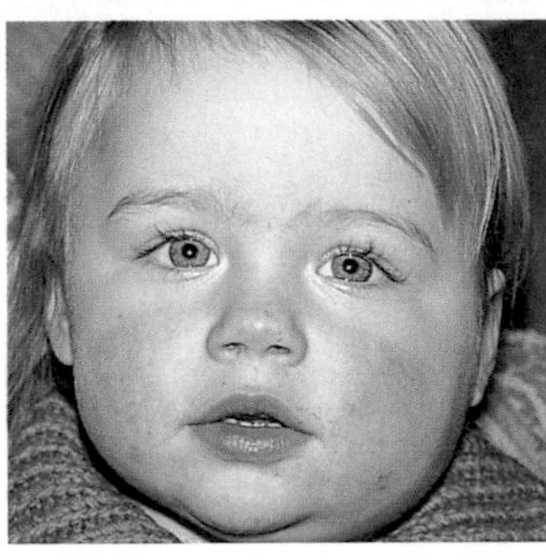

LEFT: Mumps can result in swelling of the glands just inside the angle of the jaw.

- **Measles vaccine** prevents deaths and complications from measles, a disease that can still be serious. One in 1000 children with measles develops encephalitis, and one in 2500–5000 die.

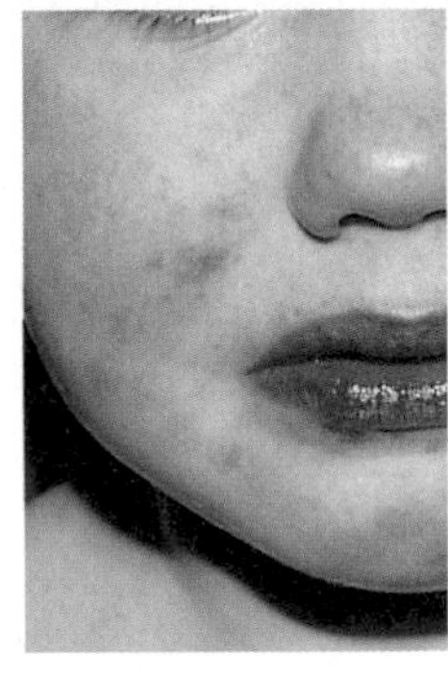

RIGHT: German measles causes the enlargement of the lymph nodes in the neck and a widespread rash.

- **Rubella vaccine** prevents mothers catching rubella while pregnant and damaging their babies while they are still in the womb. In congenital rubella syndrome, babies can be born with deafness, blindness, heart problems and brain damage.

What to expect after the vaccination

The MMR vaccine contains viruses that are very similar to those that cause the actual disease, so mild symptoms of the disease might occur after the vaccine. This shows that the vaccine is working. Often a child has no symptoms but has still responded to the vaccine.

Common reactions:

- **Redness, soreness and swelling at the site of the injection**: one in 10 children will have a very mild form of measles with rash, fever and loss of appetite about a week to 10 days after the vaccine.

- **Mild form of mumps:** slight neck swelling may occur about three weeks after the injection.

Less common and more severe reactions:

- **A rash of bruise-like spots**: this may appear about two weeks after the vaccine. It is rare and is due to the rubella part of the vaccine.

- **Fits**: one in 1000 children will have a fit after becoming feverish. This will not cause any long-term problems. A child is 10 times more likely to have a fit from measles than from the vaccine.

- **Encephalitis (brain inflammation)**: this is extremely rare, affecting about one in 1,000,000 immunised children. This is the same as the risk of a child developing encephalitis without the vaccine. In children with measles, encephalitis affects one in 5000 children.

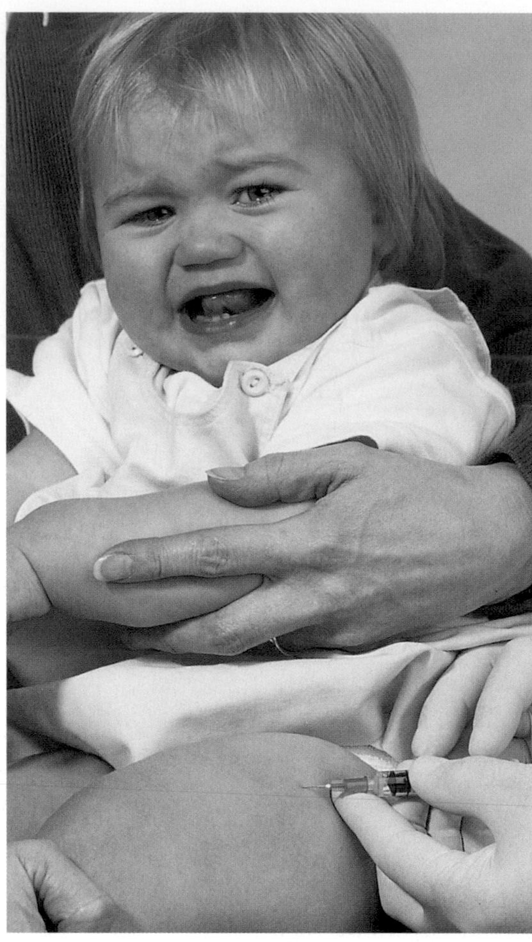

A 13-month-old baby receives her MMR vaccination. The weakened samples of the diseases boost her immune system.

When to see the doctor

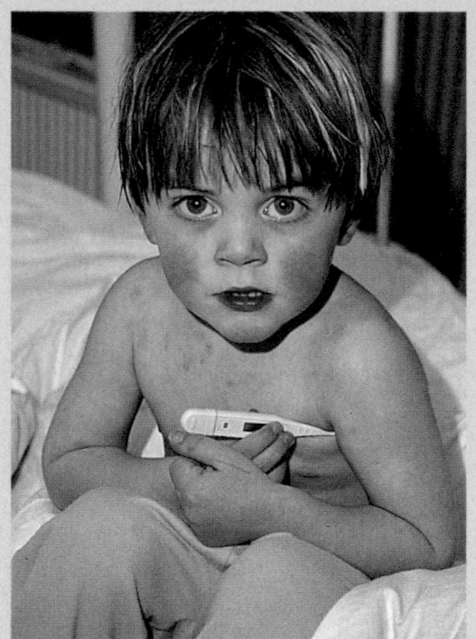

- If your child's temperature remains high for over 48 hours within a month of the vaccine, especially if there are no other signs or symptoms of infection.
- If he develops a rash.
- If he is irritable, feverish and difficult to awaken.
- If he has a fit or convulsion.

Children who should not be immunised

Although the majority of children can receive the vaccine, there are times when some children should not be immunised:

1 Certain children who are taking drugs that affect their immune system, or who have reduced immunity, cannot have the MMR vaccine. This is because it contains a live virus, albeit one that has been attenuated (tamed) to produce a very mild version of the illnesses.

2 Other children may need to delay their MMR vaccine if they have a fever or have had another live vaccine at around the same time as the MMR, such as BCG for tuberculosis.

3 Children who experienced a severe reaction to the first MMR vaccine may not be able to have the booster dose, because of the possibility that it may cause a repeat reaction.

The MMR debate

There has been concern recently that the MMR vaccine might be linked to autism and inflammatory bowel diseases such as Crohn's disease. However, there is no scientific evidence for this.

The only link between the MMR and autism is that they both coincidentally appear at around the same time – just after the first birthday. Crohn's disease is no more common in immunised people than it is in those who aren't. Therefore, there is no evidence that there is any link between measles, MMR and Crohn's disease. If less than 85 per cent of children are immunised, measles epidemics will return. Children who are not immunised in this country rely on other people immunising their children to avoid becoming infected.

MUMPS

WHAT IS MUMPS?

Mumps is caused by a virus resulting in swollen glands in the face. A relatively mild illness in children, it is more severe in teenagers and adults.

Now that most children are vaccinated against mumps, it is a much less common illness, but unvaccinated children still have a high risk of catching it. There is no treatment for mumps – it is a virus and antibiotics have no affect. However, some of the complications may be treatable with steroids.

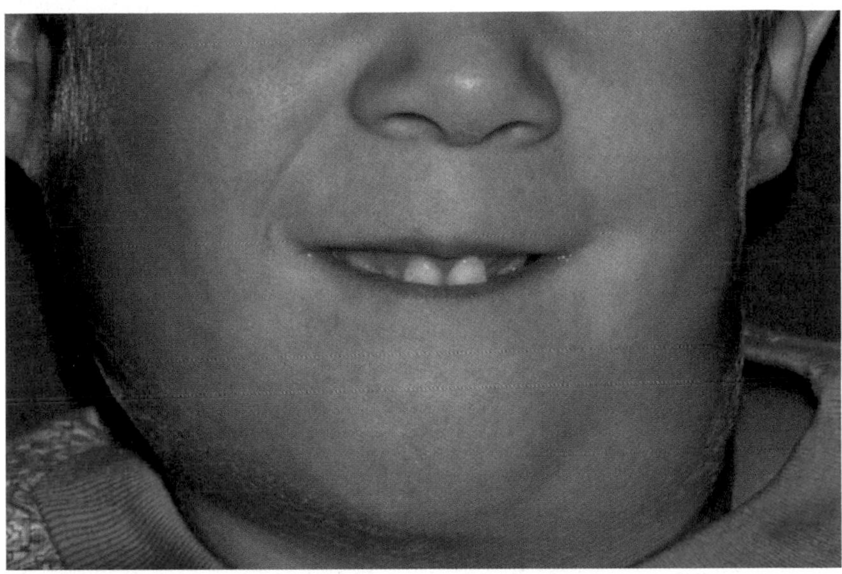

This child's parotid glands, which lie at the angle of the jaw, below and slightly in front of the ears, have become very swollen. The swelling will subside in about three days.

Symptoms

Mumps is highly contagious and is spread by coughing, sneezing and direct contact with saliva. If your child is suffering from mumps he may display the following symptoms:

- A high temperature or fever.
- Feeling generally under the weather and loss of appetite.
- Parotid glands become enlarged, tender and painful giving your child a somewhat hamster-like appearance. Often one gland may become enlarged before the other, and in a quarter of cases only one gland enlarges at all.
- Your child may have earache, which is worse when he moves his jaw, especially when chewing.
- He has difficulty swallowing.
- Other glands may also be swollen, especially around the jaw area.

When to see the doctor

Certain symptoms suggest possible complications and you should take your child to a doctor if he has:

- Severe headache
- Abdominal pain and vomiting
- Stiff neck
- Dizziness, difficulty breathing
- Extreme drowsiness
- Convulsions
- Pain and swelling in testicles
- Fever for more than four days

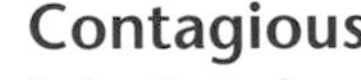

Contagious

Mumps is infectious from seven days before the symptoms appear until nine days after they have settled.

- It takes between 14–21 days after contact with the virus before the symptoms develop.
- Fever, headache and tiredness occur one to two days before the neck swelling.
- The parotid glands enlarge (sometimes on one side only) causing neck swelling for seven to eight days.
- A child who has had mumps should not go back to school until the neck swelling has gone down (usually nine days after the symptoms started).

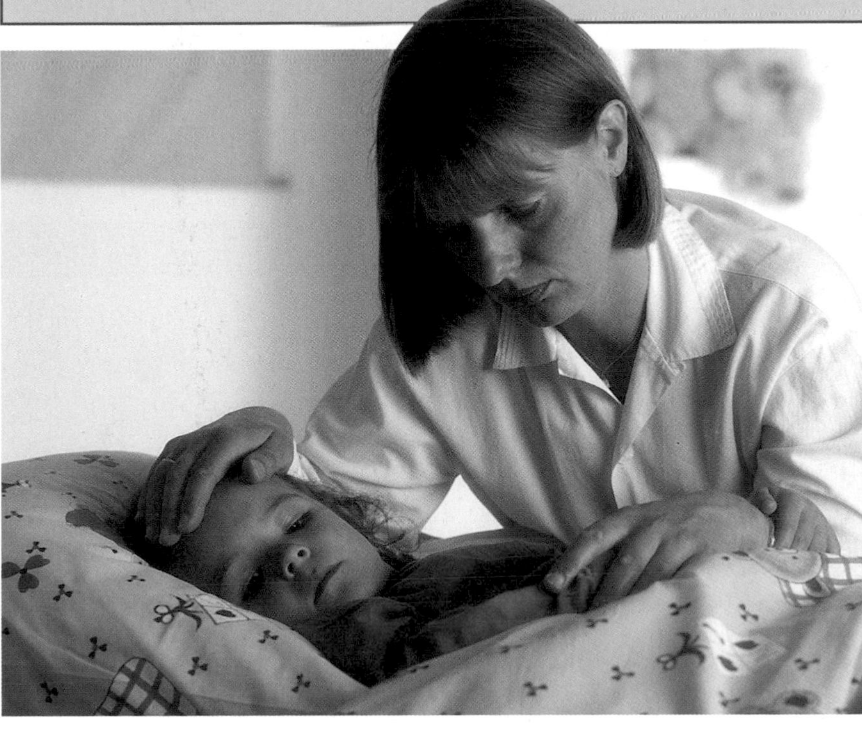

A child suffering from mumps may feel tired, have a high temperature and a headache. She may also lose her appetite as the glands around the throat will be swollen, causing her some pain when she swallows.

Vaccination

Babies between 12 and 15 months are given the vaccine by injection, together with the measles and rubella vaccines (MMR). A second dose is given between three and five years.

Occasionally, children get a very faint rash that looks a bit like measles a week or so after the vaccine. At three weeks they may also get a little swelling around the jaw glands. This will all settle with no need for medical treatment.

There are a few children who should not have the vaccine:

- Those with a problem with their immune system, e.g. with leukaemia or on drugs that are suppressing their immune system.
- Those with a serious reaction to egg, and certain antibiotics.

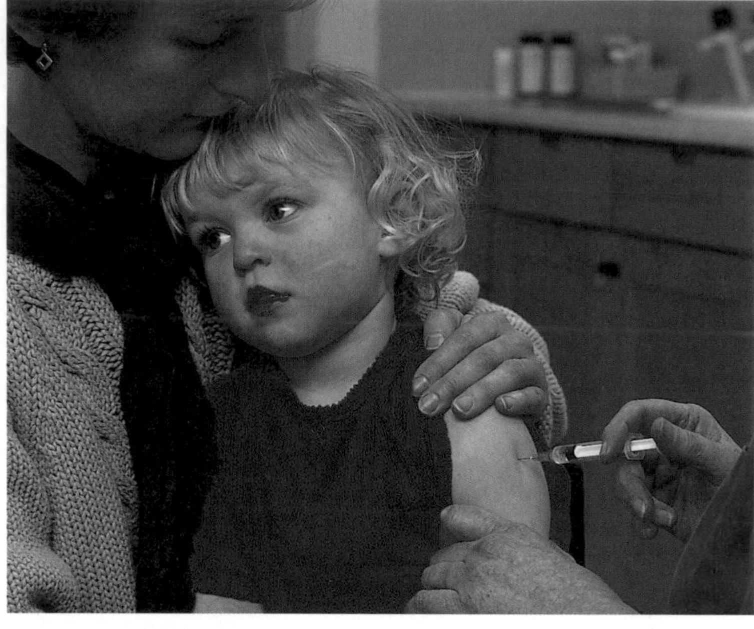

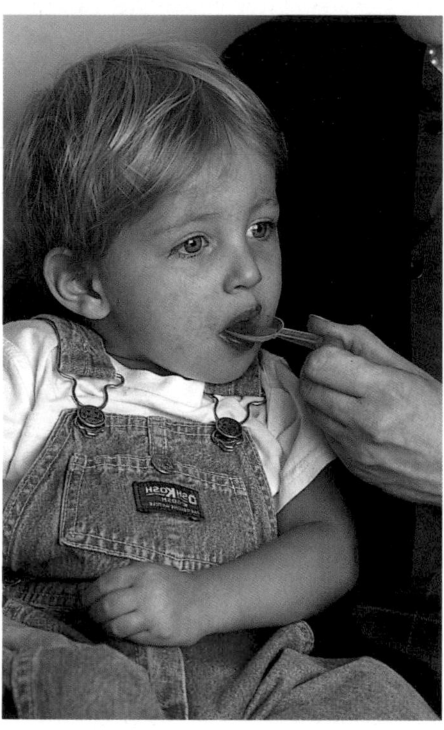

LEFT: If your child has a high temperature it can be eased with paracetamol syrup. Also ensure he is kept reasonably cool, but not uncomfortably so.

ABOVE: Mumps can be prevented by immunisation. This child is being vaccinated against mumps with a MMR (measles, mumps and rubella) injection.

How to care for your child

The symptoms will lesson in a few days but there are some things you can do to make your child feel more comfortable.

- Ease the swollen glands using either a hot-water bottle filled with warm water, or cool moist towels, whichever they find more comfortable.
- Bed rest and plenty of fluids.
- Avoid any foods or fluids that increase the flow of saliva, e.g. fruits and their juices.
- Avoid acidic foods and drinks, e.g. tomatoes and citrus drinks.
- If chewing is painful he may prefer a soft or liquid diet of soups and milky cereals.
- There is little point in keeping him isolated, as he will already have infected others in the house before symptoms developed.
- Avoid women in the first 13 weeks of pregnancy who have never had mumps or been vaccinated, as there is a risk of miscarriage.

Complications

The complications that children can develop from the mumps virus sound alarming but are usually, apart from very rare instances, very mild.

- Meningitis is quite a common complication of mumps but is usually very mild. The meningitis can develop before or after the parotid glands enlarge. A third of children have such a mild form of mumps that they develop few symptoms and no gland enlargement, but they can still develop meningitis. The child will complain that the light is hurting their eyes, called 'photophobia'. They will also have a headache and neck stiffness. They usually make an uneventful recovery with no treatment needed, but, rarely, they may be left with deafness in one or both ears.

- Inflammation of the testicles can be a very painful swelling but is almost never seen in children. However, 25 per cent of pubescent boys and adult men with mumps develop painful, swollen testes and a fever. This settles over two to three weeks and it can, rarely, cause them to become sterile.

- Encephalitis, or a swelling of the brain, is a complication of mumps but is usually mild.

DUCHENNE MUSCULAR DYSTROPHY

WHAT IS DUCHENNE MUSCULAR DYSTROPHY?

Duchenne muscular dystrophy (DMD) is one of a group of rare inherited diseases that cause the muscles to become weak.

- DMD only affects boys and is the most common type of muscular dystrophy; the condition is diagnosed in about one in 3000 babies. There are some rare types of muscular dystrophy that affect girls, but these tend to be forms of the disease that have much milder symptoms.

- Muscular dystrophy arises because of a gradual deterioration in the fibres that make up muscles.

- The condition is inherited, as parents pass on an abnormal gene to their children.

- Girls can 'carry' and pass on the abnormal gene that is responsible for duchenne muscular dystrophy.

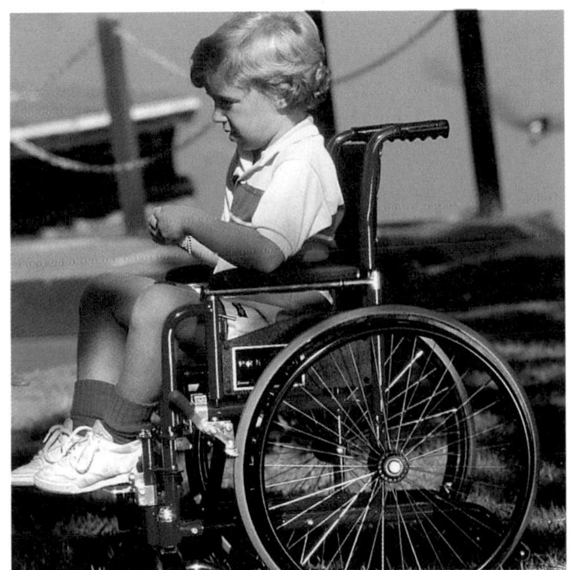

Duchenne muscular dystrophy causes the muscles to weaken, making walking progressively more difficult. A wheelchair is often necessary by nine to twelve years of age.

Other types of muscular dystrophy

These are rare and have slightly different symptoms from DMD.

1 **Becker muscular dystrophy:** this affects boys but is rarer than DMD. Although a child has the disease from birth, the symptoms may become apparent only between the ages of 11 and 15. The muscle weakness often becomes debilitating when a person is in his 40s or 50s.

2 **Childhood muscular dystrophy:** this condition can affect girls as well as boys, and is rare in the UK (more common if parents are blood relatives).

3 **Limb-girdle muscular dystrophy:** this type of muscular dystrophy is also seen in both girls and boys, but it affects different muscles in the body.

4 **Emery-Dreifuss muscular dystrophy:** this has similar symptoms to the other types, but may also affect the heart.

Initial signs and symptoms

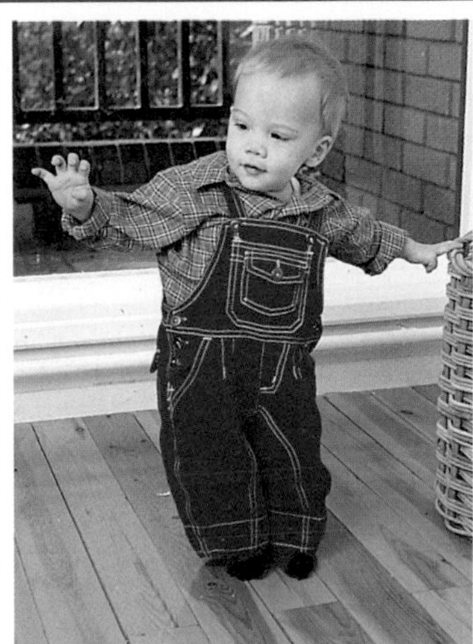

In DMD, the symptoms usually become apparent at around 18 months when the child fails to start walking. Parents may then notice signs that indicate that the child is having difficulty moving around.

1 The first clue that something is wrong may be that the child fails to meet milestones and is not starting to walk at the normal age.

2 If a child is walking, he may 'waddle' and fall over a lot more than is normal for a toddler.

Children with DMD often have difficulty reaching developmental milestones. A child with DMD may have difficulty in learning to walk, and may 'waddle' and fall over more than he should.

3 A characteristic sign of DMD is obvious when a child is getting up to a standing position from sitting on the floor. He will 'walk' his hands up his legs to achieve a standing position (doctors call this Gower's sign).

4 The muscles in the calf at the back of the leg may appear firm and slightly larger than normal, although they are in fact weak and don't function properly. Muscles in the back, legs and pelvic area are also weak.

How DMD is diagnosed

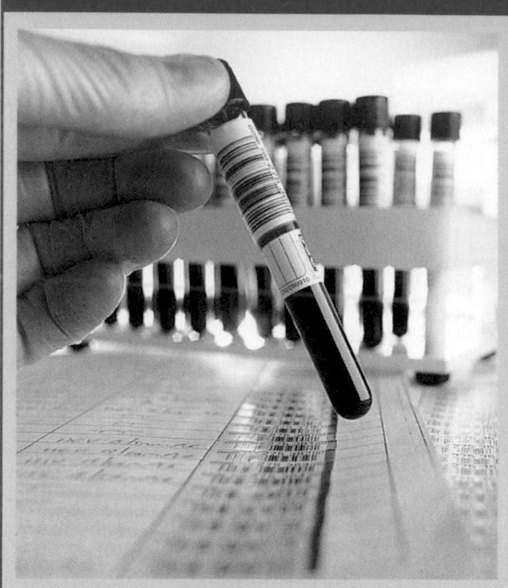

A doctor may suspect that a child has muscular dystrophy from his symptoms. He may then refer the child to a specialist paediatrician.

- **Blood tests:** an enzyme called creatine phosphokinase is normally present in healthy muscle. In muscular dystrophy, it is present in very high levels.
- **Muscle tests:** electromyography (EMG) is a test that measures the electrical activity in muscles. In a child with muscular dystrophy, the results are abnormal.

If a specialist suspects that a child has DMD, he may carry out a blood test to ascertain if the child has a higher level of the enzyme creatine phosphokinase in his blood.

- **Biopsy:** this involves examining a tiny piece of muscle tissue under a microscope. Usually, dystrophin will be seen around the muscle fibres. In DMD, there is a lack or complete absence of dystrophin. This test is usually carried out under a light general anaesthetic in babies.
- Doctors may wish to carry out tests on the heart to check whether it has been damaged.

How DMD is inherited

DMD is inherited via a faulty gene on the X chromosome.

- In almost every cell in the human body is a nucleus that contains 46 chromosomes. Within each chromosome there are thousands of genes. Chromosomes and genes are made from a substance called DNA, which passes on characteristics from generation to generation.
- Each gene contains a 'blueprint' for the manufacture of a particular protein. Proteins are the basic building-blocks of the body.
- DMD is the result of a faulty gene on the X chromosome, which is present in both males and females. This gene is responsible for producing the protein dystrophin, which forms healthy muscle.
- Girls can inherit the faulty gene, but do not usually develop the condition as they have two X chromosomes, one of which has a 'normal' chromosome that compensates for the abnormal chromosome.
- Research indicates that, in boys, the faulty gene may be the result of a change in the gene after birth, and is not necessarily inherited.

Later symptoms

As DMD progresses, the symptoms often become more severe, as the muscles become less and less able to provide normal movement.

1. The muscles in the arms can make picking up or holding objects firmly difficult.
2. Contractures develop in the muscles in the limbs and the joints become stiff. This most commonly affects the ankles, hips and knees, which often become deformed.
3. The muscles that hold the spine erect start to waste, causing it to curve (scoliosis).
4. Walking tends to progressively become more difficult.
5. Some children have learning difficulties and find it increasingly difficult to keep up at school.

What can be done to help?

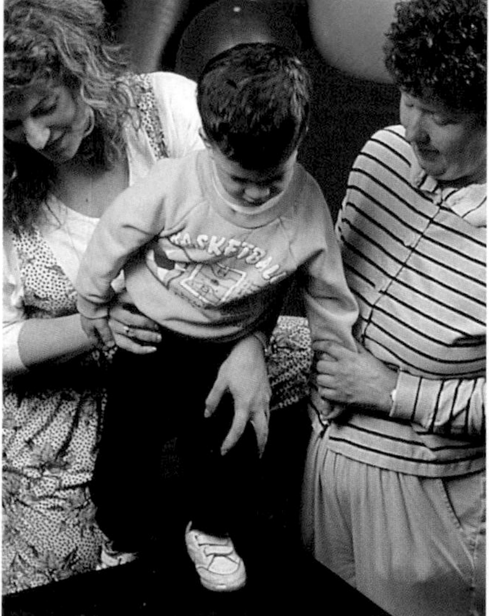

As there is no cure for DMD, emphasis is placed on encouraging the child's mobility, hence enabling him to live as full a life as possible.

There is currently no cure for DMD. Treatment involves assessing a child's ability and helping him to get the most out of life.

- Physiotherapy is vital to help a child move around and remain active, keeping limbs supple and preventing muscle wastage. Splints can be applied to limbs to prevent contractures developing, and limb exercises help to keep joints flexible and muscles strong.
- Walking aids can be beneficial to a child who is walking but is not stable.
- Occasionally, a child with muscular dystrophy has learning difficulties and may need specialist educational input.
- It is important to remember that the siblings of children with DMD may sometimes feel neglected and also need some attention.

NAPPY RASH

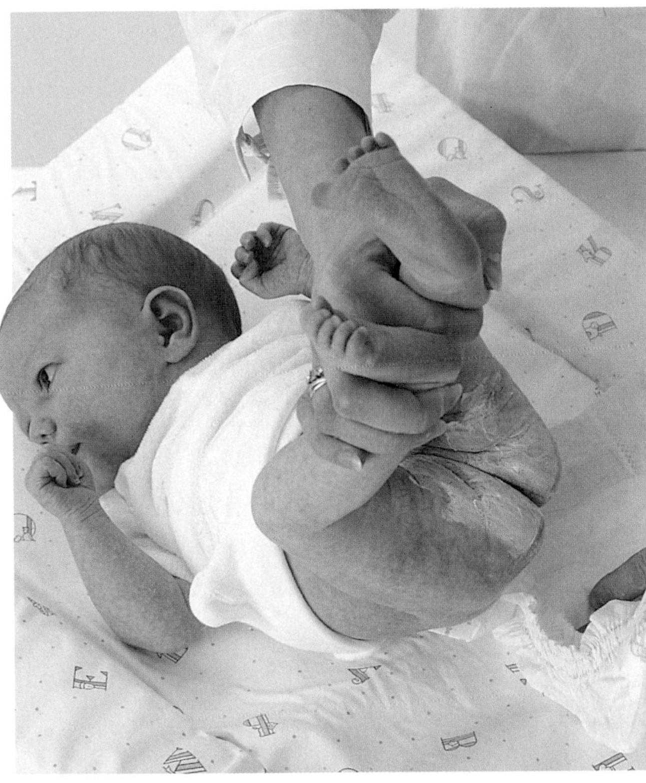

WHAT IS NAPPY RASH?

Nappy rash (napkin dermatitis) is a common skin condition affecting the area covered by a baby's nappy. It causes the baby's skin to become red, inflamed and hot to touch. Most babies develop nappy rash at some stage during their first year. The rash is not usually serious, but it may be very sore and can be distressing for the baby and her parents.

What causes it?

Nappy rash occurs when your baby's skin comes into prolonged contact with urine and faeces. Bacteria in the faeces breaks down urine to release ammonia, which causes burning and irritation.

The rash is most likely to appear if your baby's nappy region is not cleaned regularly or if she remains in a wet nappy for too long.

Your baby's skin must be kept dry, as bacteria grow best in a warm, wet environment – if a nappy stops air reaching your baby's skin, the urine will not evaporate.

Friction caused by wearing tight nappies or clothing, and some brands of soap, washing powders and baby wipes, can aggravate the soreness.

Nappy rash is caused by contact with the ammonia in urine. Good nappy hygiene can help to treat and prevent it.

What increases the risk?

All babies are prone to nappy rash, but certain factors can increase the likelihood of your baby being affected. You should be especially alert:

- A few days after an immunisation injection.
- If your baby is changing from breast to bottle or is being weaned.
- When your baby starts drinking cow's milk (once your baby is one year old).
- If your baby has a stomach upset causing frequent bowel movements or diarrhoea.
- If your baby is teething.
- If your baby is generally unwell (especially if she is taking antibiotics).

Symptoms

Nappy rash is easy to diagnose and you should notice it as soon as it develops.

- Nappy rash starts off with a slight redness on the bottom, genitals and surrounding skin.
- The skin may become sore and inflamed with red raised patches, spots and wrinkles. Groin creases are usually spared.
- If it is left untreated, the rash can worsen into open sores (ulcers).
- Nappy rash can make your baby irritable. In some cases, it becomes infected with a fungal infection called thrush.

When to call the doctor

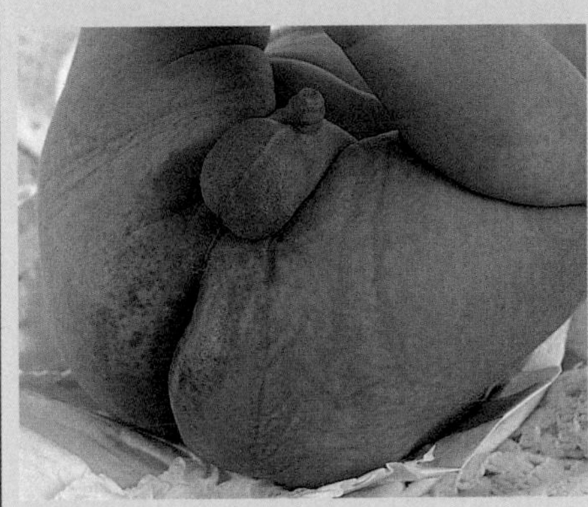

Many cases of nappy rash can be treated at home. However, severe bouts will need medical attention to make sure the rash clears completely.

- You should consult a doctor if your baby's rash is severe or lasts longer than a week or if your baby also has a fever.

Take your baby to the doctor if the skin on his genitals and bottom has red patches or spots that are sore and inflamed. Antifungals or antibiotics may be prescribed to reduce the infection.

- Occasionally, a baby with nappy rash develops a secondary bacterial infection, which needs to be treated with antibiotics.
- If your baby's skin is also red, weepy and scaly, especially in the folds, eczema may be the cause (rather than nappy rash), and this requires a proper diagnosis.

Treatment

Nappy rash needs to be treated as soon as possible. If the condition is left untreated it will leave your baby in extreme discomfort and pain.

1 At the first sign of soreness, use an antiseptic nappy rash cream, which will soothe and heal your baby's skin and prevent secondary bacterial infections. You should also use a barrier cream to protect the skin from the ammonia in urine and faeces. Trial and error is most likely the best way to find the most effective cream. Apply the cream several times a day as necessary and after every nappy change.

2 Whenever possible, you should leave your baby's nappy off to encourage the healing process. Try switching to another washing powder and using different or unperfumed baby wipes.

3 Your doctor may prescribe a mild steroid cream to soothe the inflammation, with antibiotic cream or medicine for a secondary infection. If the nappy rash is associated with thrush, an anti-fungal cream may help. The doctor will check your baby's mouth for thrush, prescribing an anti-fungal syrup if needed. If you are giving him a thrush treatment, you still need to use barrier cream on his bottom.

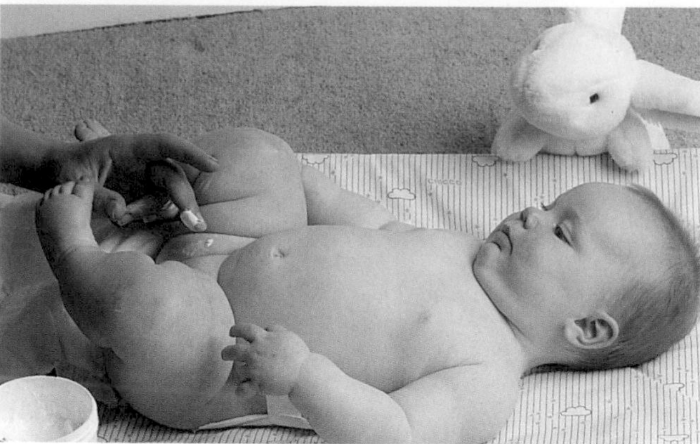

After you have cleaned your baby's bottom and genitals, apply barrier cream over the area, especially the folds of the skin. Avoid placing cream into the vagina or on the penis.

Ways to prevent nappy rash

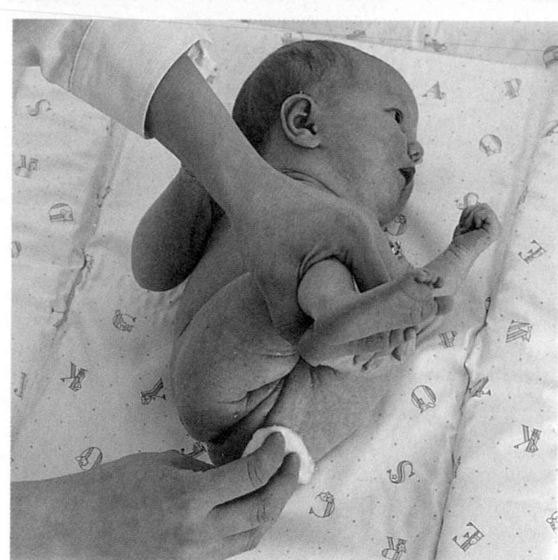

Always clean your baby's bottom carefully. For a girl, wipe from front to back, and never pull back the foreskin of a boy's penis – it will clean itself.

Most babies will get nappy rash in some form during their nappy-wearing period. However, employing a good nappy-changing routine will ensure that it is kept to a minimum.

1 Keep clean: a nappy needs to be changed as soon as it becomes wet or soiled. Use cotton wool with plain water or a special baby lotion or baby wipes to remove all traces of faeces. Then rinse with water and pat your baby's bottom dry.

2 Use a nappy cream: apply a protective barrier cream, lightly and evenly, paying attention to the folds of your baby's skin. Nappy creams protect against wetness as they contain ingredients that repel water. Talcum powder should be avoided, as this may lead to further inflammation.

3 Air your baby's bottom: lie your baby down and let her have a kick around without a nappy on for a while each day. This will keep her skin healthy and aid the healing process if she is already suffering from irritation.

4 Practise good hygiene: wash your hands before and after a nappy change, wipe your baby's bottom from front to back to avoid cross-infection, and use a separate bowl for washing your baby's bottom if you are not bathing him. You should also dispose of all used nappies hygienically.

Choosing and using nappies

Nappy rash can affect babies wearing disposable or towelling nappies.

- If your baby suffers from nappy rash, you should review the brand of nappy your baby wears or switch from towelling nappies to disposables (or vice versa).

- If you are using towelling nappies, don't use plastic pants on top, as these can stop the urine evaporating.

- Terry towelling nappies should be boil-washed to remove any trace of ammonia and also destroy harmful bacteria. Non-biological washing powders are less likely to cause irritation.

- Many disposable nappies are designed to limit nappy rash: they are extremely absorbent and seal moisture away from the skin while allowing air to circulate. Avoid using very thick nappy creams with disposable nappies as these can clog up the one-way action of the nappy.

PNEUMONIA

WHAT IS PNEUMONIA?

Pneumonia is a general term used to describe any infection of the lungs.

- In pneumonia, the lowest part of the respiratory tract – the alveoli and the tissue of the lung – is affected. The inflammation reduces the transfer of oxygen to the blood and also causes sepsis – poisoning of the tissues, which can spread to the blood (septicaemia).

- Pneumonia was once divided into two categories: lobar pneumonia, when only one lobe of a lung is affected (the right lung has three lobes and the left has two); and bronchopneumonia, when more than one lobe is affected. This distinction is rarely made nowadays. The term 'double pneumonia' is also rarely used – it merely means that both lungs are affected.

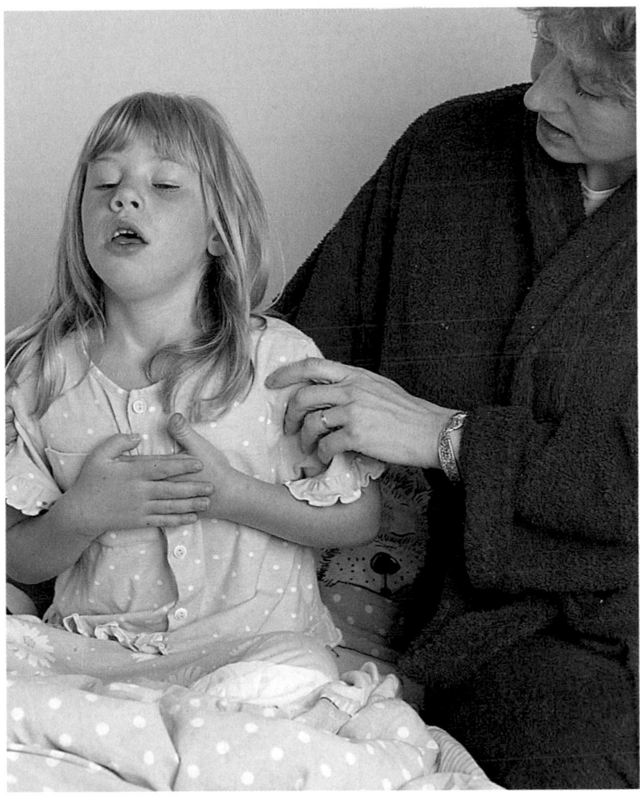

Pneumonia is an inflammation of the chest that affects the small air sacs and the lung tissue. Babies or young children suffering from pneumonia may need to be treated in hospital because their immune systems are immature.

Who is at risk?

Generally, pneumonia develops when the body's natural defences are weakened.

- The elderly are especially vulnerable, as are young children and premature babies, whose immune systems are not yet fully mature. Around four out of every 100 children under five contract some form of pneumonia each year.
- Without treatment, pneumonia can be extremely serious for children. The World Health Organisation estimates that pneumonia causes the death of about four million children under five each year.

When to call the doctor

Pneumonia can have serious consequences, so you should consult the doctor as soon as your child displays any of the symptoms of the condition. He needs emergency help if:

- Breathing is abnormally fast or is difficult and laboured.
- His temperature rises to 38.9°C (102°F) or higher.
- His lips or fingernails are turning a bluish-grey colour.
- He vomits, refuses feeds or vomits after bouts of coughing.

Take your child's temperature using a forehead strip or a conventional thermometer under the arm. If his temperature is 38.9°C (102°F) or above, call your doctor immediately.

Signs and symptoms

The symptoms of pneumonia vary according to its cause, the degree of infection and the age of the child involved.

- Neonatal bacterial pneumonia is often difficult to diagnose, because the onset of the condition is gradual and symptoms are masked by other problems. They include irritability, lethargy, feeding difficulties and hypothermia. Without prompt treatment, the condition can be fatal.
- An attack of pneumonia is often preceded by an infection of the upper respiratory tract, such as a sore throat. The symptoms start a few days after the initial infection and develop quickly.
- In both viral and bacterial pneumonia breathing becomes rapid and laboured, often with wheezing and coughing. Your child may lose her appetite and experience vomiting, chest pain and a fever. In severe cases, her lips and fingernails may turn a bluish-grey.
- The symptoms of chlamydial pneumonia include rapid breathing, a barking cough and a blocked nose. There is no fever but, in 50 per cent of cases, the child may have conjunctivitis.

What causes pneumonia?

The infective agent that causes the inflammation in pneumonia can be either a bacterium, a virus, a fungus or a micro-organism.

- Childhood pneumonia differs from adult pneumonia in that different infective agents are more common than others at different ages. For example, mycoplasma pneumoniae is thought to be the most common cause of pneumonia in children aged over five and adolescents, but only rarely affects children under five.

- Congenital pneumonia is usually caused by E. coli (Escherichia coli) or Klebsiella pneumoniae. Neonatal pneumonia is often caused by Group B Streptococcus and is picked up from the mother's birth canal. Babies born with this form of pneumonia usually have a low birthweight and need to be nursed in intensive care.

- Between the age of one and three months, bacterial pneumonia becomes less common, and other causes of pneumonia predominate. The most important of these is the micro-organism chlamydia. A chlamydia infection is a sexually transmitted disease that is becoming increasingly common, and can be contracted by the baby during the birth.

- Viral pneumonia is usually caused by respiratory syncytial virus (RSV), which also causes bronchiolitis and occurs in epidemics between mid-winter and early spring.

- The most common cause of pneumonia in children between four months and five years is respiratory syncytial virus, although influenza viruses, parainfluenza viruses and adenovirus can also be responsible. The bacteria Streptococcus pneumoniae, Haemophilus influenzae and Bordellata pertussis (the bacterium responsible for whooping cough), can cause pneumonia. Vaccinations against Haemophilus influenza (Hib) are given from the age of two months in the triple vaccine.

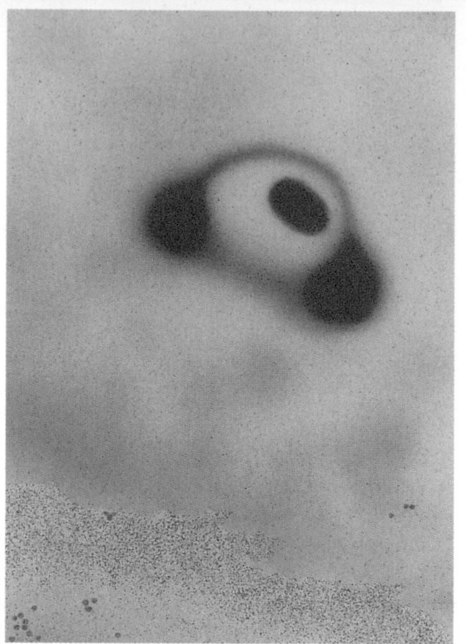

Mycoplasma pneumoniae is a common cause of bacterial pneumonia in children over the age of five and in adults. Pneumonia in children under five years is more likely to be caused by the respiratory syncytial virus (RSV).

What is the treatment?

The treatment for pneumonia depends on the infective agent that is responsible and the severity of the condition.

1 The first priority is to establish the type of pneumonia and determine what bacterium, virus or other agent is the cause. This is done by examining a phlegm or blood sample. An X-ray of the chest may be taken to determine the extent of the inflammation.

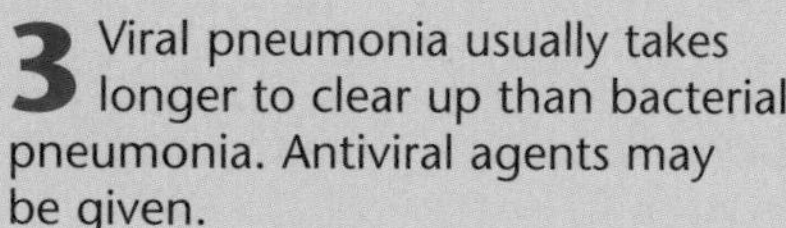

2 In the case of bacterial pneumonia, antibiotics are given. These are normally effective within one to two weeks.

3 Viral pneumonia usually takes longer to clear up than bacterial pneumonia. Antiviral agents may be given.

4 Pneumonia is usually treated at home, except in serious cases when antibiotics are given in hospital. An affected child should stay in bed, in a room with a humidifier to increase moisture, keep warm and drink plenty of fluids. The child's temperature should be monitored regularly, and a doctor called immediately if there is any deterioration in his condition.

A child with mild pneumonia will need plenty of bedrest and fluids. Cough medicines should not be given without medical advice, as coughing can help to clear the lungs.

Complications

Even if treated successfully, pneumonia may cause some complications later in life.

- A higher proportion of children who have had pneumonia suffer from asthma later in life. However, it is also believed that a significant proportion of children who have pneumonia also had undiagnosed asthma beforehand, which may have contributed to developing pneumonia. Therefore the nature of the link is unclear.

- Lung function has been found to be reduced in adults who had pneumonia when they were children. Again, however, they may have contracted pneumonia because their lungs were less efficient in the first place.

PREMATURE BABIES

WHY A BABY MAY BE BORN EARLY

A baby that is delivered before 37 weeks is classed as premature.

● Around 8 per cent of babies are born prematurely, either because the mother has gone into early labour of her own accord or because her labour has been induced for medical reasons. Exactly what triggers labour is not known, but there are various risk factors that increase the chances of a premature birth.

● A multiple pregnancy is a risk factor for a premature birth, usually because there is insufficient space in the uterus for more than one baby. Twins are usually born at 37 weeks and are often delivered earlier than this.

● Other risk factors include excessive exercise and inadequate rest. The mother who smokes in pregnancy is also likely to go into premature labour and have a low birthweight baby.

● Certain medical conditions can either trigger an early labour or make it necessary for the labour to be induced early. These include diabetes, high blood pressure, pre-eclampsia, vaginal or urinary infections and placental insufficiency.

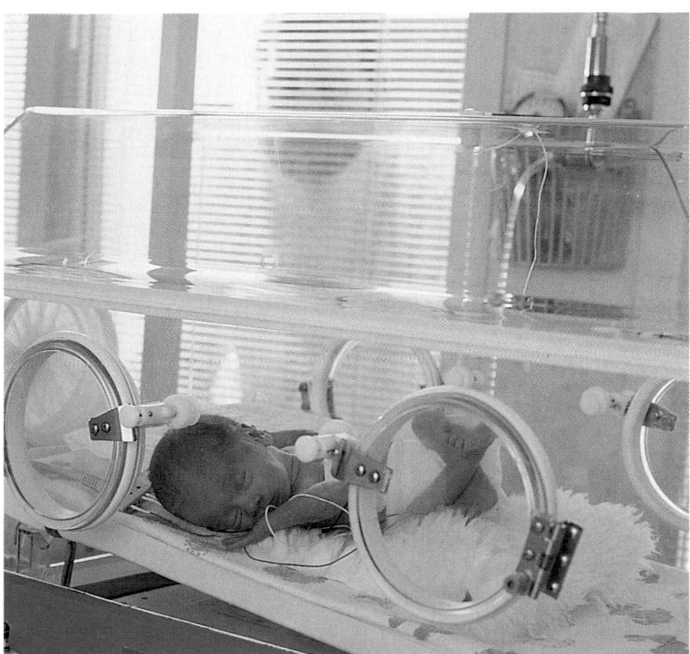

A premature baby is kept at a constant temperature in an incubator. Premature babies lack extra fat and muscle so conditions in the incubator provide them with extra warmth.

Common problems for premature babies

Premature babies tend to suffer from a variety of medical problems – some are more serious, but most can be alleviated with the appropriate equipment and care in the Special Care Baby Unit (SCBU).

● **Lack of fat and muscle:** babies lay down large amounts of fat and muscle in their last few weeks in the womb, and this helps to regulate body temperature after birth. Premature babies are often low in birthweight, under 2500g (5lb 8oz). They lack this extra fat and muscle.

● **Respiratory distress syndrome (RDS):** this is a common problem in premature babies and those born to diabetic mothers. It is caused by an inadequate supply of a chemical called surfactant. This is produced during the last trimester and lines the air sacs (alveoli) in the baby's lungs. It helps the alveoli to stay open and promotes the exchange of oxygen and carbon dioxide when breathing in and out. Premature babies do not have sufficient surfactant, and so have breathing difficulties.

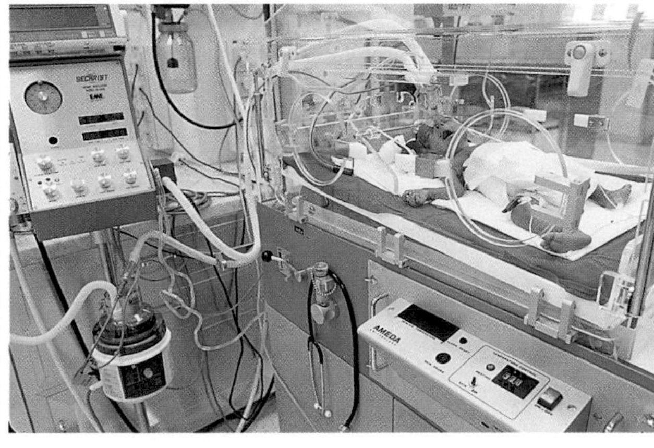

● **Hypoxia:** this occurs when there is an insufficient supply of oxygen to the tissues and low blood sugar. It can cause brain damage if it is left untreated.

● **Infection:** all premature babies have very immature immune systems and so are at risk of contracting an infection.

Breathing difficulties are a common problem in premature babies. In some cases, they may need the help of life-support equipment.

● **Jaundice:** neonatal jaundice usually wears off in a few days. It occurs because as the baby's old red blood cells are broken down, a yellow pigment (bilirubin) is released. As the liver matures, it starts to metabolise bilirubin, which is then excreted, and the jaundice fades. However, a premature baby's liver is not sufficiently mature to do this, so bilirubin builds up in the body. To combat this, premature babies may be given phototherapy treatment – ultraviolet light, which breaks down bilirubin in the skin – and extra fluids until their liver matures.

Special Care Baby Unit

Many premature babies need to be cared for in a Special Care Baby Unit (SCBU), even if only for a short time, in order to protect them and supply any necessary nutrients while they grow and mature.

- A SCBU has two sections: 'high-dependency' neonatal intensive care (NICU) for very premature or ill babies, and a section in which care is less intensive and babies are monitored once they are able to breathe and feed independently.

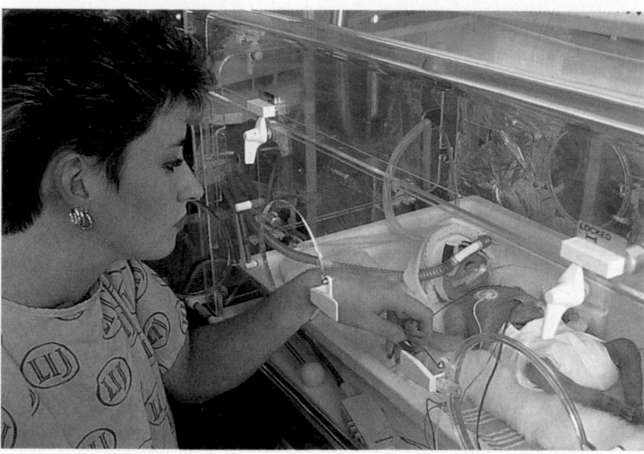

- A ventilator helps a premature baby to breathe.
- Monitors check the heartbeat, breathing rate and oxygen in the blood. An alarm alerts staff to any problem.

An incubator allows parents and SCBU staff to handle the baby without disturbing the air surrounding him.

- An intravenous drip delivers measured doses of fluids and any necessary drugs to the baby.
- A nasogastric tube may be inserted into the stomach via the nostrils to deliver milk to babies who cannot suck or swallow.
- Parents are encouraged to give skin-to-skin contact in a 'kangaroo hold', in which the naked baby is held upright between the mother's breasts. Babies have been found to thrive when held in this way.

The SCBU team

Medical staff who work in a SCBU are well qualified and dedicated to caring for babies in their charge.

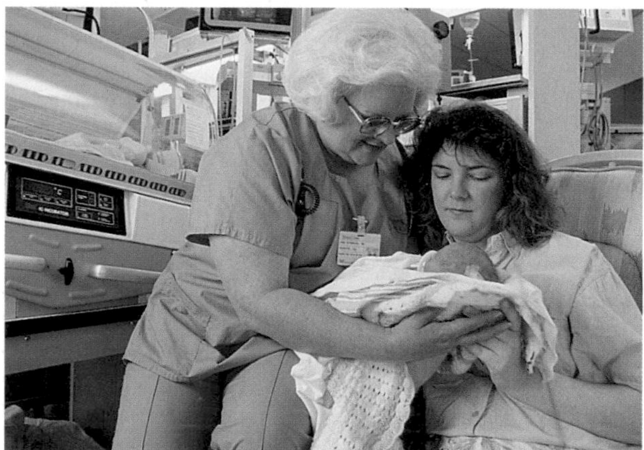

- The medical team is led by a consultant neonatologist – a paediatrician with training in treating newborn babies. Junior doctors and paediatric nurses carry out day-to-day care, under the consultant's guidance.
- The paediatric nurses will help you to look after your baby, but encourage you to take an active role in her daily care. In some units an individual nurse is allocated to care for a specific baby.

Nurses in the SCBU are there to offer specialist support to the parents of premature babies.

- Midwives ensure the mother's wellbeing after the birth and encourage breast-feeding. Milk may need to be expressed if the baby cannot suckle adequately.
- Other medical staff, such as physiotherapists, visit the unit to treat particular babies at the doctors' request.

The outlook

Though having a premature baby can be a worrying experience, the outlook is generally very good.

- Modern technology and techniques have greatly improved the way premature babies are treated and significantly increased the chances of survival of even the earliest babies.

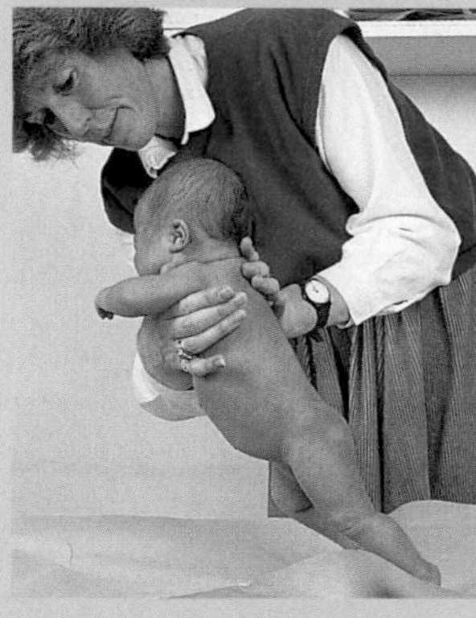

- Once a premature baby is well enough to go home, health-care professionals will monitor her progress.
- It is likely that a premature baby will be developmentally behind for the first two years. Parents should avoid comparing their premature babies with those born at term. By their second birthday, most premature babies will have caught up.

Parents should not become over anxious if a baby born prematurely takes longer to reach developmental milestones.

Useful addresses

BLISS (the National Charity for the Newborn)
Provides information and support for parents of special care babies.
Tel: 0500 618 140
www.bliss.org.uk

The Association of Breast-feeding Mothers
Provides information and help to mothers who are breast-feeding their special care babies.
Tel: 020 7813 1481
www.abm.me.uk

RINGWORM

WHAT IS RINGWORM?

Ringworm has nothing to do with worms; it is, in fact, a fungus infection that attacks the skin, scalp and nails. The fungi that cause ringworms are called dermatophytes, and there are 30 species that can affect humans.

- The condition is called ringworm because if the skin is infected a rash develops in a characteristic ring shape.
- It can affect adults, children and animals – the latter being a common source of infection for humans.
- Children are often infected on the scalp; another common form of ringworm is athlete's foot.

The rash

If a child's body is infected with ringworm, she will develop an intensely itchy, red, scaly rash.

- It takes from four to 10 days after coming into contact with the infection for the rash to appear.
- It begins as a red patch that develops into a ring shape. Within a few weeks new individual patches may form.
- It is a slow-growing rash, and does not just appear overnight.
- Unlike most other itchy rashes, only one part of your child's body may be affected.
- The dermatophytes causing ringworm are, like all fungi, living organisms. Ringworm lives off a layer in the skin called keratin and, as the fungi use up the keratin, they move outwards. This means the scaliest skin is at the outer edge of the ring where the fungi are most active. As the skin in the centre of the ring begins to heal and appears healthy, the ring itself will grow bigger.
- If the initial rash is mistaken for eczema and steroid creams are applied, the skin at the edges may appear less scaly and the whole rash less ring-like. Even without steroids, the typical ring shape may not always be present.

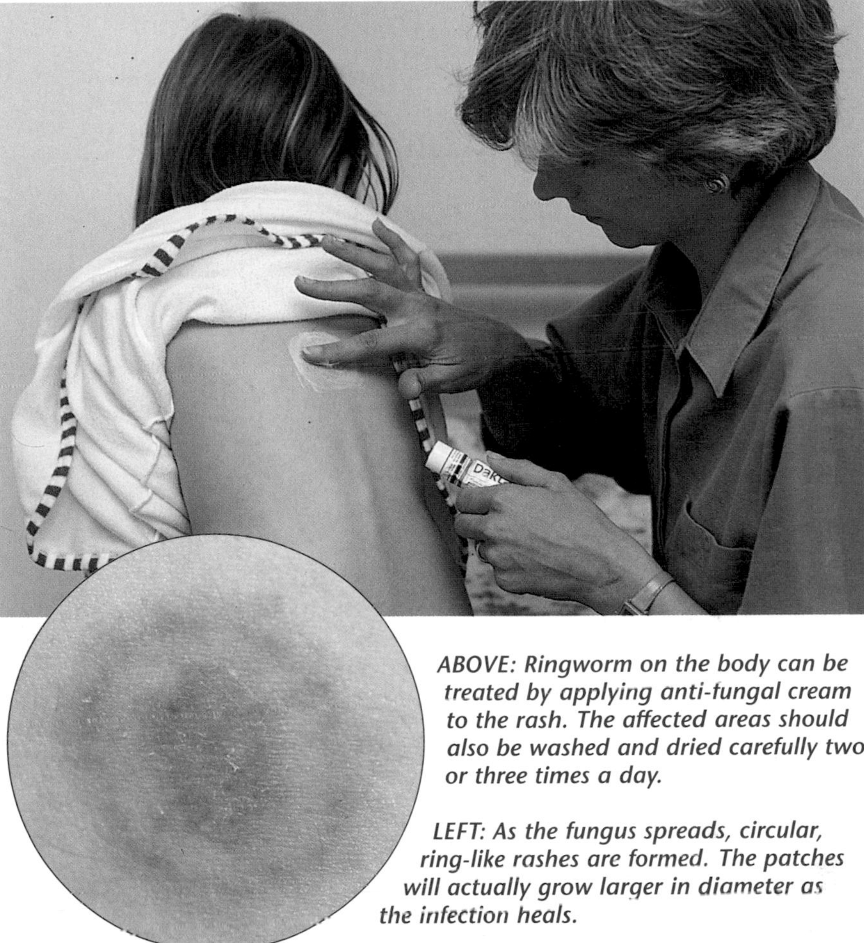

ABOVE: Ringworm on the body can be treated by applying anti-fungal cream to the rash. The affected areas should also be washed and dried carefully two or three times a day.

LEFT: As the fungus spreads, circular, ring-like rashes are formed. The patches will actually grow larger in diameter as the infection heals.

Scalp ringworm

Scalp ringworm affects mainly children; this form of the condition has become particularly prevalent in large cities.

- Children with scalp ringworm have bald patches where the skin in the patch looks red, scaly, and may be ring shaped.
- The hairs within the ring may break off, but they will start to re-grow once the skin in the centre of the ring begins to heal.
- If your child has scalp ringworm, there may be other children at her nursery with the condition, or you may notice that a family pet has also developed bald patches.

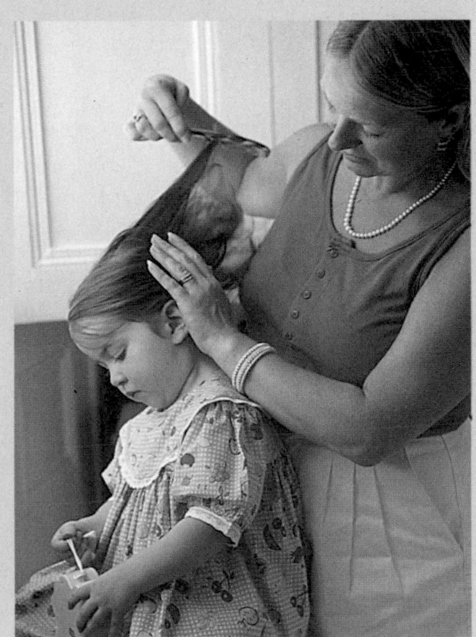

Ringworm can be spread via infected materials. So if your child's scalp is infected, it's important that her comb or brush is not used by anyone else.

How ringworm is spread

Children can catch ringworm from direct contact with the skin of an infected person or animal, or indirectly from material objects such as clothes, sheets, combs and towels. The fungal infections caught from animals tend to be worse than those passed between humans.

1 Ringworm is highly contagious and the fungi that cause it thrive on moisture and warmth.

2 It is infectious while the spores are still present and an infected child should be kept away from other children as much as possible. Once the ringworm is being treated, however, it should be safe for the child to start to re-attend school.

3 Adults can catch scalp ringworm from a child, but the fungi prefer children's hair because it has less fat in it. If you have bald patches or a sore itchy scalp, there's a chance you have the infection.

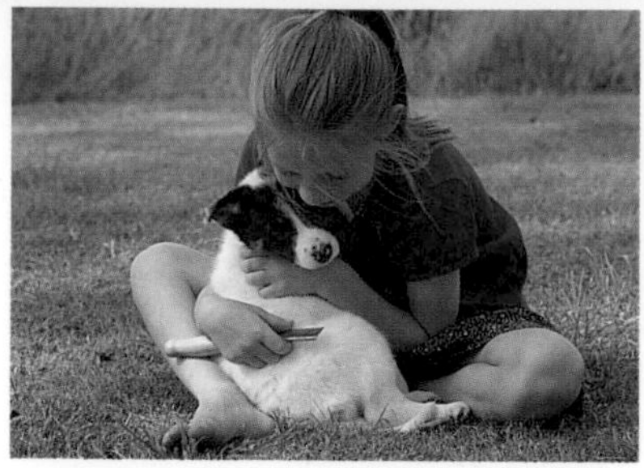

Ringworm is often spread by family pets. If you suspect that your cat or dog has the condition, take it to the vet for immediate treatment.

Can ringworm be prevented?

Ringworm can't be prevented, but you can take measures to ensure that the infection is not spread more widely.

- If your child has ringworm, inform her nursery or school so that other parents can be notified.
- Do not let an infected child share baths, clothes, towels, sheets or hairbrushes with anyone else.
- To minimise the risk of the infection being spread, clean infected materials thoroughly: wash sheets and towels in hot water and sterilise hair-brushes and combs.
- If your child has ringworm on her body, dress her in loose-fitting cotton clothes to keep the infected areas cool and dry. The fungi are less likely to thrive in these conditions.

Microsporum persicolor is just one of 30 species of fungi that can cause ringworm; this particular variety will live in the scalp. The fungi feed on keratin, which is a protein found in the hair, nails and outermost layers of the skin.

Diagnosing ringworm

- Ringworm is diagnosed by analysing a scraping of skin under a microscope. Leaving the sample for a few days allows the fungus to grow and may reveal different fungi. Hair samples can also be used to identify scalp ringworm.
- Another test used by dermatologists to diagnose skin conditions is to shine a Woods light on the affected area. This is an ultra-violet light that fluoresces a particular colour; for example, it goes green if there is a fungal infection.

Treating ringworm

On the body: this form of ringworm responds well to anti-fungal creams or ointments. Some examples of these are Canestan, Daktarin and Ecostatin. The infection must be treated for at least four weeks. This should include treatment for two weeks after the rash has disappeared because the fungus may still lie in the skin cells, and the extra two weeks will make sure it is completely eradicated.

Scalp ringworm: this is more of a problem than body ringworm as it doesn't respond to ointments and creams. The patient will be seen by a paediatric or dermatology specialist, who will need to take scrapings of the infection to make sure it is ringworm. If scalp ringworm is diagnosed, an oral medication called terbinafine may be prescribed, which needs to be taken every day for one month.

Recognising other skin conditions

Eczema: this may be very itchy, but the rash is usually behind the knees, in front of the elbows, in front of the ankles, and under the chin.

Psoriasis: this is rarely seen in children under three years old. The rash forms very thick disc-like patches on the scalp or body, usually covered in a silvery coating.

Cradle cap: this scalp condition is common in young babies. It causes dry, flaky skin which may develop into a greasy, yellowish-brown crust, covering the scalp.

RUBELLA

WHAT IS RUBELLA?

Rubella, also known as 'German measles' or 'three-day measles', is a contagious illness caused by a virus that invades cells of the skin and lymph glands.

- The term 'German' does not indicate any connection with Germany. It probably comes from the old French word 'germain', which means 'similar to' or 'alike'. Thus the term 'German measles' simply means 'like measles'.

- It is a much milder disease than measles and does not usually cause any serious problems, except for pregnant women.

- The incubation period is 14–21 days, the average being 18 days. Infection usually requires fairly close contact with an infected person and the rubella virus is passed on in droplets from the nose and throat. A person is contagious from one week before until one week after the rash appears.

- The virus is also present in the blood and stools of the infected person, but transmission in this way is unlikely.

- Rubella occurs more frequently in winter and spring.

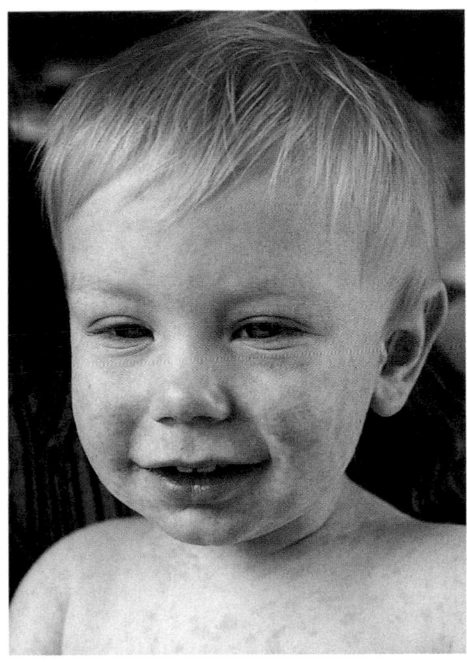

One of the symptoms of rubella is a non-itchy rash that starts on the forehead and moves down the face to the body. This usually lasts for one to five days.

Symptoms

Up to half of those who contract rubella show no symptoms at all, and children and small babies are usually the least affected. Children with rubella usually recover within a week, although adults can take longer. This is why it can be difficult to detect and diagnose.

- **Fever:** rubella may begin with one or two days of mild fever, with a body temperature of 37.2–38.8°C (99–102°F) and with symptoms similar to those of influenza.

- **Swollen glands:** along with the fever there may be swelling of the glands at the back of the child's neck or behind the ears.

- **Rash:** after two or three days a non-itchy rash spreads from the child's forehead down the rest of the body. This can be the first symptom of rubella in small children. The pink or red spots are about 2–3mm (up to ⅛in) in diameter and may merge to form patches. The rash can last for any period of time between one to five days. As it spreads down the child's body, the affected skin may be shed in flakes.

- **Other symptoms:** a child with rubella may complain of aching joints and a stuffy or runny nose.

Rubella and pregnancy

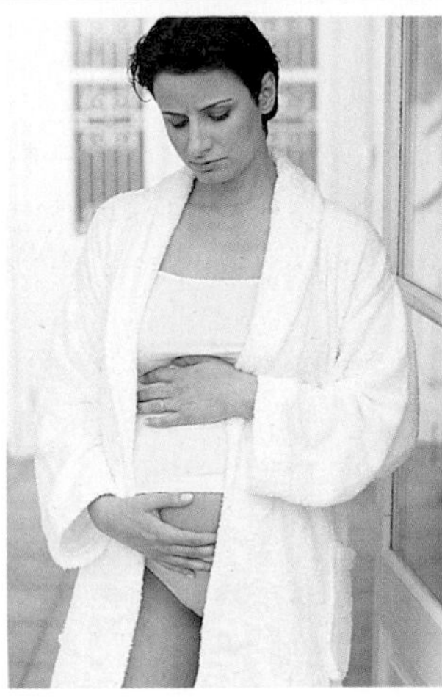

Rubella is a harmless illness in children. However, doctors pay special attention to it because the disease can cause defects in an unborn baby if it is caught by a pregnant woman who is not immune to rubella.

- It is very important to ensure that neither the patient nor any contacts who are not immune to rubella come into contact with a pregnant woman.

Pregnant women should avoid contact with anyone who has rubella. It is possible for the virus to cause serious foetal defects if the woman isn't immune.

- Babies infected with rubella during their early development in the womb may suffer from serious defects, including growth retardation, malformations of the heart, eyes and brain, deafness and problems with the liver, spleen and bone marrow.

- The risk of damage is very high during the first 10 weeks of pregnancy; at least 50 per cent of foetuses that come into contact with rubella develop abnormalities.

- Only 10–20 per cent of foetuses are damaged during weeks 10–16.

- After the 16th week of pregnancy, damage is rare.

When to call the doctor

It is important for a diagnosis to be made as soon as possible.

1 A doctor should be called if the child develops a fever of over 38.3°C (101°F) or if the child appears to be unusually ill for what is normally considered a mild disease.

2 If you suspect your child has rubella, you should not take him into a crowded surgery. If you have to visit the surgery, telephone first to tell them that you are bringing in a child with suspected rubella. This way an appointment can be arranged where your child does not come into any contact with pregnant women.

3 A pregnant woman who comes into contact with rubella and is not sure if she has immunity should seek medical advice immediately.

Home nursing

Very little treatment is necessary. The disease is normally very mild in children and the symptoms are resolved within a few days.

- A child should be kept off school until he is well again, and as a general rule for at least seven days after the appearance of the rash.
- The child's temperature should be taken regularly.
- Keep the child cool by reducing the amount of clothing or bedding.
- Depending on how ill the child is feeling, he should be encouraged to rest.
- There is no specific reason to keep children away from the patient – in fact it may be beneficial for children, particularly girls, to get rubella as this can confer immunity in later life.

One of the first symptoms of rubella can be a high temperature, so this should be closely monitored.

- Rubella cannot be treated with antibiotics. To relieve minor discomfort, liquid paracetamol can be given. Children with a fever should not be given aspirin.

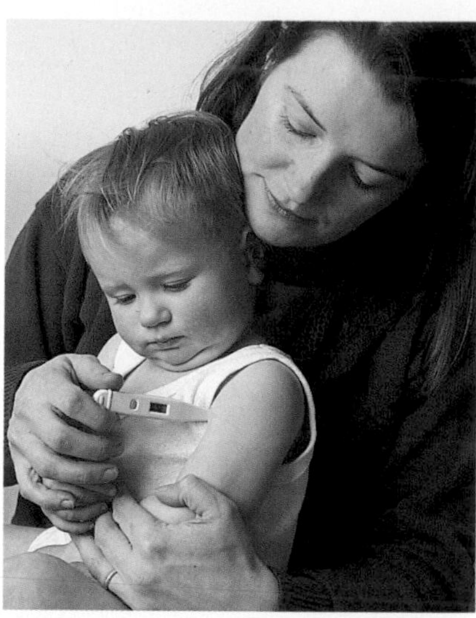

Immunisation

Anyone who is not immune to the rubella virus may catch rubella. A simple blood test can establish whether or not someone is immune.

- Until the late 1980s, girls were routinely inoculated against the rubella virus when they were in their early teens.
- Today a vaccine known as MMR is given at the age of 12–15 months, with a booster at three to five years of age.
- The MMR vaccine is a combined vaccine that protects against mumps, measles and rubella.

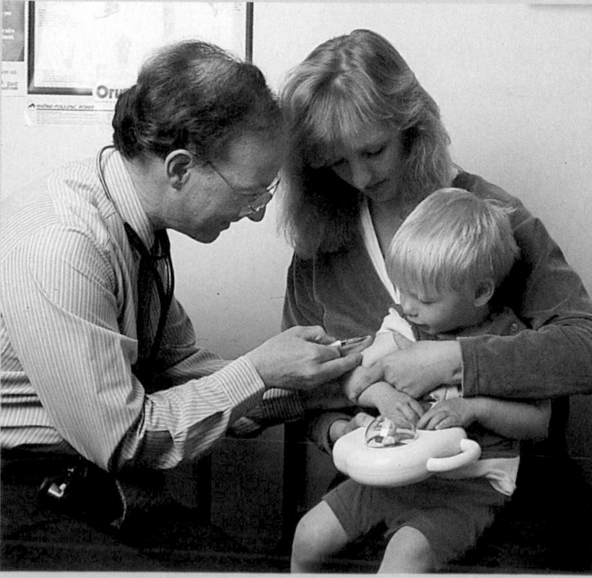

- Rubella vaccine normally, but unfortunately not always, provides immunity for life.
- The MMR vaccine is not given to pregnant women or to women likely to become pregnant within three months of vaccination.
- Actually having the disease usually confers lifelong immunity. The disease causes the body to produce antibodies that remain in the blood for life, preventing any later infection.
- Testing of pregnant women for rubella immunity is accurate. However, people's memories of past illnesses can be inaccurate and some women may mistakenly think they have had rubella in the past and that they are immune to the virus.
- If a non-immune pregnant woman is exposed to the rubella virus, she will be given blood tests over the following one to three weeks to establish whether or not she has developed the rubella virus.
- It is thought that if the use of the vaccine were to become sufficiently administered worldwide, the disease could be successfully wiped out in the same way that smallpox has been eradicated.

Your child will be given a combined vaccine that protects against mumps, measles and rubella. This usually provides immunity for life.

SEPTICAEMIA

WHAT IS SEPTICAEMIA?

Septicaemia is the medical term for blood poisoning.

- It is caused by harmful germs, such as bacteria, entering the blood through a wound or infection and multiplying rapidly.
- It is more common in very young children, as their immune systems are not as developed as those of adults, making them vulnerable to infection.
- Some of the symptoms include fever, chills, rapid, shallow breathing, a fast heart rate and delirium.
- Septicaemia progresses rapidly, so it is critical that the signs are recognised as soon as possible and potentially life-saving treatment given.

Septicaemia can be caused in newborn infants by E. coli infection, and in any age by the meningococcus bacterium.

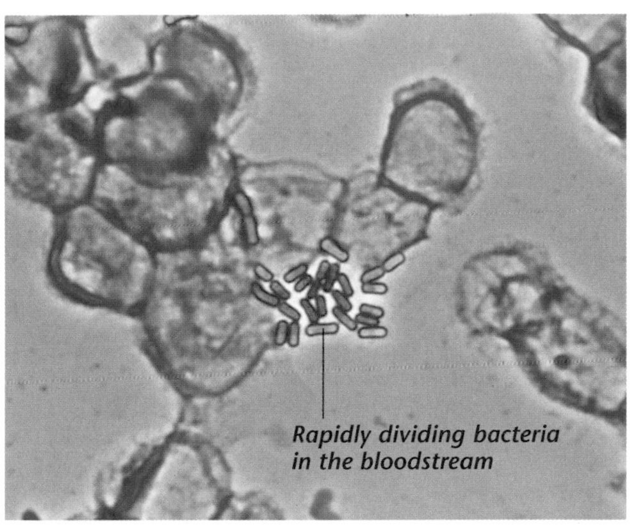

Rapidly dividing bacteria in the bloodstream

Signs and symptoms

Septicaemia can spread very quickly. Recognising the signs early is crucial to effective treatment.

- Septicaemia begins with flu-like symptoms. The child will feel unwell, and will have a lack of energy.
- He may also complain of pains in his muscles and joints.
- The child may have stomach pain, vomiting and/or diarrhoea.

The child will become rapidly unwell, showing a range of symptoms:

- A very high temperature, more than 39.4°C (103°F).
- Listlessness and a lack of appetite.
- Extreme shivering.
- Cold, pale hands and feet.
- Rapid, shallow breathing.
- A fast heart rate.
- The toxins released by the bacteria damage the blood vessels causing a rash, known as a haemorrhagic rash, to develop. Literally, this means that there is bleeding under the skin.
- The rash first appears as a cluster of tiny spots, which resemble pinpricks in the skin. The spots gradually enlarge to look like multiple bruises, which join together to form large areas of purple skin damage.
- Septicaemia can develop very quickly and, in some cases, the rash can literally spread in front of your eyes.
- Delirium and loss of consciousness can also occur.

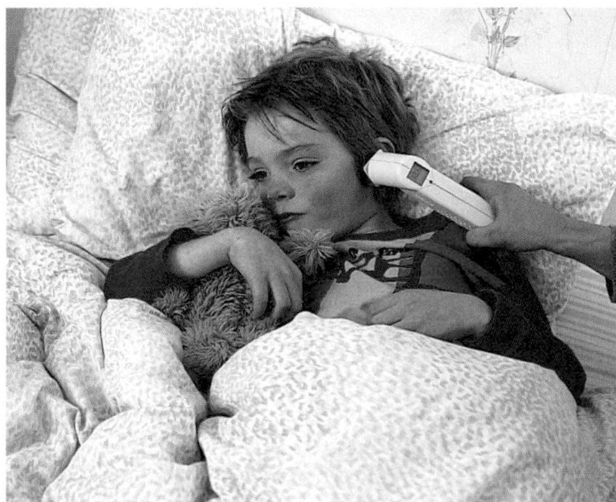

A very high temperature is one symptom of septicaemia and can be accompanied by a rash. It is crucial to recognise the signs as early as possible.

Causes

Septicaemia is caused by harmful germs (typically bacteria) entering the blood.

- These germs commonly enter the bloodstream through small sites such as a cut or through the mouth, but are usually destroyed by the immune system.
- However, if germs enter the bloodstream in large numbers from a major source of infection such as a kidney infection, blood poisoning can occur.
- Septicaemia can develop as a result of a complication of any serious infectious disease.
- The toxins released by the germs cause a cascade of reactions in the body, leading to widespread cell and tissue damage, low blood pressure (shock), organ failure and ultimately death.
- Although bacteria are the main cause of septicaemia, other germs such as viruses and even fungi may be a cause.

Diagnosis

If a child appears to have septicaemia, doctors must work fast to treat the child and prevent circulatory collapse (shock). They will also try to establish the organism which is responsible for the infection and where it has entered the body.

- A medical history will be taken and the doctor will ask the parents whether the child has had any recent infections, such as a kidney infection, which might have spread.
- The doctor will carry out a physical examination, looking for any wounds.
- Samples of body fluids such as blood and urine will be taken. These will be examined in the hospital laboratory in order to identify the germs that may be causing the infection.
- Tests will be carried out to monitor the level of oxygen in the blood. If this drops too low the child's life is at risk.
- A sample of spinal fluid may need to be taken for analysis by inserting a needle into the lower back.
- In many cases, the condition may deteriorate too rapidly for tests to be carried out. The doctors will make a diagnosis of septicaemia and emergency treatment will proceed accordingly.

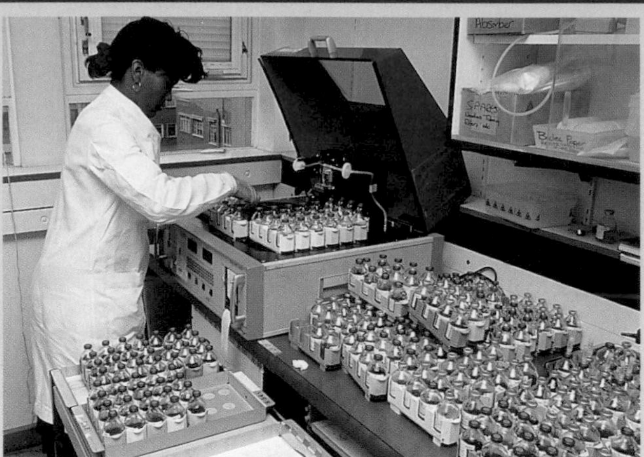

In order to discover the germs responsible for causing septicaemia, a number of tests, such as examining samples of body fluids, may be carried out.

Treatment

It is critical that treatment begins as soon as possible to prevent further damage to the body. If a doctor suspects that a child has septicaemia, the child will be admitted to the hospital intensive care unit for immediate treatment.

1. Intravenous antibiotics will be delivered into the bloodstream to combat harmful bacteria.
2. Once the precise bacteria has been determined by blood tests, a more specific antibiotic will be given.
3. Intravenous fluids will be administered to prevent shock and to maintain the delivery of essential nutrients to the organs, and the delivery of oxygen to the tissue.
4. Drugs may be given to restore blood pressure.
5. Oxygen may be given if the child has low oxygen levels or signs of shock.
6. Abscesses will be drained, or any dead or severely infected body tissue will be removed.
7. Blood pressure, blood oxygen levels and heart rate are monitored.

How can it be prevented?

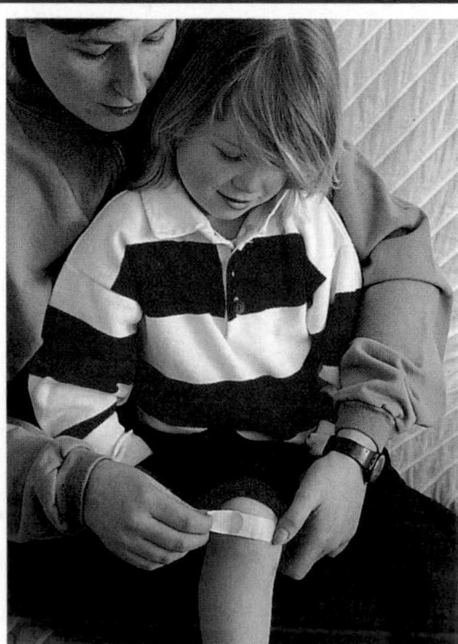

Septicaemia usually develops quickly and without warning. However, there are a number of measures which may prevent it in the first place.

1. Prevent infection of wounds by keeping them sterile at all times. Use plasters to prevent bacteria entering minor wounds and ensure that the wound is clean underneath by cleaning with cooled boiled water or a dilute antiseptic lotion such as TCP.
2. If it looks infected, the wound will be treated with oral antibiotics.

Septicaemia can be caused by germs passing into the bloodstream via a wound or cut. For this reason, it is important to clean wounds thoroughly and to cover them with a plaster.

3. Follow antibiotic courses carefully, making sure that your child takes the correct dosage and completes the course. This will help to prevent existing infections spreading to the bloodstream.
4. Recognise the early signs of infection, such as flu symptoms or an upset tummy and aching muscles and joints.
5. Septicaemia is prevented in hospitals through control measures, such as isolation and barrier nursing, that prevent the spread of infection from one patient to another.

SICKLE-CELL ANAEMIA

WHAT IS SICKLE-CELL ANAEMIA?

Sickle-cell anaemia is an incurable genetic disorder that can only be passed on from parent to child. Sickle-cell disease mainly affects people of African and Caribbean origin (about one in 200). It also occurs in people of Indian, Middle Eastern and Mediterranean origin – all places where malaria has been prevalent in the past.

- Sickled cells (the cells are curved in a sickle shape) are thought to have evolved as a natural defence against certain types of malaria.
- There are an estimated 6000 sufferers of sickle-cell anaemia in Britain, and as many as 30,000 people may be carrying the sickle-cell gene.

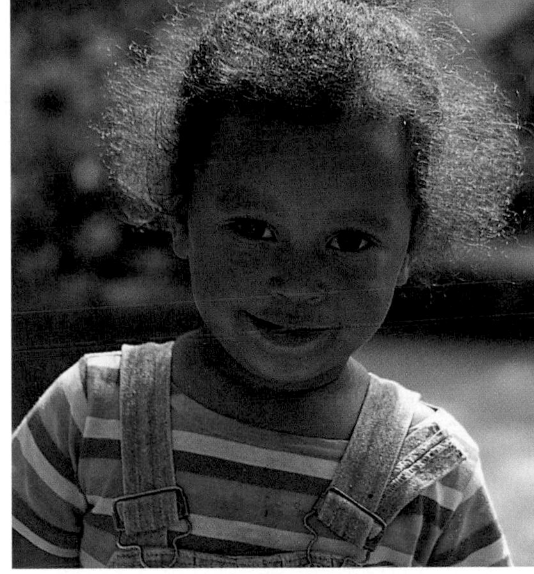

Sickle-cell anaemia is an hereditary disease that can affect people of African, Mediterranean, Indian or Middle Eastern descent.

Why it occurs

Sickle-cell disease is caused by a disorder of the haemoglobin (a protein contained in the red blood cells), which circulates oxygen around the body.

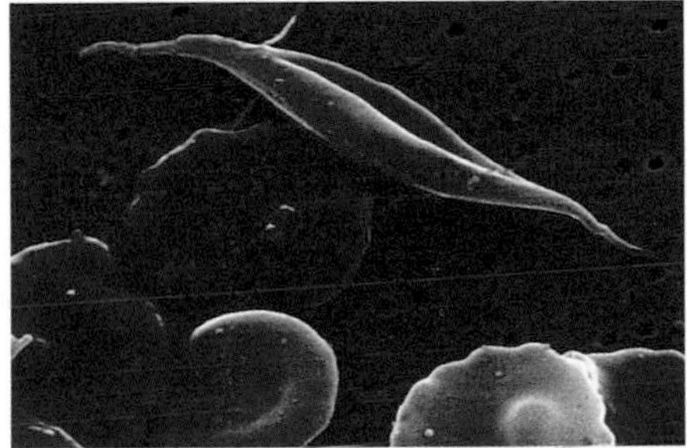

Sickled cells have difficulty passing through small blood vessels because of their long, sickle shape. This hinders the movement of oxygen through the blood.

- After releasing the oxygen, 'sickled' haemoglobin molecules stick together to form rigid rods, giving the red blood cells a sickle or banana shape (unlike normal red blood cells, which are flexible and doughnut-shaped). This hard sickle shape makes it difficult for these blood cells to squeeze through small blood vessels.
- Severe blockages can result, which cause intense pain and can damage internal organs. These blockages are known as 'sickling crises'.
- Sufferers often have chronic anaemia, because 'sickled' red blood cells do not live as long as normal cells. This makes sufferers easily fatigued and more susceptible to infection. They may also have headaches, disturbed sleep, palpitations and cuts that are slow to heal.

Sickle-cell trait

Sickle-cell disease can only be inherited by people whose parents both carry the sickle-cell trait.

- People who have one sickled haemoglobin gene and one normal haemoglobin gene will not develop full sickle-cell disease, but may have the sickle-cell trait. In this case, the normal gene keeps the red blood cells sufficiently flexible to avoid sickling crises. However, extra care must be taken in situations where oxygen is restricted, for example, under general anaesthetic, at high altitudes or when scuba-diving.
- If both parents have the sickle-cell trait, their children will have a one in four chance of inheriting the full disease. If only one parent has the sickle-cell trait, their offspring will inherit at least one non-sickled haemoglobin gene and will not suffer from the full disease.

Symptoms

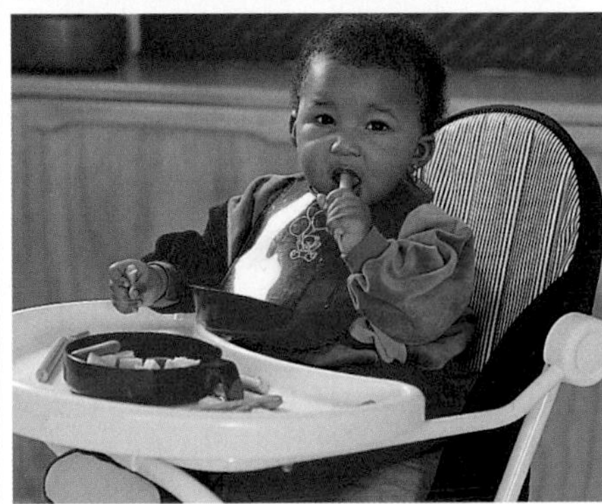

The symptoms of sickle-cell anaemia don't usually become apparent before the age of four to six months. Most sufferers, or 'sicklers', can lead a completely normal life in between crises.

The symptoms of sickle-cell anaemia can vary in frequency and intensity.

- One of the first signs is often a painful symmetrical swelling of the hands and feet, known as 'hand and foot syndrome', or dactylitis.

Other symptoms include:

- Frequent infections
- Mild jaundice (yellowing of the whites of the eyes)
- Delays in growth
- Frequent bedwetting
- Extreme tiredness
- Pain in the limbs, back and stomach (in older children)
- Painful joints

Testing for sickle cell

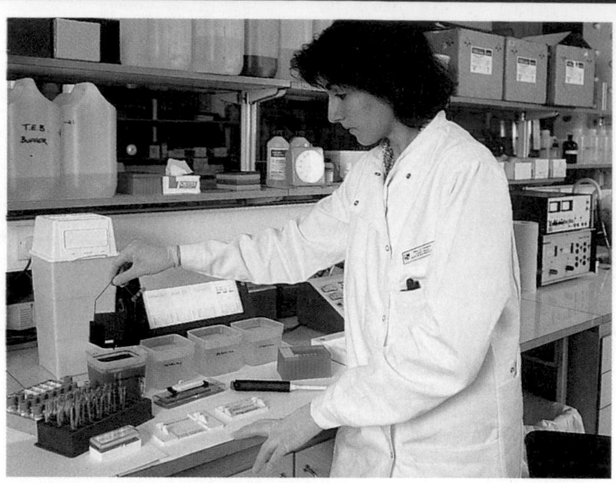

A blood count and a test called a haemoglobin electrophoresis are necessary to assess whether sickle-cell trait or disease is present.

- Unborn babies can be tested for sickle-cell disorder while in the mother's uterus, by an amniocentesis test or chorionic villus sampling (CVS).

The heel prick (Guthrie) blood test done on babies at six to nine days of age is used to screen at-risk populations.

- In an amniocentesis test, a needle is inserted into the woman's uterus to obtain a sample of amniotic fluid. The results are available in three to four weeks.

- In a CVS test, a small sample is taken from the placenta, via the cervix or a needle into the uterus. The results are available within one week.

Preventing a sickling crisis

Sickling crises are most commonly triggered by dehydration, lack of warmth or exhaustion. Other triggers vary from person to person.

1 It is vital that your sickler child drinks 1–1½ litres of fluid each day. This can be partially supplied by soups and fruit.

2 Your child should be kept warm and dry whenever possible.

3 He should have regular dental check-ups. Make sure that your dentist knows he has sickle-cell disease.

4 Complaints of tiredness should be taken seriously and your child should be allowed to rest.

5 Cuts and infections should be treated promptly.

6 Encourage regular exercise, as it helps strengthen your child's heart and circulation. A sufferer should swim in heated pools or warm wateronly.

What medication may be given?

Sickle-cell disease cannot be cured, but certain medications can ease some of the symptoms.

- Sickle-cell sufferers are advised to take regular doses of penicillin as a preventative measure against infections that can cause sickle crises.

- Folic acid, found in green leafy vegetables and available in tablet supplements, can help chronic anaemia sufferers.

- Painkillers such as paracetamol are needed to reduce pain experienced during crises. However, it is essential that the correct dose is given, especially in young children.

- Blood transfusions may be necessary in severe crises.

Treating a sickling crisis

Try to recognise the signs of an impending crisis. These may include a headache, drowsiness, severe chest or abdominal pain or stiffness in the neck. If your child has a sickle-cell crisis, make sure he is as comfortable as possible.

- Try to support painful areas.

- Young children should be held or gently rocked.

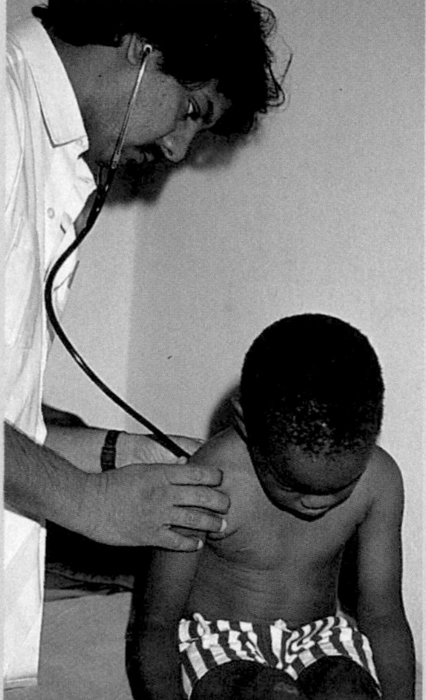

- Increase circulation and body warmth by rubbing and massage. Hot-water bottles and deep-heat creams can also be helpful.

- Encourage complete rest and relaxation. Deep breathing exercises can reduce anxiety and help to relieve pain.

- Administer painkillers in safe doses according to the age of your child. Ask your doctor for advice on dosage.

- In any crises, call your GP. Hospital treatment may be necessary in severe cases.

A child with sickle cell will need to have regular health check-ups and blood tests to monitor the condition.

Useful address

- The Sickle Cell Society can be contacted at 54 Station Road, Harlesden, London, NW10 4UA.
Tel: 020 8961 7795
Fax: 020 8961 8346 E-mail: info@sicklecellsociety.org

- The Sickle Cell Society has an informative website at www.sicklecellsociety.org. It also has links to Planet Sickle, a website where junior sicklers can meet and share their experiences of the disease.

SPINA BIFIDA

WHAT IS SPINA BIFIDA?

Spina bifida is a congenital abnormality in which one or more of the vertebrae (the bones which form the backbone) fails to form properly, leaving part of the spinal cord exposed.

- Spina bifida occurs most commonly in the lower back but it may affect other sections of the spine. The severity of the condition depends on how much of the nerve tissue is exposed.

- Due to the general use of screening and prevention programmes and the use of termination following antenatal scans, spina bifida is rare. However, each year in the UK, about 1200 pregnancies are affected by neural tube defects, resulting in around 175 babies born with spina bifida.

- Although the precise cause of spina bifida is unknown, vitamin deficiency seems to be one of the main factors involved. Folic acid supplementation prior to conception appears to reduce the risk of spina bifida in pregnancy.

- Spina bifida is a defect present at birth and is only partially hereditary. However, once there has been an affected pregnancy, there is an increased risk of further spina bifida pregnancies.

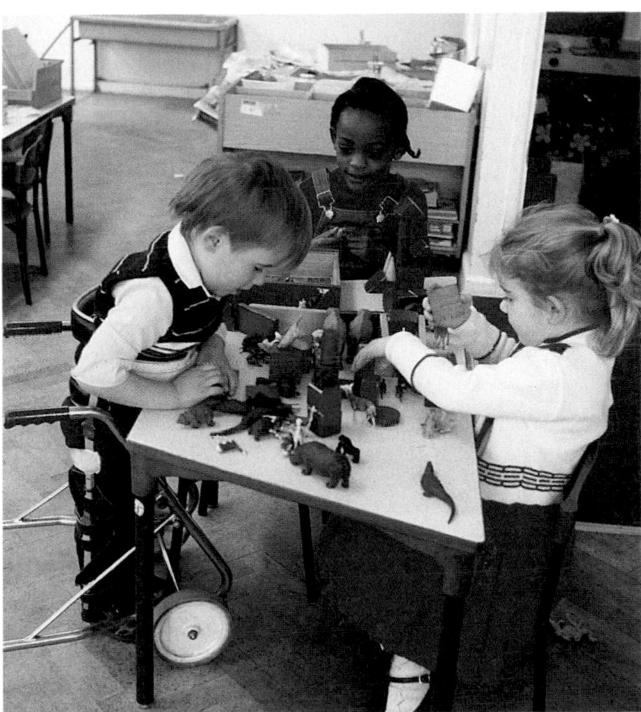

Spina bifida, which develops in the baby during pregnancy, is a gap in the backbone. The condition can cause paralysis of the legs.

Types of spina bifida

There are two main types of spina bifida: spina bifida occulta and spina bifida cystica. A third kind, cranium bifida, is extremely rare.

1 Spina bifida occulta: this is the most common and the least serious form of spina bifida in which there is only a slight deficiency in the formation of one of the vertebrae. The majority of people suffering from spina bifida occulta have no symptoms or problems; one in 1000 may be more severely affected and experience significant difficulties.

2 Spina bifida cystica (cyst-like): in this type, the bone defect is greater. The visible signs are a sac or cyst on the back covered by a thin layer of skin. There are two forms: meningocele and myelomeningocele. In meningocele, the sac contains the tissues that cover the spinal cord and cerebrospinal fluid (which bathes and protects the brain and spinal cord). The nerves are not usually damaged and are able to function, therefore there is often little disability present. Myelomeningocele is the most severe form of spina bifida. Here the sac not only contains the meninges and cerebrospinal fluid but also nerves and a malformed spinal cord. This child is likely to be severely handicapped.

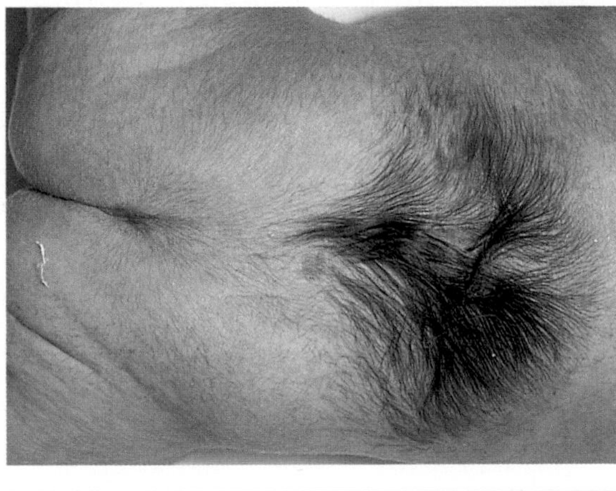

As many as one in 10 people suffer from spina bifida occulta. In the more severe cases there may be a birthmark, hairy patch or dimple over the affected area.

Symptoms

In spina bifida occulta there are often no symptoms or problems, but in spina bifida cystica symptoms can include:

- Partial or complete leg paralysis, with loss of sensation in all areas below the defect.

- Hip dislocation and other leg abnormalities.

- Hydrocephalus (excess cerebrospinal fluid in the skull) is common and without treatment may result in brain damage. Associated abnormalities include cerebral palsy, epilepsy, learning disabilities and visual problems.

- Bladder problems: paralysis of the bladder leads to incontinence or retention of urine, infections and eventual kidney damage. The anus may also be paralysed causing chronic constipation and leakage of faeces.

How is it detected?

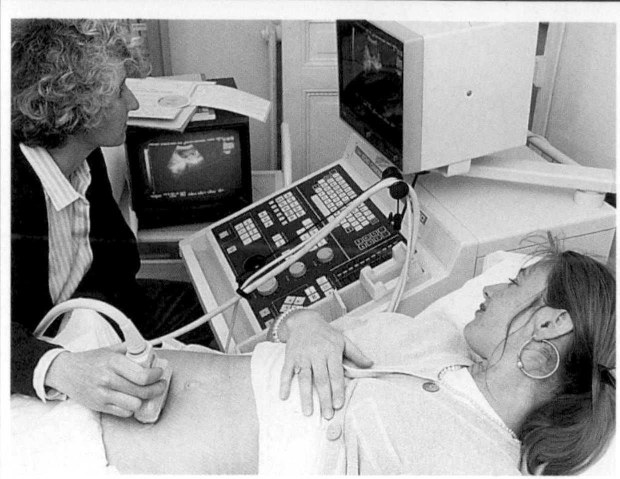

Neural tube defects such as spina bifida can be detected by routine tests during pregnancy.

- A neural tube defect can often be identified at an early stage in the pregnancy by ultrasound scanning.

- High levels of alpha-foetoprotein (AFP) in the maternal blood or amniotic fluid during amniocentesis may indicate spina bifida.

An early scan can identify a severe spinal defect in an unborn baby. The parents must then decide whether to continue the pregnancy.

- After birth, spina bifida cystica is easily recognisable by the protruding sac on the baby's back. Spina bifida occulta can be diagnosed by an X-ray of the spinal column, but this is often only performed if symptoms such as bladder and bowel problems develop in later life.

Treatment

1 If the spinal abnormality is not severe, surgery can correct the defect. This should be done within the first few days of life.

2 If the defect is more severe, surgery may be performed to save the child's life but may not be able to prevent severe physical or mental disability.

3 In a child with hydrocephalus, a shunt (a tube and valve mechanism) is inserted into the brain to relieve the build-up of fluid.

How to prevent spina bifida

To prevent her baby developing spina bifida, a woman should increase her intake of folic acid.

- Take a 400 microgram folic acid supplement for at least one month before you plan to conceive, and up to 12 weeks into the pregnancy.

- Eat more foods that are naturally high in folic acid, such as granary bread and green vegetables, and do not overcook them!

- If you have had a pregnancy affected by spina bifida, you should seek genetic counselling before trying to conceive again. You will be given a higher dose of folic acid before you conceive and the AFP levels in your blood will be closely monitored.

Make sure you eat plenty of food that is rich in folic acid, such as broccoli, sprouts and spring greens.

Living with spina bifida

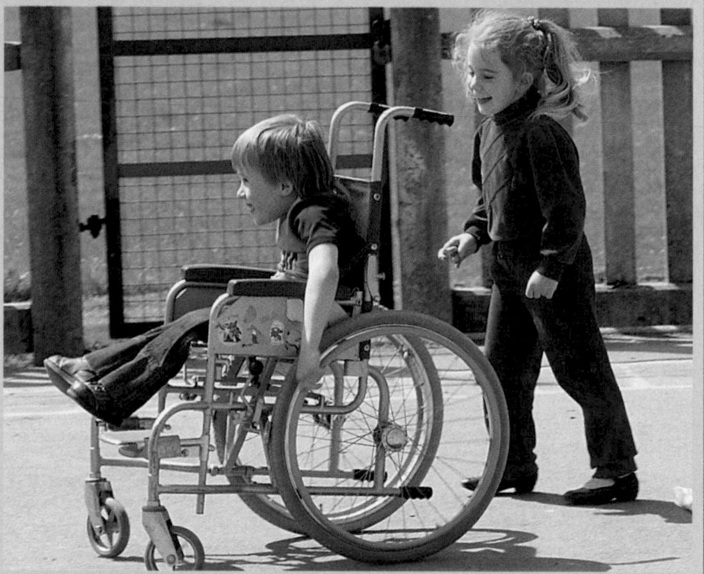

- Most people with spina bifida have some degree of neuropathic bladder and bowel – when nerve damage affects the functioning of the bladder and bowel. Urinary retention or incontinence may be relieved by the insertion of a catheter into the bladder. Chronic constipation may also be a problem and laxative drugs may be needed. The child should drink plenty of fluid to prevent urinary infections and constipation. He should also be encouraged to eat food with a high fibre content, such as cereals, prunes and puréed fruits.

Children with spina bifida can lead relatively normal lives (40 per cent attend mainstream schools). However, they may need special schooling depending on their disability.

- Frequent hospital visits may be necessary, especially if a child has hydrocephalus. Parents will receive specialist training to help them identify any complications in their child's condition.

- Physiotherapy encourages mobility and independence. Wheelchairs and other mobility aids may be required for more severely affected children.

THALASSAEMIA

WHAT IS THALASSAEMIA?

Thalassaemia is a rare inherited blood disease. An affected child inherits one or more faulty genes from a parent and as a result develops anaemia that ranges from mild to severe.

- There are two main types of thalassaemia – alpha-thalassaemia and beta-thalassaemia.
- Beta-thalassaemia is by far the more common form of the disease.
- Thalassaemia mainly affects people from Mediterranean countries, the Middle East, Southeast Asia and Africa.
- Couples from these countries who are considering starting a family may be offered genetic counselling to discuss the likelihood of their children being affected by the disease.

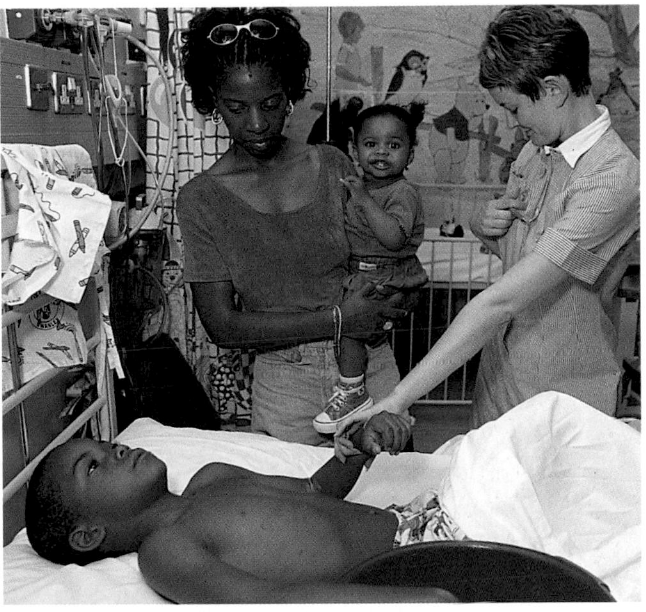

Thalassaemia is a rare blood disease that causes anaemia. A child with this condition will be given regular blood tests and, in severe cases, blood transfusions.

What causes the condition?

Haemoglobin is a pigment in the red blood cells, which carries vital oxygen around the circulation and delivers it to all the cells in the body. In thalassaemia, a child has low levels of haemoglobin – a condition known as anaemia – and this means that there is not enough oxygen available for the body's tissues to function properly.

- **Alpha chains:** in each normal haemoglobin molecule there are four 'chains' of protein – two alpha chains and two beta chains. In thalassaemia, an inherited defect means that one or more of these chains of protein is missing, so that a child has defective haemoglobin molecules in the red blood cells. Because the haemoglobin is not normal, the red cells are broken down prematurely by the spleen.
- **Alpha-thalassaemia:** this rare form of the disease occurs when one or more of the four genes that create the alpha chain is absent.
- **Beta-thalassaemia:** this more common form of thalassaemia occurs when the responsible genes are present but are faulty. The severity of the condition will be determined by the number of genes that are affected.

How is thalassaemia passed on?

Every individual has thousands of genes – normally there are two copies of each gene, one from each parent. These genes are made up of DNA, a substance that provides instructions on how the body will develop and function. If one of the genes is missing or faulty, it can sometimes cause a disease or a birth defect.

1 Beta-thalassaemia: if a child inherits the thalassaemia gene from only one parent, then the symptoms may be absent (the child is a carrier only and can pass the disease on) or very mild. If, however, the gene is inherited from both parents, then the condition is more serious and is known as beta-thalassaemia major.

2 Alpha-thalassaemia: between one and four of the alpha chain genes are lost when the mother's and father's genetic material is mixed during egg fertilisation.

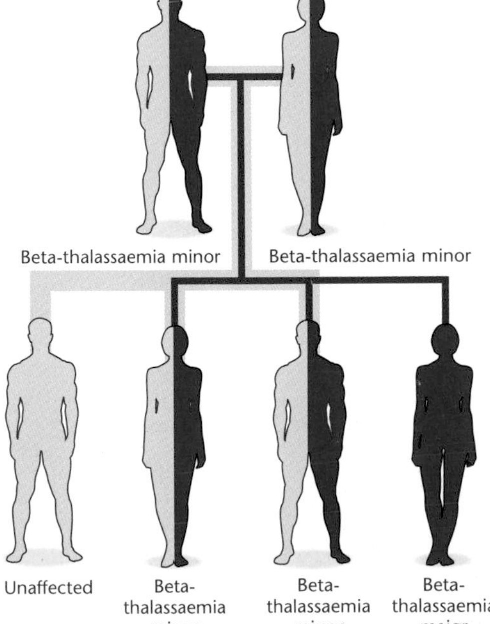

People with beta-thalassaemia minor carry one normal gene and one thalassaemic gene, each of which they can pass on to their offspring.

KEY
- Normal gene
- Thalassaemic gene

Symptoms

The symptoms of both alpha- and beta-thalassaemia vary from being so mild as to be undetectable, to very severe. In the worst form of alpha-thalassaemia, the affected foetus dies. There are two sub-divisions of beta-thalassaemia; beta-thalassaemia minor (children usually have no symptoms and the condition may only be discovered by chance during a routine blood test) and beta-thalassaemia major, which is very serious and can be life-threatening.

1 A child affected with the blood disorder may appear lethargic and pale.

2 He may have a poor appetite and fail to gain weight.

3 A blood test will show anaemia, which could vary from mild to severe.

4 The skin may have a yellow tinge (jaundice).

5 The child's abdomen may seem swollen due to an enlarged spleen. This happens because the spleen is working overtime to destroy abnormal red blood cells. It then grows bigger to cope with the increased workload.

6 As a child gets older, the bones, especially those in the head and face, become thicker and enlarge. This is because the body is trying to compensate for the lack of haemoglobin by producing more blood cells, making the bone marrow work overtime and expand.

7 If the type of alpha-thalassaemia occurs where all four genes are missing, the baby will die before birth.

Treatment

The only treatment for thalassaemia is to keep haemoglobin levels within the normal range. There is no cure for the disease itself.

- A child with thalassaemia will have regular blood tests to check the levels of haemoglobin. Regular blood transfusions are essential in the more serious forms of the disease and are carried out in the hospital, usually in a day-care unit.

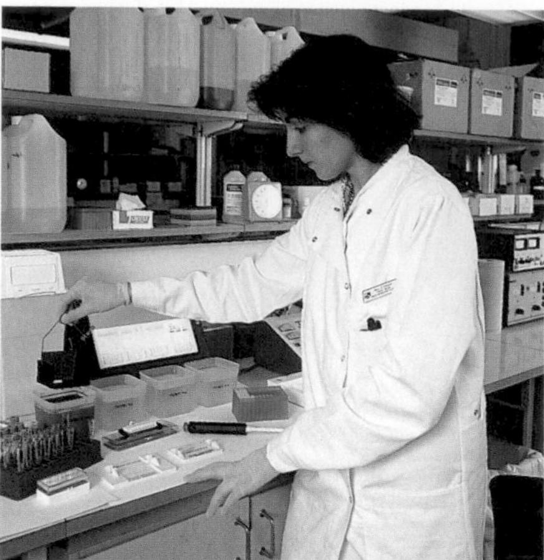

A child with thalassaemia needs to have regular blood tests to monitor his levels of haemoglobin. He may also require regular blood transfusions.

- Regular blood transfusions can lead to an accumulation of iron in the body, which is toxic to the vital organs. To combat this, a drug called desferrioxamine is given either directly into the bloodstream or through a small pump that gradually injects the drug just under the skin.

- Occasionally, it is necessary to remove the spleen of a child with thalassaemia. If this is the case then the child's ability to fight infection will be reduced as the spleen also plays a role in the immune system. Doctors may prescribe long-term antibiotics.

- In some children, a bone marrow transplant is possible from a healthy sibling with a compatible tissue type.

Detecting thalassaemia antenatally

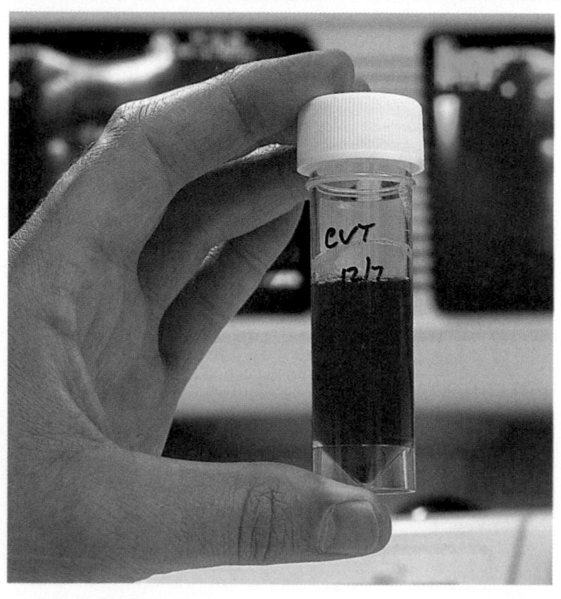

There are two ways that thalassaemia can be diagnosed before birth. However, these tests are only usually carried out if it is known that the parent is a thalassaemia carrier – they can pass the abnormal gene on to their children but do not themselves have symptoms of the disease.

- In a chorionic villus sampling (CVS) test performed in the third month of pregnancy, a small sample is taken from the placenta, via the cervix or a needle into the uterus. The results are available within one week.

To determine whether or not an unborn baby has thalassaemia, chorionic villus sampling (CVS) may be carried out.

- During the second three months of pregnancy, a blood sample can be taken directly from the baby's circulation and analysed for the abnormal gene.

- Both these procedures carry risks for the baby and consequently are not undertaken unless it is absolutely necessary.

THREADWORM

WHAT IS A THREADWORM?

A threadworm is a parasitic roundworm that invades humans and lives in their intestines, surviving on the nutrients in the faeces.

- Its scientific name is enterobius vermicularis, which is why the threadworm infection is sometimes called enterobiasis.
- Threadworm infection occurs all over the world, but is particularly common in temperate and cool climates, such as Europe.
- Because of the way it is spread, threadworm infection is more common in children, and in people living in crowded living conditions, institutions or communities.

The threadworm inhabits the human intestine, can grow up to 12mm (about ½in) long and lays eggs around the anus which causes itching. It is very common in children, but is usually easily treated.

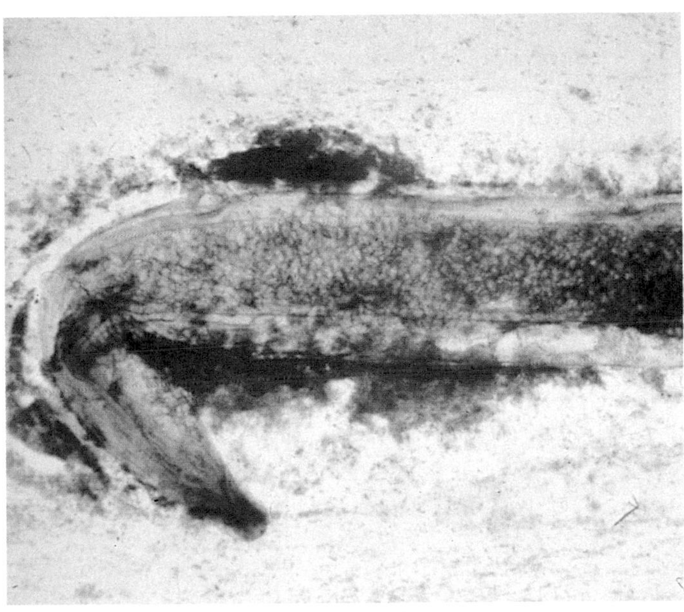

What is a parasite?

A parasite is a creature that lives in or on another living organism, such as a human being.

- Parasites get their food and shelter from their host, and do not provide any benefit to the host in return.
- The types of parasites that affect humans are fungi (such as those that cause athlete's foot), viruses, bacteria, 'protozoa' (single-celled organisms that can cause illnesses such as malaria) and, lastly, 'helminths' (worms).
- There are three main types of helminths: nematodes (roundworms), cestodes (tapeworms) and trematodes (flukes, or flatworms). Threadworms are a type of nematode. Nematodes are distinguishable from other helminths as they have cylindrical bodies that are unsegmented.

Symptoms

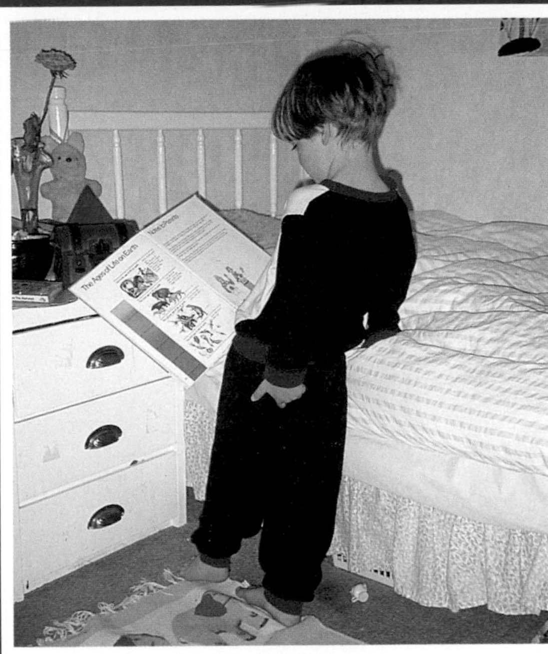

A child with a threadworm infection will experience itching around the anal area, which in turn may become uncomfortable and sore.

The problem with threadworm is that it often has few, if any, symptoms and therefore frequently goes undetected. It is important to be aware of the signs though, to enable you to catch it early and stop the infection spreading.

1. When symptoms develop, they are usually first detected when a child complains of persistent itching in the anal area, which can lead to it becoming very sore.
2. In girls, the itching can spread to the vulval area.
3. You may notice tiny white thread-like worms in the stools, and on examination of the anal area at night.
4. Itching is particularly noticeable at night as this is when the worms become active around the anus.
5. A child may become irritable and overtired as a result of broken sleep.
6. Very rarely, if the infection is extremely severe, the worms can cause superficial damage to the lining of the intestine. In these cases, abscesses can develop.

How threadworm is spread

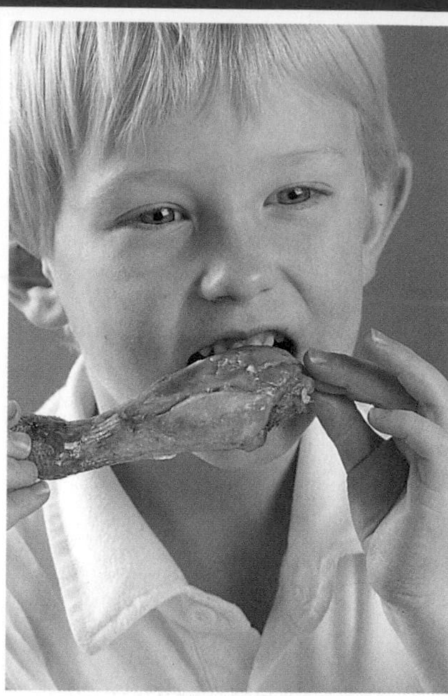

Humans are the only hosts for the threadworm. It is unable to survive outside the body, although its eggs can. The threadworm has a distinct life cycle and children can continually re-infect themselves and, by the same means, each other.

1 The first step in the cycle occurs when a child with the infection scratches his bottom and consequently eggs become tucked under the fingernails.

2 The next stage occurs as the child then either puts his fingers in his mouth or he handles food, which he then eats – along with the eggs.

A child who has the threadworm infection can easily re-infect himself, commonly by scratching and then handling food. This process is called auto-infection.

3 The eggs are easily spread from one person to another through the child sharing his food or eating utensils with family members, classmates or friends.

4 Eggs will often find their way on to bath towels, which are then shared.

5 Once the eggs are in the intestine, they hatch into worms.

6 To complete the cycle, the mature worms move to the anus at night-time where they lay their eggs.

Diagnosing threadworm

Even when your child complains of itching, and threadworm is suspected, it may be difficult to diagnose the condition, because the worms remain in the intestine for most of the time. It is only by seeing them or their eggs that a definite diagnosis can be made.

- The GP will want to check that there is no other reason for your child's itching, for example a localised infection or an allergy to soaps or washing powders.

- At night, the female worms move down the intestine to the anus and lay thousands of eggs. They use special 'glue' to stick the eggs on to the skin so that they are secure. It is during sleep, therefore, that the worms can be detected.

- The doctor may suggest examining the anal area in a sleeping child. Sometimes the worms are visible to the naked eye – they resemble tiny white pieces of thread or cotton about 5–10mm (up to ½in) long.

- If the worms are not visible to the naked eye, a piece of clear tape can be applied to the anal area. When the tape is removed and examined under a microscope, the eggs can be seen.

Treating and preventing threadworm

Once discovered, the threadworms need to be killed to avoid re-infection. Threadworms are easily treated and your doctor will prescribe a simple and effective medication.

- A single dose of a drug called mebendazole is usually all that is needed to eradicate the worms. The drug is taken as a single tablet, which is then repeated a fortnight later to make absolutely sure that the worms have been killed.

- Mebendazole is not suitable for children under two years of age and so an alternative treatment is available. This drug is called piperazine and it works by paralysing the worms in the gut, so that they are naturally passed out in the faeces.

- It is vital that the entire family are treated to avoid re-infection, so your doctor will prescribe enough drugs for everyone.

- You should thoroughly wash all your linen and towels as eggs can linger in these places. You should also ensure that your child washes his hands thoroughly before eating.

It is recommended that you vacuum often and regularly to pick up any stray eggs. Threadworm is highly contagious and all the eggs must be killed to prevent re-infection.

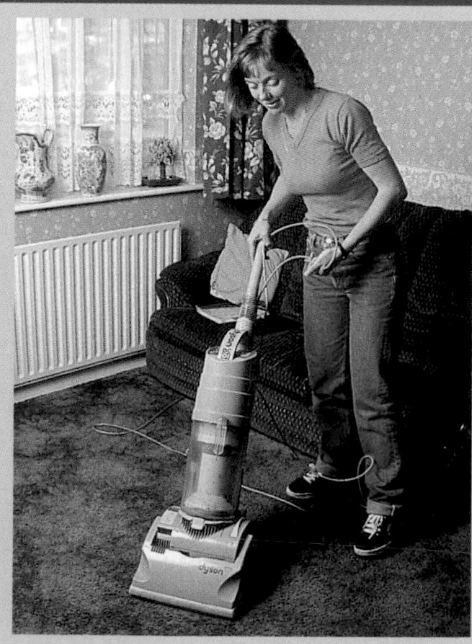

TONSILLITIS

WHAT IS TONSILLITIS?

The tonsils are a pair of small glands that lie at the back of the throat, above the tongue. Their job is to protect the body from harmful bacteria and viruses that may try to enter through the nose and mouth.

- Tonsillitis is the name given to an infection of the tonsils. It occurs when the tonsils become overwhelmed by harmful germs that infect both of the tonsils and the surrounding throat.

- Tonsillitis is most common in young children, but adults can get it too.

- The most common cause of tonsillitis is a viral infection. However, about one in five cases will be due to a particular type of harmful bacteria called streptococci. Other causes, which include glandular fever, are rare.

- Tonsillitis can be contagious – the germ is spread through coughing, sneezing and touching. This means it can be a particular problem where there is close contact between children, such as in nurseries or schools.

- In the past, bacterial tonsillitis sometimes led to serious conditions, such as rheumatic fever and kidney disease. This is now rare because of treatment with antibiotics.

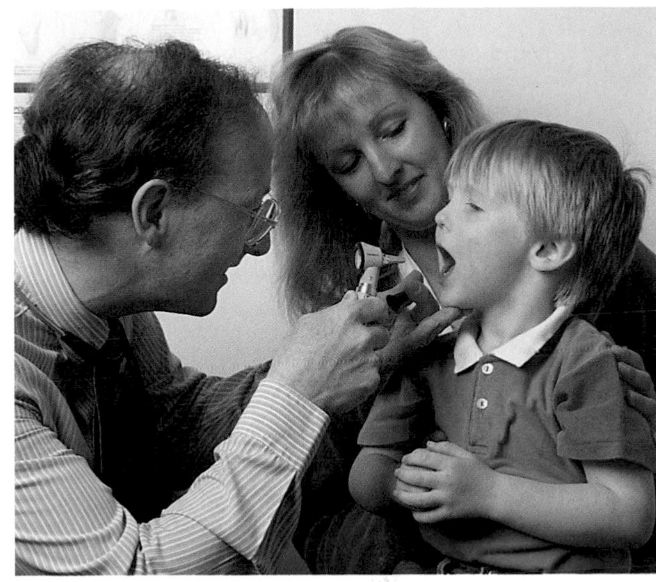

- Around 50,000 tonsillectomies are performed each year in the UK, mainly for recurrent tonsillitis.

If a child has suspected tonsillitis, the doctor will examine his throat to check whether the tonsils are red or inflamed.

Symptoms

These can range from a mild sore throat to side-effects that cause your child to feel poorly. Signs that your child has tonsillitis include:

- **Sore throat:** ranging from a tickle to pain when swallowing.
- **Difficulty swallowing:** can lead to drooling in a young child, and a reluctance to eat or drink.
- **Fever:** a temperature of 37.5°C (100°F) or above, lasting a few days.
- **Hoarse voice:** results from the sore throat.
- **Inflamed throat:** your child's throat may look red and sore. The tonsils may appear swollen, with white purulent areas.
- **Headache:** may be accompanied by a general feeling of being unwell.
- **Tender glands:** the glands in the neck and around the jaw may be tender and swollen.
- **Tummy ache:** common sign, sometimes accompanied by nausea and vomiting.

When to call the doctor

If your child has a sore throat, but does not seem too unwell, then simple steps such as giving paracetamol may be all he needs. However, you should take your child to the GP if:

1. Swallowing is becoming more difficult, especially if he is finding it hard to drink.
2. He has trouble breathing through his mouth, which often begins as noisy breathing.
3. Your child's temperature rises above 39°C (102°F) or if it stays above 37.5°C (100°F) for longer than two days.
4. He is very poorly and distressed by his condition.
5. This is a recurring problem and your child is spending a lot of time away from school or nursery.

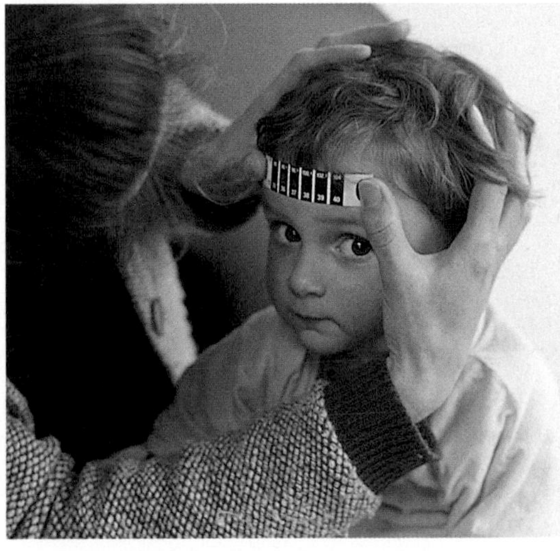

If your child has severe throat problems or repeated bouts of tonsillitis, your GP may refer him to an ear, nose and throat (ENT) specialist.

Many bouts of tonsillitis are mild, but monitor your child's temperature if you suspect that it is more serious.

What the doctor will do

You should probably make an appointment to take your child to the doctor if he has a sore throat, but bear in mind that most sore throats are due to viruses and cannot be cured by antibiotics. To diagnose and prescribe treatment for tonsillitis, the GP will do the following:

- The GP will ask you questions about your child's symptoms, especially whether he has had difficulty swallowing and breathing.
- He will look inside your child's mouth with a small torch – you can help by reassuring your child and holding him still on your lap.
- The GP may want to take a swab that can be examined at the hospital laboratory. The swab, a piece of sterile cotton wool on a stick, is gently rubbed against the infected area inside the mouth.
- If a diagnosis of bacterial tonsillitis is likely, an antibiotic will probably be prescribed. Inform your GP if you think your child is allergic to penicillin, because this is the most effective antibiotic in the treatment of throat infections.
- Your child will be referred to a specialist if a tonsillectomy is needed. But there may be a waiting-list for an appointment and the operation.

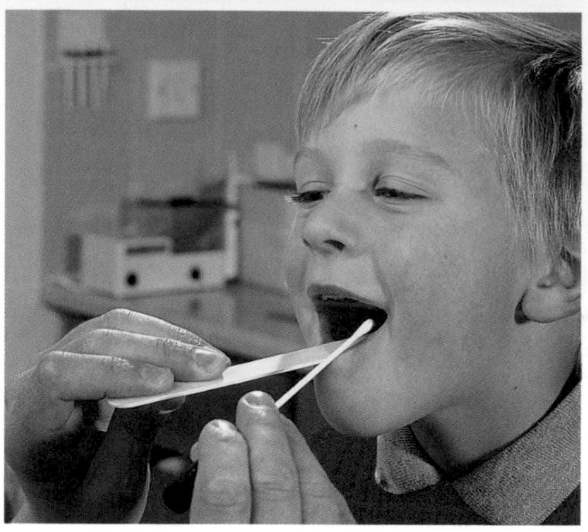

If your child has recurrent sore throats, the GP may take a sample from his throat with a swab. This is to identify the micro-organism that has caused the infection and should not be painful.

Home nursing

Tonsillitis can be very distressing for a young child, however mild the bout, but there are steps you can take to make him more comfortable and ease any pain.

1 Give paracetamol syrup, such as Calpol. This will relieve the pain of a sore throat as well as helping to lower a raised temperature.

2 Make sure your child drinks plenty of liquids.

3 Give nourishing liquids, such as soup and milkshakes, if your child finds it difficult to swallow.

4 If antibiotics have been prescribed, make sure that your child takes the whole course, even if he seems well again. If the antibiotics are stopped too soon, the infection may come back.

5 Encourage your child to rest quietly while he is feeling unwell or if he has a raised temperature.

6 Avoid contact with other children and wash your own hands well after tending to him.

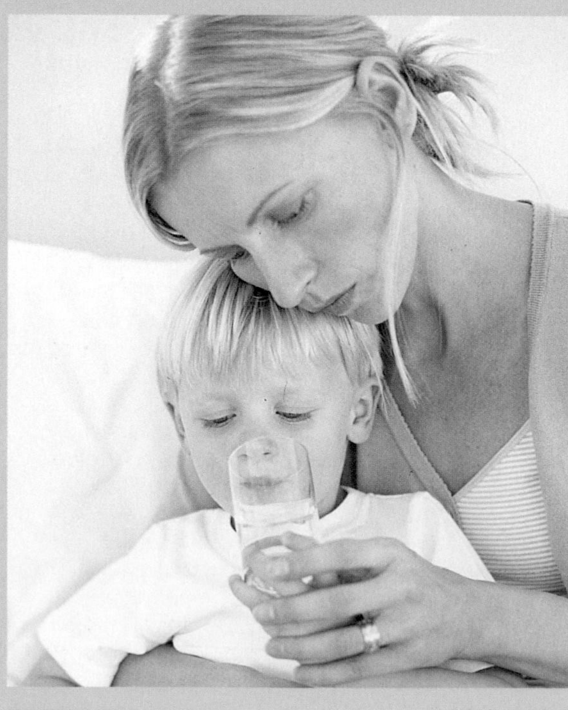

Increasing your child's fluid intake is a very effective way to relieve the symptoms of mild tonsillitis. If he isn't responding to steps you are taking at home, seek medical advice.

A tonsillectomy

Most simple cases of tonsillitis are treated with antibiotics, and surgery is only used in certain circumstances.

- It used to be very common for children to have their tonsils removed, with an operation known as a tonsillectomy, in the days before reliable antibiotics were available.
- Now the operation may be performed when the child has repeated bouts of tonsillitis over a period of time; usually where the child has four to six episodes of tonsillitis each year for two to three years. This is because being repeatedly ill may adversely affect a child's schooling.
- A tonsillectomy may also be performed when the tonsils are too large and cause problems with breathing and swallowing.
- Sometimes the operation is necessary due to the presence of an abscess on the tonsil.

TRAVEL SICKNESS

WHAT IS TRAVEL SICKNESS?

Travel sickness is the general term used to describe nausea associated with any form of transport – usually cars, ships or planes. It can range from that slight queasy feeling when you try to read a map in the car, to the incapacitating vomiting and dehydration that may affect ship passengers on their way through choppy waters.

A more accurate name for travel sickness is motion sickness, and the symptoms are numerous. These include increased salivation, pallor (looking pale), sweating, headache, lack of energy, yawning and hyperventilation (rapid breathing).

While the thought of a long journey with a child who's prone to sickness may seem daunting, it need not be impossible. There are effective treatments available from your local pharmacy, who can advise you. Follow the travel tips overleaf to help reduce symptoms.

Travel sickness is often worse on a ship. Staying outside in the open air, rather than in a stuffy cabin, can help relieve your child's symptoms. Standing in the middle of the ship on a low deck also helps – that is where there is least movement.

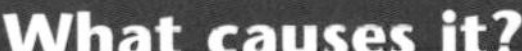

What causes it?

There are two main theories as to why people suffer from travel sickness. One puts it down to over-stimulation of the body's balance mechanism in the inner ear by unaccustomed types of movement, e.g. the side-to-side swaying of a ship.

The second theory attributes it to a conflict between the messages received by the brain from the balance mechanism in the ear, and the information it gets from the eyes. If you're sitting on a ferry in a gale, the balance mechanism in your ears tells you that you are being moved from side to side. Your eyes, however, are telling you that you're really sitting still reading your magazine. This conflict triggers the area of your brain that controls vomiting.

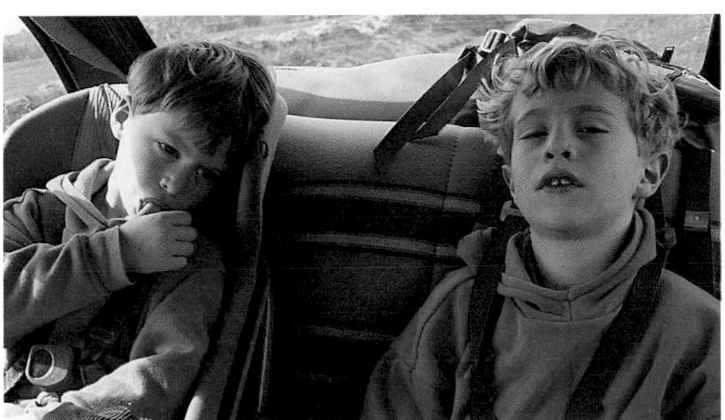

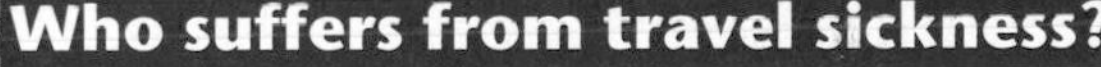

Who suffers from travel sickness?

Children are far more likely to suffer from travel sickness than adults. It rarely affects children before the age of two, and those between the ages of three and 12 are the most likely to suffer. Thankfully, most do seem to grow out of it as they get older.

Whether child or adult, surveys suggest that females are more susceptible to motion sickness than males. The reason for this isn't clear. Perhaps females are more ready to admit to having symptoms; on the other hand, hormones may play a part. Women are most susceptible during menstruation and when they're pregnant.

The type of journey, whether a child is excited and even what they have had to eat, can also affect symptoms. A child who has no problems in the car on a trip to the supermarket may react differently on a long drive home from the seaside, especially if they've stuffed themselves full of ice cream and candy floss!

Long car journeys, particularly along winding roads, can easily induce nausea. Try to encourage your child to concentrate on the road ahead – reading can make things worse.

What treatments are available?

A variety of travel sickness remedies are available from your local pharmacy. All need to be taken before your journey starts – some a couple of hours before, others the previous night. Don't wait until the symptoms of travel sickness occur before reaching for your remedy – by then it may be too late.

- **Travel sickness remedies** generally fall into two main groups: hyoscine, which is probably the more effective, and antihistamines, which are usually better tolerated. Hyoscine hydrobromide (such as Joy-Rides or Kwells) is probably the most effective remedy, but it is relatively short acting and carries a higher risk of side-effects. These may include drowsiness, a dry mouth, blurred vision and urinary retention. However, these are not generally a problem at the low doses used here. The earlier types of antihistamine, developed to treat hay fever, can be used to treat travel sickness. Examples include cinnarizine (Stugeron), dimenhydrinate (Dramamine), meclozine (Sea-Legs) and promethazine (Phenergan). These brands are equally effective but differ in how long they act, the age they're intended for and how much drowsiness they may cause.

- **When choosing** a travel sickness remedy, you'll need to consider the length of your journey. A remedy that's effective for four to six hours is no good for an overnight ferry crossing. Drowsiness as a side-effect may be acceptable with young children. However, it's not such a good idea for dad to take the same remedy if he'll be doing the driving when you reach your destination. Ask your pharmacist for advice.

- **For a non-drug method** of treating travel sickness, try Sea Bands. These are elastic bracelets that put pressure on an acupressure point called the P6 or Nei-Kuan point on the inner wrist. They are inexpensive, easy to use, safe and free from side-effects. However, they may need adjusting to fit very young children.

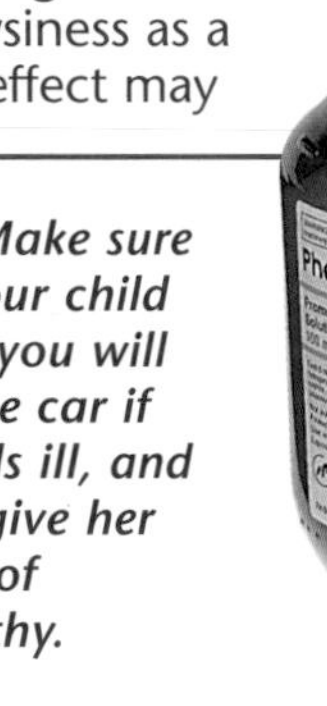

LEFT: Make sure that your child knows you will stop the car if she feels ill, and try to give her plenty of sympathy.

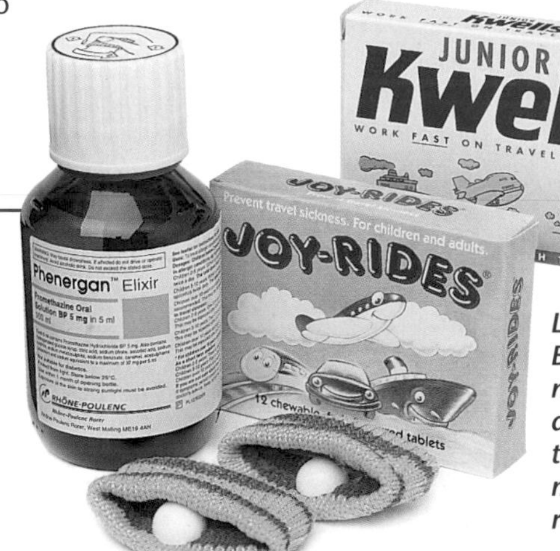

LEFT: 'Sea Bands' are a non-drug alternative to traditional motion sickness remedies.

How to keep sickness at bay

There is a lot you can do to help reduce the likelihood that the little ones in your party will feel ill on your journey.

- Opt for sensible food: greasy foods such as fish and chips can aggravate travel sickness, but an empty tummy can also be trouble.

- Offer frequent, light snacks when travelling, but not acidic fruits such as oranges. Ginger is one of nature's anti-nauseants so pack ginger biscuits to nibble. Avoid fizzy drinks – plain water or non-acidic fruit juice is best.

- Get some fresh air: a hot, stuffy environment can make things worse. Open a window in the car or take a walk on the ship's deck. Avoid smoking areas, restaurants and the duty-free perfume shop.

- Choose your seat carefully: a good view when travelling can work wonders. Adjust car seats so that toddlers can see more than just the back of the seat in front. On a boat, sit by a window and keep watching the horizon.

- The swaying on a ship is less apparent on a low deck in the middle. On a plane, a seat over a wing is where the aircraft is most stable. An aisle seat offers quick toilet access!

- If possible, schedule your travelling for when your child usually takes a nap, or go at night.

- If all else fails, be prepared. Take a sick-bag (plastic ones with the zip on the top work well), plenty of wipes, an air freshener in the car and a change of clothing!

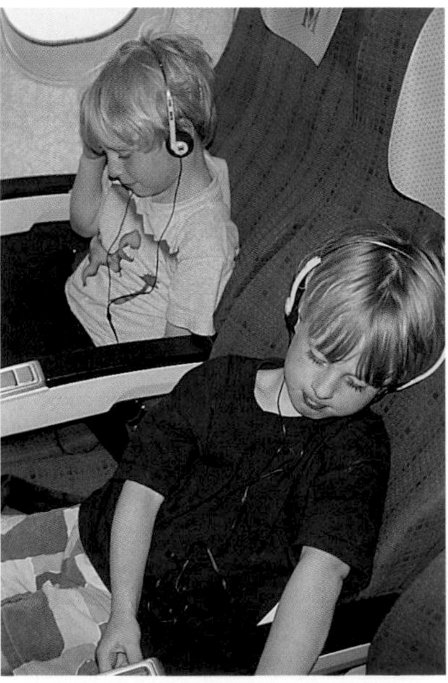

Once a child starts to feel sick, the sensation is unlikely to go away. Distractions, such as listening to tapes or playing travel games, can help ease discomfort.

TUBERCULOSIS

WHAT IS TUBERCULOSIS?

Tuberculosis (TB) is a disease caused by a rod-shaped bacterium known as mycobacterium tuberculosis.

- TB is a serious but slow-acting disease that has affected the human population for thousands of years. It can cause permanent damage to lungs and other organs of the body.

- As a result of infection, tubercles form in the lungs. A tubercle begins as an area of inflammation that develops into a small abscess. As the body's immune system works on the bacteria, the tubercle has a central zone of destroyed tissue surrounded by an area of inflammation and healing. Eventually, the tubercle reduces to a small scar.

- TB was formerly known as consumption, epidemics of which have swept across Europe many times. It became especially common during the Industrial Revolution as people began to congregate in cities.

- Until the 1940s, when drugs for treating the disease were discovered, about half of those who contracted TB died.

- It was believed that the disease had been eliminated in the UK, but the number of reported cases started to rise in 1987. It remains fairly rare but still affects about one in every 9000 people annually.

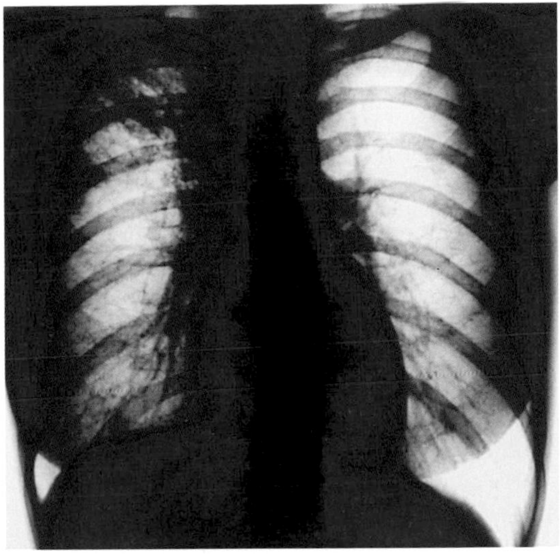

Tuberculosis can be detected on an X-ray. Here pulmonary tuberculosis can be seen in the red areas, caused by the TB bacterium spreading via the lymph nodes. If untreated, TB can cause permanent organ damage.

How tuberculosis is contracted

The disease can be spread in a number of ways, mainly through contamination or infection via exposure to TB bacterium.

1 The tuberculosis bacterium is almost always breathed in with droplets of mucus in the air produced when an infected person coughs or sneezes.

2 The disease can also be acquired by ingestion of contaminated food.

3 The bacteria can survive in a dry state for a long time in dust, particularly dark corners.

4 The TB bacterium multiplies very slowly and in practice it takes many bacteria for the disease to take hold. Thus repeated exposure to the disease is more likely to lead to infection than a single exposure.

5 A baby may acquire TB before or during birth by swallowing infected amniotic fluid.

Symptoms

Infection with TB usually causes no immediate problems, and the disease can remain latent for some time. The disease may not appear in an adult patient for weeks, months or even years.

- An infection usually appears about six weeks after inhalation of the bacteria. With a healthy immune system, the bacteria are usually dormant but if the immune system is weakened, the disease can reactivate.

- In about a third of cases the first sign is fluid in the space between the pleural membranes, leading to shortness of breath.

- Early symptoms of TB include heavy coughing, spitting up mucus and tiredness.

- As the infection progresses the patient may cough up blood and have trouble breathing. There may also be chest pains, loss of appetite and weight, together with fever and sweating.

- In a new infection, bacteria may infect and enlarge the lymph nodes that drain the lung. These may start to compress the bronchial tubes, causing a brassy cough and, occasionally, a collapsed lung. If the infection spreads and enlarges the lymph nodes in the neck, the infection may break through the skin of the neck, discharging pus.

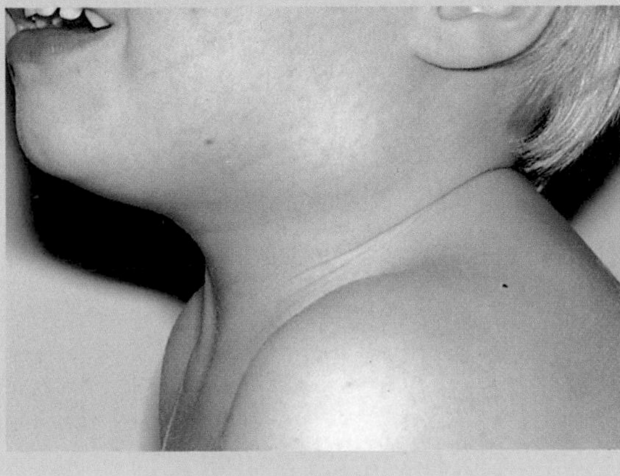

Swollen lymph glands are one of the main symptoms of TB. Other signs include a brassy cough and breathing difficulties.

Who is most vulnerable?

The TB bacterium is killed by ultraviolet light present in sunlight, but thrives in dark, damp conditions. Poverty is closely associated with the disease.

- Those at risk include the homeless and those living in poor social conditions. Babies, young children and pregnant women are also vulnerable, as well as people with bronchitis and asthma. People with HIV are at risk because of their severely weakened immune systems.

- People over 65 are vulnerable to TB, partly because many people of this age became infected when they were younger and TB was more widespread; also because of the effects of ageing on the body's immune system.

- In the US, TB began to increase during the 1980s due to the increasing incidence of AIDS, plus the overcrowded and unsanitary living conditions of some urban areas. The epidemic is now declining.

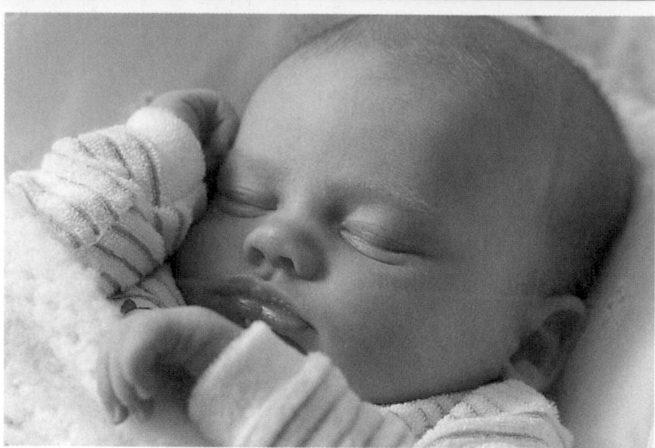

Babies are considered to be vulnerable to tuberculosis because their immune systems are not sufficiently developed to fight off the disease. Others who may be at risk include old people and pregnant women.

How the body is affected

TB can affect any part of the body, although it usually starts in the lungs.

- Apart from the lungs, the most common sites of infection are the bones and kidneys. Infection of other sites is called extrapulmonary tuberculosis.

- In men, infection may spread to the prostate gland, seminal vesicles and epididymis; in women, to the ovaries and fallopian tubes, resulting in sterility. Infection can also spread from the ovaries to the abdominal lining, which can cause acute pain. In children, the bacteria may infect the vertebrae of the spine and the arm and leg bones.

- Tuberculous meningitis – the infection of the base of the brain – is extremely dangerous. The drowsiness it causes can lead to coma. Miliary tuberculosis – massive spread of the infection throughout the bloodstream – frequently leads to meningitis and is common in infancy.

Diagnosis and treatment

TB is highly contagious and the patient should be isolated until the treatment has lasted two weeks.

- **X-ray:** the disease can often be detected by a chest X-ray. Diagnosis is confirmed by a sputum smear test, which involves growing the bacteria on a culture medium. This takes four to six weeks, although a quicker method is being developed.

- **Medication:** a combination of antibiotics is used. It takes a long time to kill all the bacteria present and a course of treatment takes several months. Some patients develop multidrug resistance, usually the result of poor medical supervision and poor compliance by the patient. It is essential that the combination of prescribed drugs is taken.

- **Surgery:** when drug resistance is present and the disease is confined to one or two lung lobes, surgical removal of the lobes may be best.

Prevention

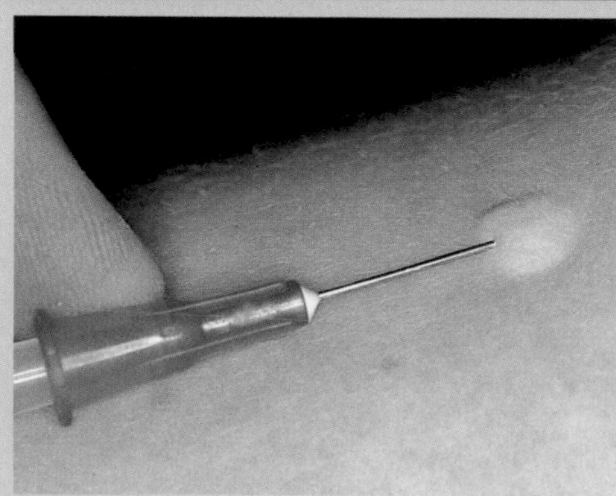

TB is prevented by vaccination and screening of contacts.

- Vaccination does not completely protect against TB. However, it is a great help to the body's own immune system in fighting off infection caused by the TB bacterium.

Although vaccinations, now compulsory in most schools, do not completely protect against TB, they do greatly help the immune system to fight it off.

- BCG (Bacillus Calmette-Guérin) vaccine contains weakened bacteria, derived from the cattle tuberculosis bacterium. In western countries nearly all children are given the vaccine.

- X-ray screening and testing of all contacts of a child or adult with TB can detect the disease. The disease can be detected before symptoms appear.

TUMMY ACHE

A COMMON COMPLAINT

Children often complain that their tummies hurt, and recurring bouts of stomach pain are one of the most common childhood ailments.

- Although there are over 80 causes of tummy pain in children, only a few are common. Some stomach disorders, such as appendicitis, can cause problems in any age group, whilst other conditions, such as blocked bowel, affect particular age groups.
- Most children with tummy ache never see a doctor, and those that are admitted to hospital are often discharged with a diagnosis of 'non-specific abdominal pain', because no underlying cause is found.
- Children cannot localise pain very well. They frequently complain of tummy ache even if the underlying problem is an ear, throat or urine infection.

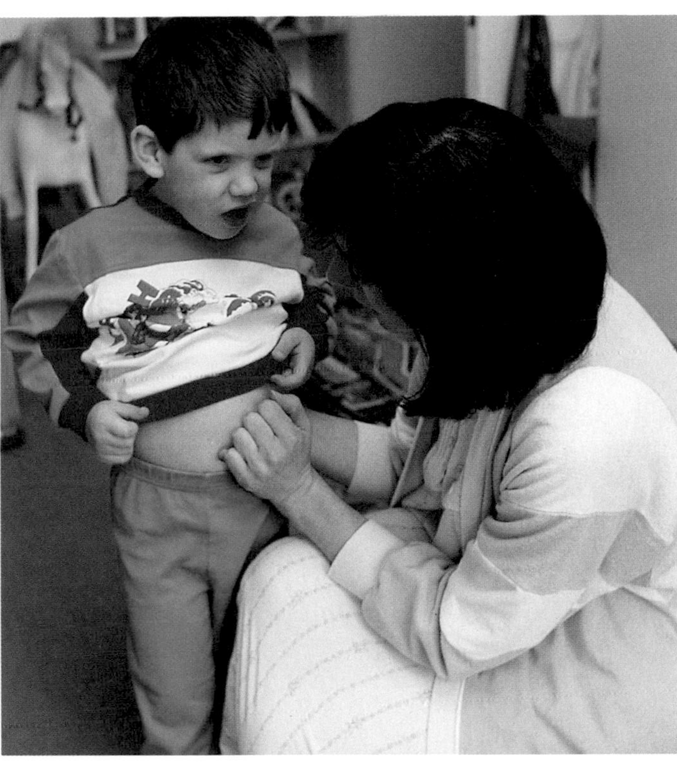

Your child may just point to his belly button if you ask him to show you the site of the pain. If he points elsewhere, it is a useful indicator of what might be causing the pain.

How to tell if the pain is serious

If your child complains of tummy ache, it can be difficult to know whether it's attention-seeking behaviour or the symptom of an illness.

Site of the pain
- Pain over the right or left of the abdomen, going through to the side of the back, is called 'loin pain' and could be a sign of a kidney infection.
- A pain that settles on the right-hand side may be appendicitis.
- Pain that is very low down, near or in the testicles, could be a twisted testicle.

Nature of the pain
- Sudden, severe stomach pain should be taken seriously.
- Some pain is a constant ache causing a child to lie very still.
- Pain in the gut and kidney area often comes and goes, making a child writhe about.
- 'Non-specific abdominal pain' is usually vague, around the belly button.

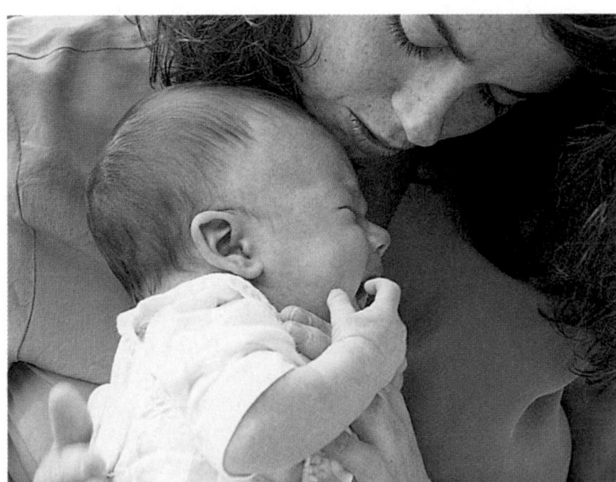

If your baby is distressed and draws up his knees, especially after a feed, he may have colic. The condition usually disappears without treatment.

Other symptoms

If your child has any of the following symptoms, as well as a tummy ache, there could be a more serious problem:

1. A change to his bowel movements, for example, constipation or diarrhoea.
2. A high temperature – an indication that the pain should be treated seriously.
3. Vomiting – a sign that the pain is serious. He may have gastroenteritis.
4. Green or yellow bile in the vomit – the gut may be blocked.
5. Bloody stools – this may be due to an infection or a blocked bowel.

NOTE: a child with a history of abdominal surgery may have scarring that will block the bowels.

When to see the doctor

- If there is sudden, severe stomach pain that has not settled with paracetamol.
- If your child's tummy looks distended, that is, blown out as if filled with air.
- If you notice a lump in your child's tummy or groin.
- If there is vomiting, a high fever and loose bowel motions that do not ease the pain.
- If your child's vomit is stained green (bile).
- If there is blood in your child's stools.

Treatment and diagnosis for tummy ache

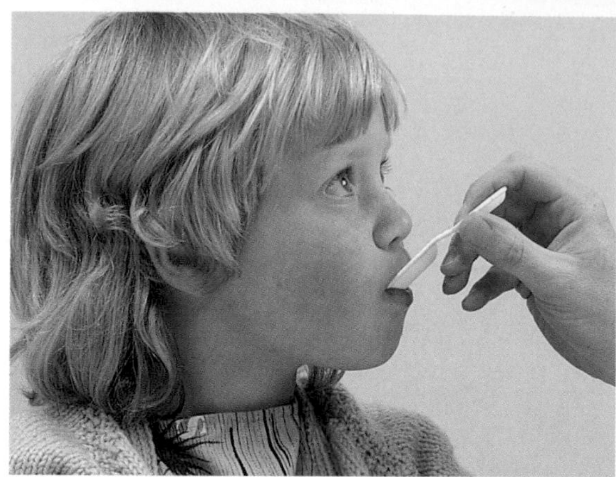

Minor tummy ache can be treated at home with liquid paracetamol. However, if the pain persists, make sure that your child is examined by your GP.

Home nursing

- Try giving your child some paracetamol medicine.
- If your child has diarrhoea, continue offering normal meals but include extra fluid, ideally oral rehydration sachets, which you can buy from a chemist.
- Get your child to sit on the toilet in the hope that he will open his bowels and relieve any constipation. This may be all that is needed to ease the pain.

Medical tests

- A urine test will be very helpful in exploring the possible causes of the pain. Infection can often be identified using a simple urine test.
- A blood test might show a higher than normal white cell count and this may increase the suspicion of appendicitis.
- Although an X-ray of the tummy will not usually identify stomach problems, it may reveal previously unsuspected constipation.
- A rectal examination is sometimes carried out.
- A stool test is advisable if a bowel infection is suspected.

Conditions that cause tummy ache

CONDITION	SYMPTOMS
Appendicitis: inflammation of the appendix	The 'typical' appendicitis pain starts in the area around the navel, and then moves to the lower right-hand side of the tummy. Your child may have a high temperature, vomiting and her tummy may be tender to the touch.
Colic: due to wind in the intestines, linked to feeding	Young babies will sometimes be very upset after a feed and draw up their knees while crying inconsolably for hours.
Constipation: extremely common and is often the reason for tummy ache	Constipation often follows a feverish illness, and any change in diet or environment may lead to infrequent stools, or stools that are difficult to pass.
Gastroenteritis: inflammation of the stomach due to a viral or bacterial infection	This can start suddenly, causing symptoms of vomiting, cramping pain in the stomach and fever.
Hepatitis: this is usually caused by a viral infection of the liver	Symptoms include nausea, vomiting, fatigue, jaundice and pain in the right-hand side of the tummy.
Hernia: caused by a part of the small intestine bulging through a weak part of the abdominal wall	A hernia may become twisted and stop the bowel working, causing severe pain and vomiting.
Intestinal obstruction: lack of bowel movement caused by partial or total blocked bowel	There may be severe tummy pain and vomiting. The blockage must be removed immediately.
Intussusception: when one segment of the gut folds inside another	A child may draw up her legs into a frog-like position and cry from the pain. She will vomit, and may pass a stool containing blood and mucus.
Malabsorption: this occurs when the gut cannot absorb essential nutrients	Causes diarrhoea, weight loss and cramping pains in the stomach.
Mesenteric adenitis: seen in children with colds and viral infections, affecting throats and ears	Lymph nodes in a child's tummy become swollen, causing vague, griping tummy pain.
Psychological pain: children will focus on their tummies when they are worried, anxious and stressed	This will usually be a dull ache, as opposed to a particular area being tender in the case of something more serious.
Urinary infection: an infection in the urinary tract	May cause tummy pains as well as vomiting, a high temperature, drowsiness and a burning sensation when urinating.

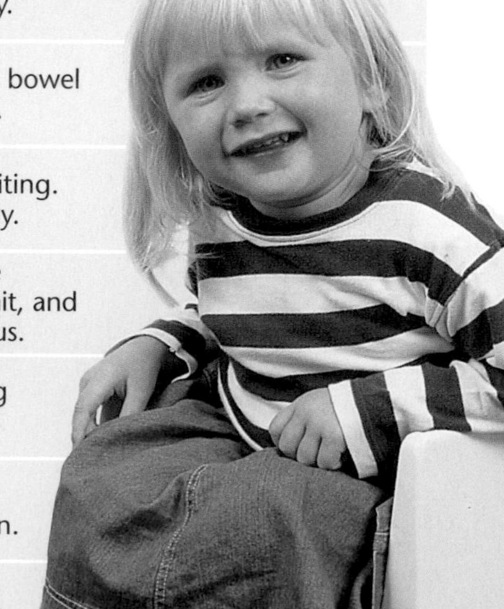

UNDESCENDED TESTICLE

WHAT IS AN UNDESCENDED TESTICLE?

An undescended testicle, also called cryptorchidism, is a common problem in which only one testicle is present in an infant's scrotum. It occurs when the normal process by which the testicles reach the scrotum fails.

- During the fifth week of pregnancy, each testicle starts to form near a kidney inside the abdominal cavity of the male foetus. In the following months, a fold of tissue (the process vaginalis) and the cremaster muscle push down into the abdominal cavity and grow towards the scrotum. In the sixth month of pregnancy, the processus vaginalis joins the inguinal canal, which leads directly to the scrotum.

- During the seventh month of pregnancy, the mother's hormones and male hormones produced by the maturing testicles stimulate each testicle to move, with the help of the cremaster muscle, down to enter the scrotum. The processus vaginalis closes off after the testicle has passed through it.

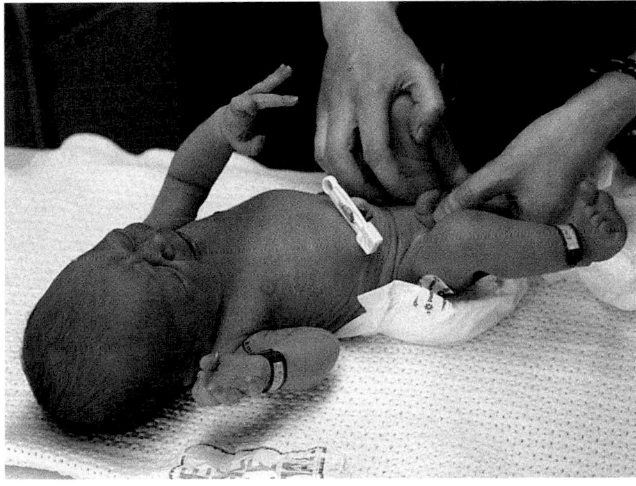

A boy's testicles are examined at birth to check that they are both in the correct position. If they haven't dropped naturally within the first year, surgery may be required.

What causes it?

It is not known for certain why a testicle fails to drop. There are a number of possibilities.

1 A weakness in the cremaster and other muscles means that the testicle fails to move down and stays in the abdomen.

2 The testicle may follow the wrong path and end up in the groin area but not in the scrotum – the testicle is said to be 'ectopic'.

3 A fibrous growth may form in front of the testicle, blocking its path.

4 The maternal and foetal hormones may fail to trigger the testicle's descent.

5 The undescended testicle may fail to mature properly.

How is it detected?

An undescended testicle is normally detected during the routine medical check carried out immediately after birth.

- The first test for an undescended testicle is to feel the scrotum. Once an undescended testicle has been diagnosed, it is important to find out at which stage of the descent process the testicle became stuck.

- If the testicle cannot be felt in the groin, it can usually be detected by an ultrasound examination.

- In more complex cases a laparotomy – an internal examination – may be necessary. This examination may be combined with an operation to correct the problem.

Why is it a problem?

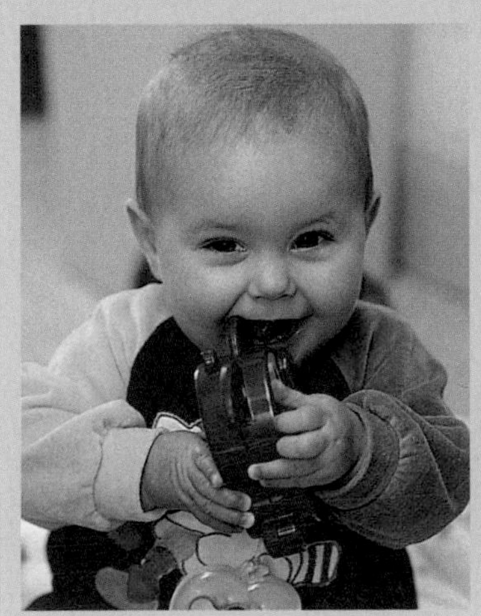

An undescended testicle can have a significant impact on your child's future health and fertility.

- Sperm cells start to die at the higher temperature inside the body.

- The risk of developing testicular cancer in an undescended testicle is about one in 2500. It is thought that the risk decreases if the testicle is placed in the scrotum.

- An undescended testicle will leave disrupted tissues in the area through which it should have passed, increasing the risk of an inguinal hernia.

- Having only one testicle in the scrotum may have psychological repercussions.

As long as the testicle is repositioned, the baby should go on to lead a normal, healthy life.

What does the treatment involve?

If the testicle does not drop naturally, treatment will usually be given when a child is aged between one and three years old. There are various options, depending on where the undescended testicle lies.

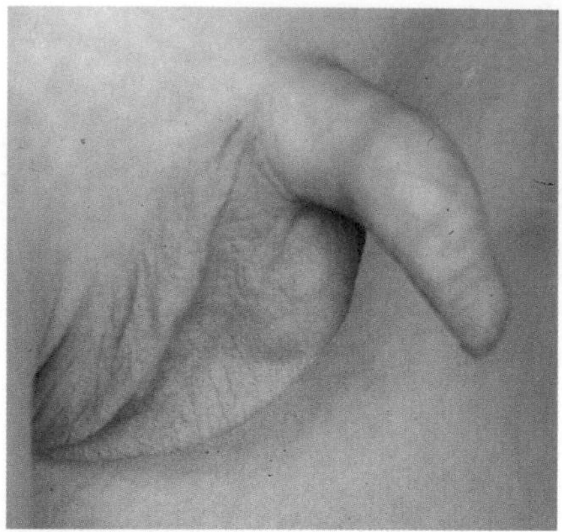

Approximately 3 per cent of full-term babies and around 10 per cent of premature babies have an undescended testicle. Surgery will be necessary if the testicle does not drop naturally during the baby's first year.

- In around 70 per cent of cases the testicle descends spontaneously, usually by the fourth month after birth. However, the chances that this will happen reduce considerably by the time the baby is six months old and are practically non-existent by the end of his first year.

- If the testicle can be felt in the groin area, near to the scrotum, the treatment of choice is likely to be an operation called a low orchidopexy. A small incision is made in the groin and scrotum and the testicle is freed from the surrounding tissues and eased into its correct position. Stitches may be used to anchor the testicle to the wall of the scrotum. The procedure is carried out under general anaesthetic, but your child won't need to stay in hospital.

- Sometimes an inguinal hernia develops in the area through which the testis should have passed. This can be repaired at the same time as the testicle is brought down.

- If the testicle is high up in the abdomen, a more complex operation, called a high orchidopexy, is required. This is performed by means of a laparoscope – a fibre-optic tube – placed inside the abdomen. The technique is still being developed and refined, and the operation is performed by experienced paediatric surgeons only.

Complications of surgery

There are few serious complications after an orchidopexy.

- There is normally pain and swelling in the groin and scrotum for a few days after the operation.

- As with any operation, there is a risk of infection and bleeding.

- The surgery requires great precision to prevent the delicate testicles, especially immature ones, from being damaged.

- Sometimes a laparoscopy detects that the testicle thought to be undescended is, in fact, missing, so the operation comes to an end. In other cases, the testicle is found to be underdeveloped and is removed (an orchidectomy) if the other testicle is healthy.

Caring for your child after the operation

Recovery following an orchidopexy is normally quick and trouble-free, but a few precautions should be taken.

- Children's paracetamol can be given to ease any pain in the groin and scrotum during the first few days after the operation.

- Many doctors recommend that the affected area is sponge-washed for the first few days. Baths and showers should be avoided.

- Monitor your child's temperature regularly to reduce the risk of serious infection. Contact your GP if your child's temperature rises above 39°C (102°F).

- Your child should avoid strenuous activities for two weeks.

Your baby's groin area will be very sore following the operation. He can be given children's paracetamol to ease the pain and discomfort.

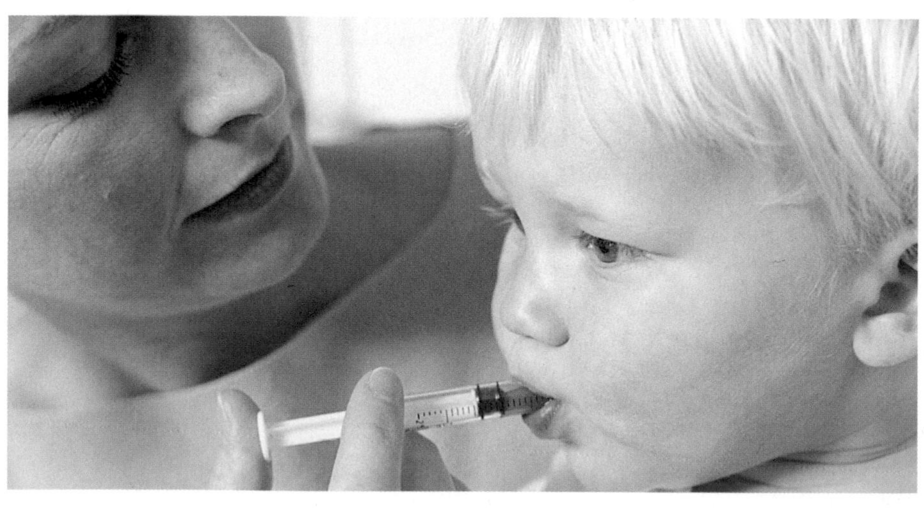

URINARY TRACT INFECTIONS

WHAT IS A URINARY TRACT INFECTION?

The urinary tract consists of those parts of the body concerned with the formation and removal of urine – the kidneys, ureters, bladder and urethra.

- When bacteria or other organisms invade part of the urinary tract they cause infections (UTIs).

- Urethritis is an infection or inflammation of the urethra, the duct through which urine passes from the bladder to the outside; cystitis is an infection of the bladder, the organ in which urine is temporarily stored; uretitis is an infection of one or both of the ureters, the ducts through which urine passes from the kidneys to the bladder; pyelonephritis is an infection of the kidneys, the organs that produce urine.

- Urinary tract infections occur in about 1 per cent of boys and 3 per cent of girls up to the age of 11. In a few cases there are physical abnormalities that predispose towards infection. Vesico-ureteric reflux occurs when the one-way valves at the lower ends of the ureters do not work properly, and allow urine to return from the bladder to the kidneys.

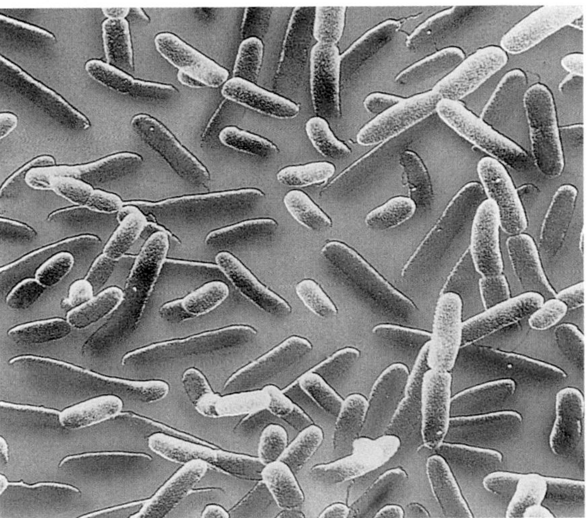

The bacterium commonly known as E. coli is found in human intestines. It is normally harmless but can cause urine infections.

How infections are contracted

Bacteria in the bloodstream may enter the kidneys and pass down into the ureters and bladder; or bacteria may enter the lower opening of the urethra and pass to the bladder.

- In very young infants urine infections are usually the result of a more generalised infection of the body.

- In older children and adults, infections are most commonly caused by the bacterium Escherichia coli. These may enter the urethra and cause urethritis and cystitis.

- Because girls have shorter urethras than boys, and their urethras open in the crotch rather than at the end of a penis, girls are more prone to contracting urinary tract infections than boys.

- Older girls may acquire UTIs as a result of wiping their bottoms from back to front.

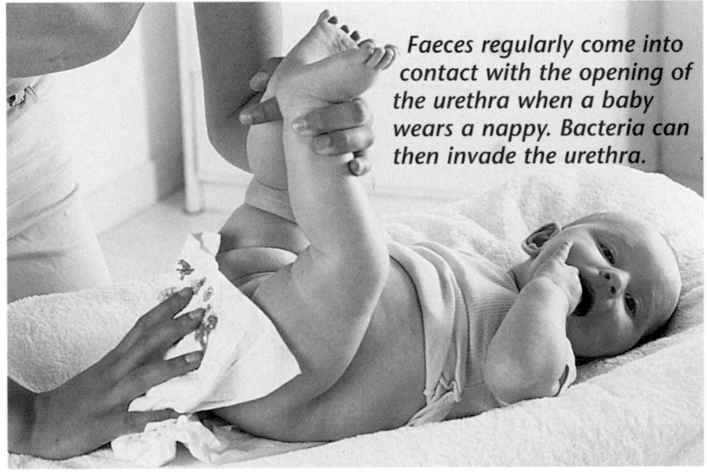

Faeces regularly come into contact with the opening of the urethra when a baby wears a nappy. Bacteria can then invade the urethra.

How the body prevents urine infections

Urine is one of the body's waste products. Normal urine contains water, inorganic salts, glucose, urea and other organic compounds. It has only a faint smell and is sterile while it is in the body.

1 The construction of the urinary tract normally prevents bacterial invasion. When urine is not being passed, the urethra and the lower opening of the bladder are squeezed shut, creating a natural barrier.

2 The bladder is a long way from the outer opening of the urethra, and the act of urination itself tends to flush out bacteria that enter the urethra. Because the bladder is completely emptied during urination, any bacteria that do find their way into it are also normally flushed away.

3 One-way valves at the lower ends of the ureters normally prevent urine from passing back up the ureters, thus helping to prevent any infection that is present in the bladder from reaching the kidneys.

NOTE: the chemical content of urine makes it a good medium for bacteria to grow in, and urine that has been left exposed to the air acquires an unpleasant smell. This is because the action of air and bacteria breaks down the urea into ammonia.

Symptoms

The symptoms of UTIs depend on where the infection is and the age of the person affected.

- **Urethritis:** usually produces a burning sensation when urinating, especially just at the start. After this initial stage many of the bacteria in the infected urethra are flushed out with uncontaminated urine.

- **Cystitis:** sometimes, but not always, produces a burning sensation at some stage during urination. Other possible symptoms include fever, lower abdominal pain, or the urine may have a strange smell or appearance; it may be dark, cloudy, or even tinged with blood.

- **Pyelonephritis:** often shows itself as a lower back pain, and can sometimes be accompanied by fever and septicaemia (blood poisoning). Damage and scarring may occur to the filtering system. If this becomes extensive and is left untreated, and if both kidneys are damaged, there's a chance of kidney failure.

Diagnosis

A doctor may diagnose a UTI from the symptoms, but the only certain way is to test a sample of urine.

- Bacteria are present on the skin and can therefore be washed into the sample by the urine itself. A 'clean catch' sample involves cleaning the genital area, urinating a small amount into a toilet to flush out any bacteria and then filling a cup.

- In small children the only sure way of getting a clean sample is to insert a needle into the bladder to collect a supra-pubic aspirate (SPA). This is usually done in hospital.

- If pyelonephritis is diagnosed, the extent of any kidney damage may be checked. A radioactive chemical is injected into the bloodstream. A gamma camera picks up the radiation and follows the course of the chemical through the kidneys to check they are functioning properly.

- For recurrent infections, doctors may test for urinary tract abnormalities. Scans can reveal any abnormalities in the bladder and kidneys.

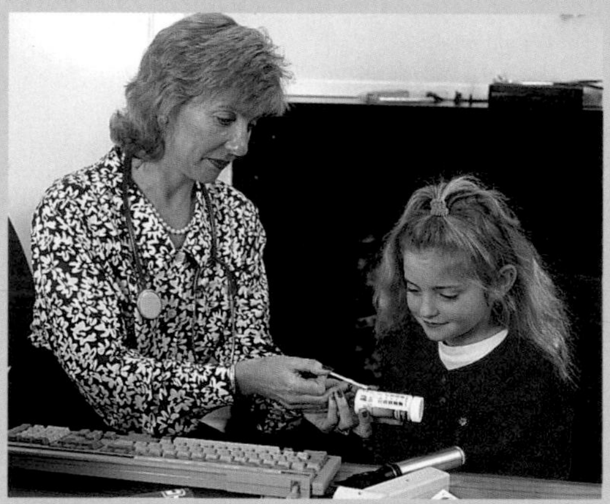

- A baby boy who has a urinary tract infection needs to be tested to ensure he doesn't have a rare but serious condition of the valves in the urethra, which can lead to kidney damage.

To analyse a child's urine a doctor may do a Uristix urine test. This is where a stick is dipped in the child's urine and then checked against a reference chart.

Treatments for infections

Antibiotics are the only effective treatment for a UTI. If you suspect that your child has any of the symptoms of urine infection, make an appointment to see a doctor immediately.

1 If the symptoms are fairly obvious, a course of antibiotics will be usually prescribed at the same time as the urine sample is taken.

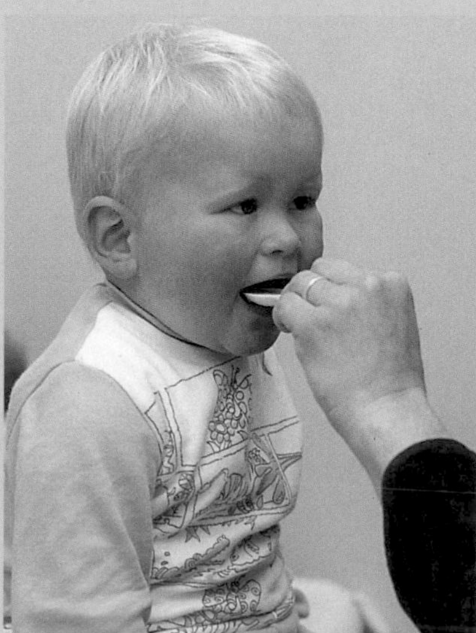

However, when the type of bacteria in the urine sample has been established, it may be necessary to change the antibiotic.

2 A repeat sample may be taken three to five days after antibiotic treatment has been started, to confirm that the bacteria are being killed.

3 Another sample taken soon after the course of treatment has been completed confirms that the infection has been removed.

NOTE: it is important that a course of antibiotics is completed, even if the symptoms have disappeared.

Antibiotics are the best treatment for urinary tract infections, and a doctor will usually prescribe a course at the same time as taking a urine sample.

Reducing the risk of infection

The best way of minimising the risk of infection is to ensure that sensible routines of washing and hygiene are followed.

- The genital and anal regions should be washed at least once a day.

- A baby's nappy should be changed frequently, immediately the presence of faeces is suspected. The genital area should be cleaned.

- A child should be taught to wipe her bottom from the front to the back, to prevent faeces being wiped over the genitals. This is particularly important for girls.

VOMITING

WHAT IS VOMITING?

Vomiting is a reflex action in which the diaphragm contracts and the muscles at the stomach entrance relax, causing the contents of the stomach to be ejected through the mouth.

- Most young children will suffer from vomiting at some point, and in the majority of cases it is not serious, is short-lived, and can be managed at home. However, there are times when it is a symptom of a condition requiring medical treatment.

- There is sometimes confusion between vomiting and possetting in babies. Possetting is when a small amount of milk is regurgitated by a baby after a feed, often when wind is brought up. Unlike vomiting, it isn't forceful, and you won't see your baby retching. Possetting is quite normal in babies and, more often than not, is unlikely to be a cause for concern.

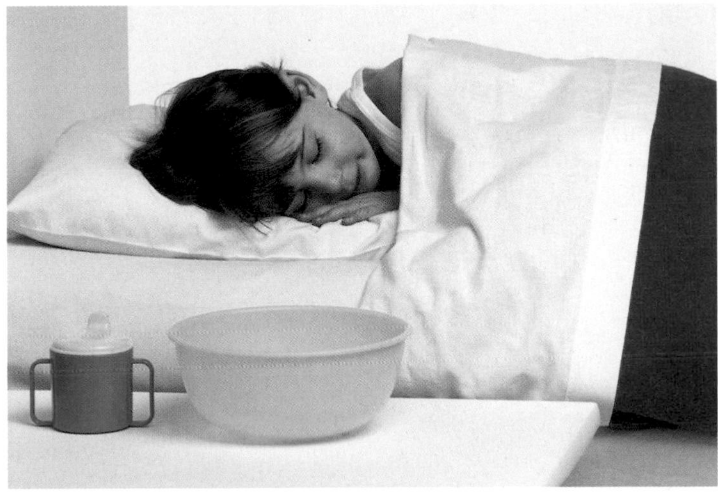

If your child has vomited, encourage her to rest. Provide a bowl in case of a further attack and some water to rinse out her mouth and prevent dehydration.

Causes in babies

If your baby vomits regularly, seek advice from your health visitor or GP to identify the cause.

1 **Rapid feeding:** many babies will vomit after consuming a large volume of milk very quickly. If your baby isn't hungry after feeds, is gaining weight, and seems otherwise well, there is probably nothing to worry about.

2 **Gastroenteritis:** this 'tummy bug' is caused by an infection in the gut. There may also be diarrhoea.

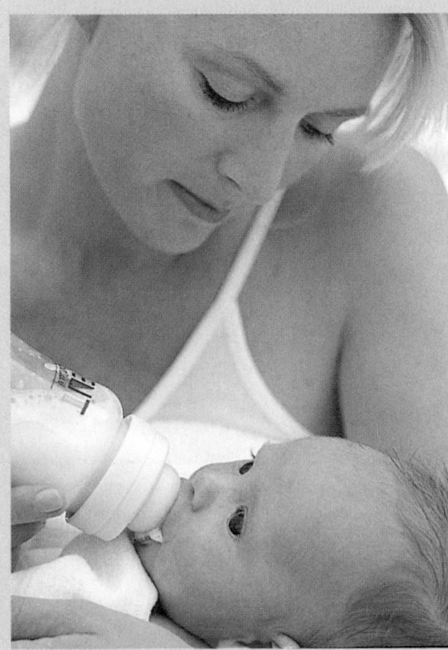

3 **Milk intolerance:** if your baby is formula fed, seems colicky and vomits shortly after each feed, a milk intolerance may be the cause.

4 **Pyloric stenosis:** a baby with pyloric stenosis has projectile vomiting during or after each feed, and is usually hungry after a feed. You may also notice waves of contractions across your baby's tummy during a feed as the stomach tries to push the milk through an obstructed opening into the intestine.

5 **Infection:** your baby may also have a fever and be off feeds.

6 **Coughing:** severe coughing fits can result in vomiting.

7 **Other medical conditions:** any condition causing obstruction of the gut can result in vomiting.

8 **Meningitis:** vomiting is often a symptom.

Your baby may drink milk too rapidly and vomit after a feed. If she seems otherwise healthy, this is probably nothing to worry about.

Causes in older children

It is important to check for other symptoms and seek medical help if necessary.

1 **Gastroenteritis:** this 'tummy bug' is a common cause of vomiting in children.

2 **Milk intolerance:** tummy ache and vomiting after eating dairy products may indicate a cow's milk intolerance.

3 **Poisoning:** for example, through drinking household cleaning fluids, or eating undercooked or out-of-date food.

4 **Food allergy:** a child may vomit after eating certain foods and it is important to seek medical help to identify these.

5 **Infection:** vomiting may be one of the symptoms of an infection.

6 **Appendicitis:** your child would also have severe abdominal pain and could have a mild fever.

7 **Meningitis:** though it is not a common cause, vomiting is one of the symptoms of meningitis.

When to call the doctor

Don't hesitate to seek medical help in the following circumstances.

Baby

- If your baby has a fever with vomiting.
- If vomiting persists for six hours, especially if your baby also has diarrhoea.
- If your baby is showing any signs of dehydration: has a dry mouth and lips; is not passing much urine and has darker urine than usual; is lethargic (drowsy); has a sunken fontanelle – the soft spot on top of the head.
- If your baby seems to be in pain and is vomiting, or the nappy contains blood or mucus.
- If the vomit is gritty brown or if it contains blood; or if the vomit is bile stained (green/yellow).

Older child

- If vomiting is severe and persists for six hours or more.
- If your child has abdominal pain and is vomiting.
- If the vomit is gritty brown, contains blood or is green/yellow.
- If your child has any signs of dehydration, such as darker urine or a dry mouth and lips.
- If you know or suspect your child has taken something poisonous, she should be taken straight to hospital. You should tell the doctor exactly what you think your child has taken. If possible, take a sample of what she has swallowed or the container with you.

Treatment for vomiting

It is important that your child drinks small, regular amounts to prevent dehydration. Babies, in particular, are at greatest risk of rapid dehydration because of their small size.

Baby

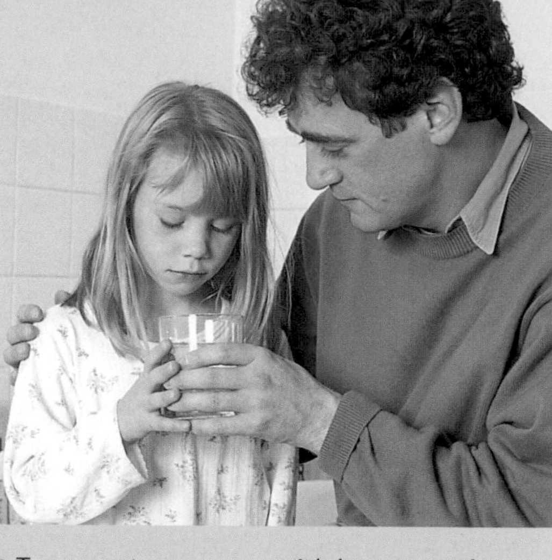

- You should continue to breast-feed your baby, offering feeds more frequently than usual. If your baby is bottle-fed, offer small amounts more frequently – for example, half the usual amount twice as often.
- A GP may prescribe an oral rehydration solution for your baby to be given as well as the usual feed.

Older child

- Soothe your child – she may be distressed.
- Have a bowl and some tissues within reach and stay with your child while she is vomiting. Offer a damp cloth to wipe her face afterwards and a sip of water so that she can wash her mouth out.
- You can give solid foods little and often, but avoid fatty foods as your child may not be able to tolerate these.

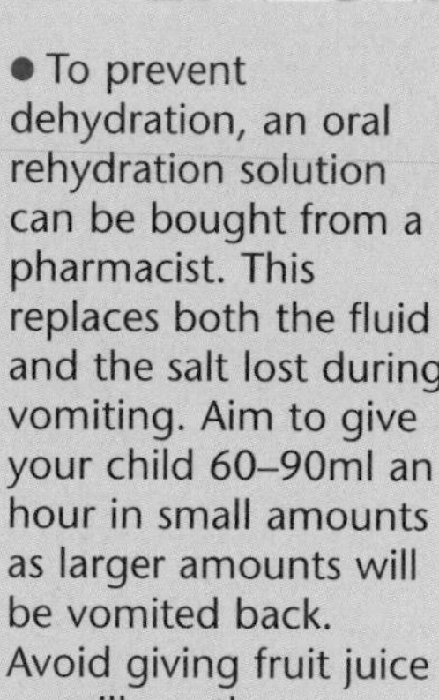

- To prevent dehydration, an oral rehydration solution can be bought from a pharmacist. This replaces both the fluid and the salt lost during vomiting. Aim to give your child 60–90ml an hour in small amounts as larger amounts will be vomited back. Avoid giving fruit juice or milk, as these are not well tolerated.
- As the vomiting subsides, you can very slowly introduce food again, starting with plain, dry snacks such as a plain biscuit.
- Aim to reintroduce a light, bland diet within 24 hours. If your child is feeling hungry, this is usually a sign that she is recovering.

It's important that your child keeps up her fluid intake to avoid becoming dehydrated.

Good hygiene

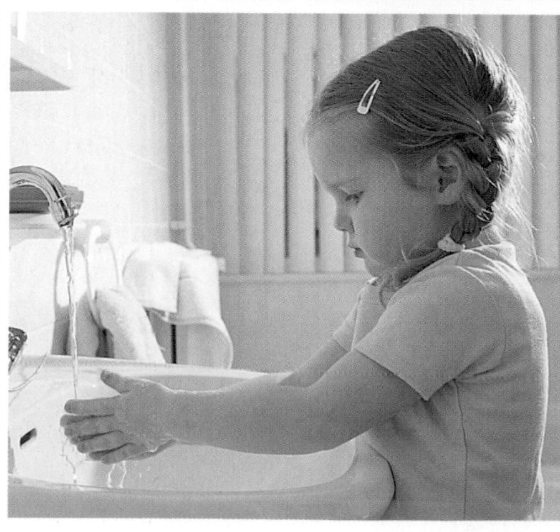

To prevent the spread of germs that can cause tummy bugs, it's important to teach your child good hygiene.

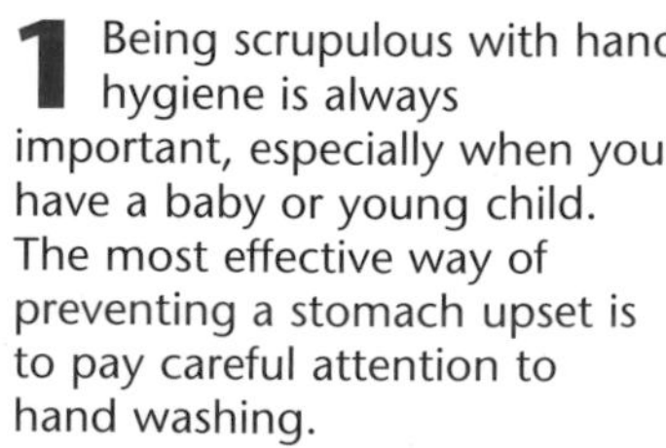

1 Being scrupulous with hand hygiene is always important, especially when you have a baby or young child. The most effective way of preventing a stomach upset is to pay careful attention to hand washing.

To help prevent the spread of germs, encourage your child to wash her hands thoroughly in warm, soapy water after using the toilet and before eating.

2 Young children should be encouraged to be diligent about washing their hands after using the toilet, before helping to serve food and before eating.

3 It is important to wash feeding bottles and beakers thoroughly in hot soapy water after use (bottle teats should be sterilised for the first year). This is to ensure the removal of all traces of old milk, which can harbour germs.

WHOOPING COUGH

WHAT IS WHOOPING COUGH?

Whooping cough is a serious childhood infection of the lower respiratory tract, which is highly contagious. It is caused by a bacterium called bordetella pertussis and spread by breathing in infected air passed from someone with the infection who has coughed or sneezed.

- The incubation period after contact with the bacteria to contracting symptoms is usually seven to 10 days, but may be up to three weeks.
- The child is infectious from seven days after exposure to three weeks after the typical cough develops, and the most infectious period is during the early cold symptoms.
- Before immunisation became available in the 1950s, there were around 100,000 cases of whooping cough in England and Wales each year. Due to the whooping cough vaccine, the condition is now extremely rare; in 2000 only around 650 cases were notified.
- The condition is diagnosed by analysing a swab taken from the back of the child's nose (a per-nasal swab).

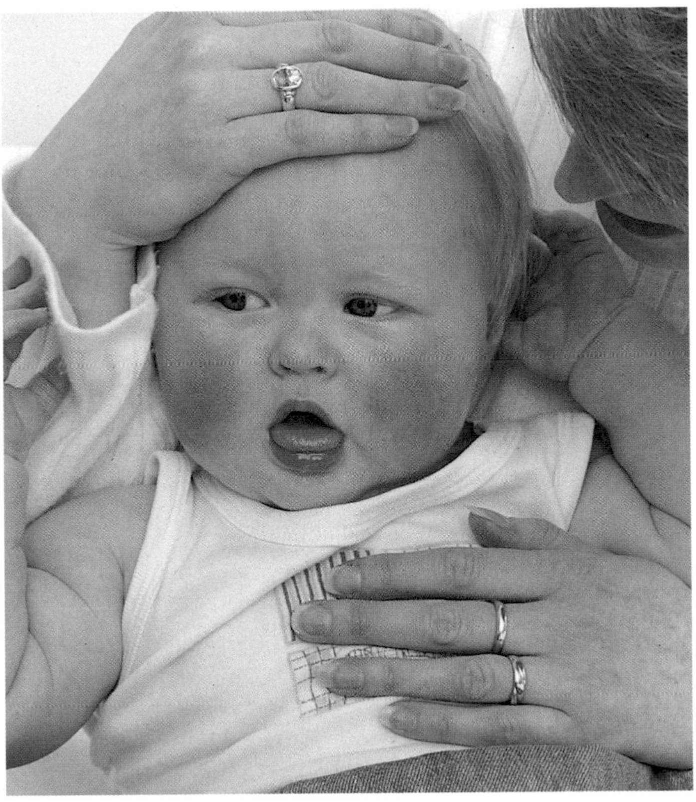

RIGHT: The cough becomes increasingly severe and is accompanied by a 'whoop' sound. It is exhausting for a baby or young child.

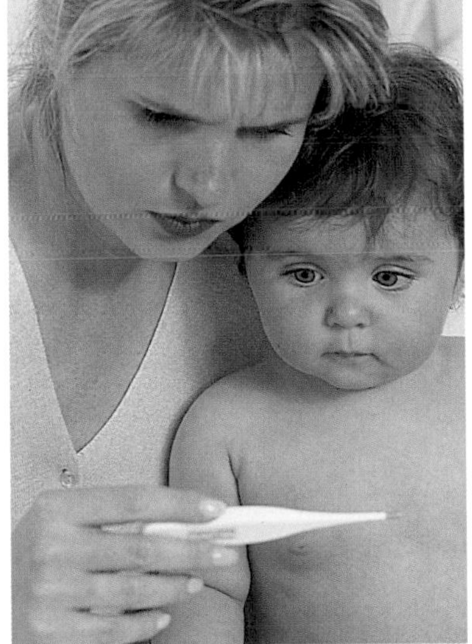

A temperature increase is one of the first signs of whooping cough in a child. A digital thermometer placed under the arm will give a fairly accurate reading.

Symptoms

The typical 'whooping' sound occurs when the child struggles to take in a breath after a coughing bout, but in very young babies the 'whoop' may not be present, which can make diagnosis more difficult.

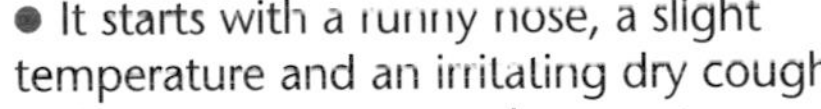

- It starts with a runny nose, a slight temperature and an irritating dry cough.
- After one to two weeks symptoms worsen with severe bouts of coughing and vomiting.
- Attacks of coughing may be worse at night or after a feed, making the child blue or grey due to lack of oxygen.
- In very young babies there may only be a cold with episodes of apnoea (where breathing stops for a few seconds) after coughing.
- After two or three weeks, the coughing episodes should lessen, but the child may have a persistent cough for two to three months.

Who is susceptible?

Whooping cough is highly infectious. On average, two-thirds of unimmunised people in a family who come into contact with an infected child are likely to catch the disease.

1 Children who have not been immunised are at greatest risk of developing whooping cough.

2 The illness is most severe in young babies, which is one reason why vaccines are now started when a baby is two months old. Babies whose older siblings have not been immunised are most vulnerable.

3 Adults and older children can get whooping cough, but the symptoms are usually much milder. It is therefore much less likely to be diagnosed correctly, particularly if they have been previously immunised.

4 The danger of whooping cough in adults or older children is that they may be a source of infection for unimmunised babies.

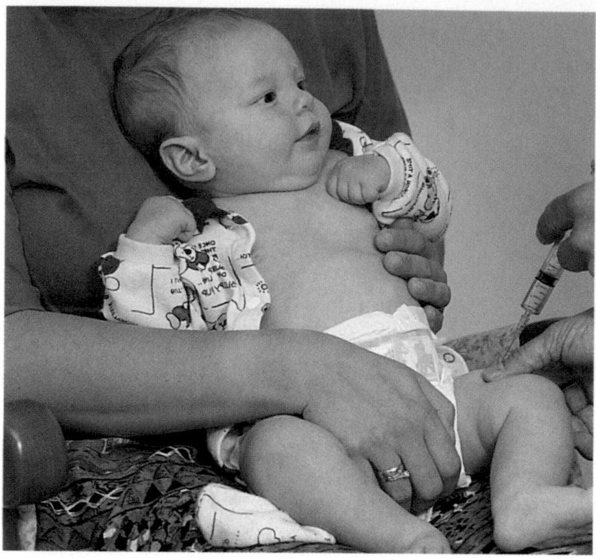

The immunisation is given in three doses at two, three and four months of age, in a combined vaccine with diphtheria, tetanus, Hib and meningitis C.

Immunisation

A full course of the whooping cough vaccine is highly effective in 80 per cent of cases and in the rest the disease is far milder than in unimmunised children.

- The vaccine has few known side-effects. Some children have a mild local reaction with an area of redness at the injection site. Babies may cry and become irritable, or develop a fever within the first 24 hours after the injection. It is important to tell the nurse giving the next injection about previous reactions.
- Only a severe reaction would be a reason to withhold future doses and specialist advice will usually be given. If a child is unwell and has a temperature, the vaccination should be postponed until he is better.
- In the 1970s, there was a scare about a rare possible risk of brain damage associated with the vaccine. This led to a marked drop in the number of immunisations, resulting in two large whooping cough epidemics over the next few years. The brain damage risk has never been proven and the vaccine is now thought to be very safe. The risks of the disease are certainly greater than any tiny theoretical risk from the vaccine.

Home nursing

If your baby or child has whooping cough, you should monitor and care for her as follows:

Medication: regular doses of paracetamol suspension are needed if she has a temperature. Don't give her cough linctuses as these are unlikely to be effective.

Breathing: if your baby has difficulty breathing or her lips or tongue become blue during coughing bouts, then you should seek urgent medical help.

Vomiting: it is very important to keep your child well hydrated by giving her plenty of fluids. Meals should be small and frequent to reduce the risk of vomiting and prevent weight loss.

Specialist care: young babies under six months will usually be admitted to hospital for observation.

Your baby may develop a fever in the first 24 hours following the whooping cough vaccination:

Treating a fever

- Try to keep your baby cool and ensure that she is comfortable.
- Give your baby the recommended dose of infant paracetamol. If her temperature is still high after a second dose four to six hours later, then contact your GP for advice.
- If there is a personal or family history of febrile convulsions then extra care should be taken to prevent a fever. You may want to seek medical advice earlier.

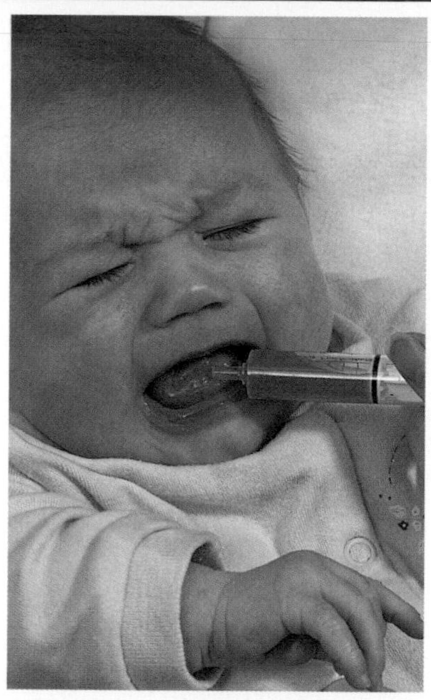

Infant paracetamol can be used to help treat a fever. Use a syringe, available from pharmacists, to squirt the medication into her mouth.

Medical treatments

Antibiotic treatment is not very effective and the symptoms are usually treated as they arise.

1 Although antibiotics aren't effective, the antibiotic erythromycin is often given because it may reduce the period of infectivity.

2 If hospital admission is needed, the child's breathing will be monitored and complications such as pneumonia will be treated.

3 Supportive treatment may be needed, such as suctioning of mucus secretions from the respiratory tract and oxygen therapy.

Complications

Babies aged under six months are at greatest risk of serious complications from whooping cough.

- Before immunisation, the most common cause of death from whooping cough was from bronchopneumonia, a secondary infection.
- There is a risk of brain damage from the severe coughing spasms that can deprive the brain of oxygen. These spasms can also cause small haemorrhagic spots on the baby's cheeks.
- If there is repeated vomiting, this can result in significant weight loss.
- A rare long-term effect is damage to some of the bronchi within the lung (bronchiectasis), leading to a chronic cough.

Chapter Three
First Aid

ACHES & PAINS

A SERIOUS SYMPTOM?

Aches and pains usually come and go quickly, but are sometimes a sign of a more serious condition. However, it can be difficult for parents to know if a child's tummy ache, for example, is serious.

- A young child may have difficulty describing the pain and where it hurts.
- It is important to look for other signs and symptoms and, if you're concerned, you should take your child to a doctor to be properly examined.
- Children often say they have a tummy ache when they are worried about something, such as going to school, or are generally seeking attention.

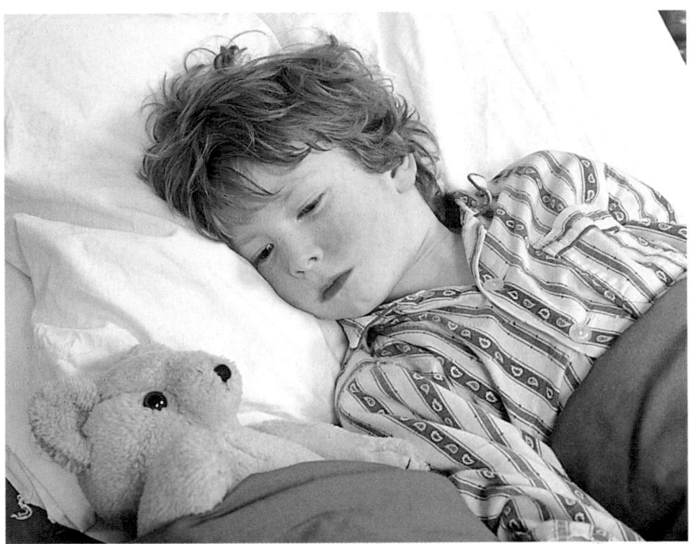

When a child complains of a tummy ache, it can be a sign of something more serious, from a kidney infection to an underlying anxiety.

When to call the doctor

Young babies under four months should always be seen by a doctor when they are unwell. If the problem persists or worsens in older children, or any of these symptoms are shown, call your doctor:

- A high temperature – over 37.5°C (100°F) – for a prolonged period
- Vomiting and nausea
- An unexplained rash
- Floppiness or lethargy
- Complaining of a severe sharp pain
- Persistent diarrhoea
- Persistent constipation
- Blood in the stools
- Blood in the urine
- A distended stomach
- Pain when urinating
- A tender area in the abdomen that becomes worse on coughing or moving
- A dislike of bright lights and loud noises

Basic home nursing

When children have minor aches and pains, loving care and attention is sometimes just as effective as medication.

- Pay close attention to what your child is saying – or trying to say – to find out about the pain. Give reassurance that all is well and try cuddling up to your child with a hot-water bottle and his favourite toy.

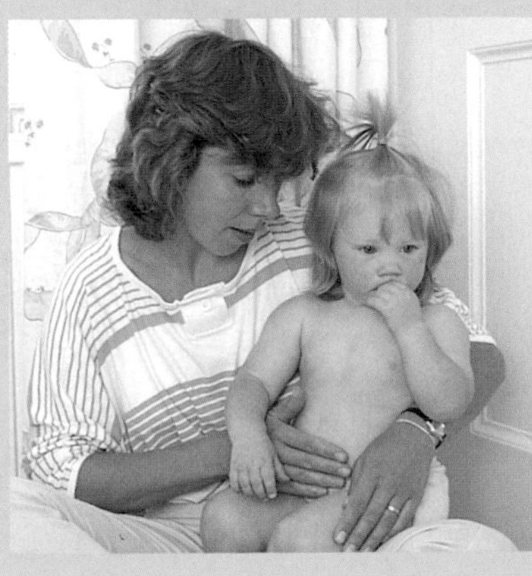

- Give plenty to drink and use oral rehydration sachets if your child has diarrhoea or has been sick.
- Give paracetamol as a painkiller and to lower temperature.
- Encourage your child to open his bowels if you suspect constipation – it may help to give him fresh fruit juice to drink.
- If the pain seems vague and you suspect it may be caused by an underlying anxiety, try to discover the cause and give reassurance.

'Rubbing it better' may be effective when your child has a tummy ache. The power of soothing touch is often very therapeutic.

Painkillers for children

There are guidelines about the use of painkillers.

- Never give a baby under six months any medicines unless on the advice of your GP or health visitor.
- Do not give children under 12 aspirin or any medicine that contains them. These can cause Reye's syndrome, which can lead to liver failure. Give junior paracetamol or ibuprofen instead and always read the label carefully.
- No carer can give your child any medication without your permission, so ensure that you can always be contacted or leave clear instructions.
- Likewise, you must not give medication to another child without parental permission.
- If your child's condition does not improve after 24 hours, or worsens, call a doctor and say what medicine has been given and in what dosage.

Stomach ache

Stomach ache is a very common condition in babies and young children.

- **Colic:** this common condition is caused by wind trapped in the intestines. An attack can be eased by infant colic drops or gripe water.

- **Constipation:** one cause of stomach aches in young children is constipation. This may be due to inadequate fluids.

- **Diarrhoea:** this can cause stomach ache in babies and young children. With babies, try introducing small quantities of new foods at first. Children can be susceptible to food poisoning, so always cook all foods hygienically and thoroughly.

- **Appendicitis:** the pain is below and either side of the navel, later moving to the right. There may be vomiting and a high temperature. The pain is made worse when the area is touched. Seek urgent medical attention.

- **Gastrointestinal/urinary/kidney problems:** consult your doctor immediately if your child has griping stomach pains with a high temperature and vomiting and has constipation or diarrhoea.

NOTE: young children are very poor at identifying correctly where the pain is, or may just feel generally unwell.

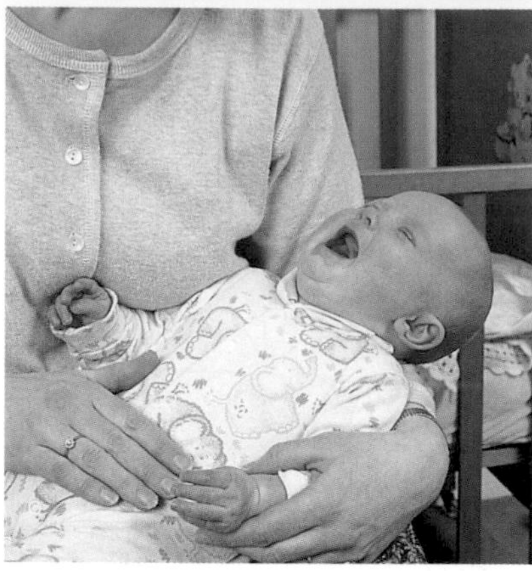

Colic, which is caused by trapped wind, may be soothed by rubbing your baby's tummy and back.

Toothache

Toothache can be very painful and distressing, but it is not always what it seems.

- **Toothache:** this occurs when bacteria found in dental plaque turn the sugar in foods to acid, which attacks a tooth until the nerve endings become exposed. The best treatment for toothache is preventive – a healthy diet that is low in sugar, regular and effective toothbrushing and regular visits to the dentist. Apart from giving paracetamol, all that can be done is to make an emergency dental appointment.

- **Sinusitis:** this can easily be confused with toothache in the upper back teeth when the cheekbone sinuses are infected. Treatment is similar to that for the common cold – junior paracetamol and plenty of fluids. Antibiotics may be needed to treat any secondary bacterial infection.

Headache

A variety of causes may lead to headaches, but if other symptoms are present they may indicate a dangerous condition, such as meningitis. Always seek a doctor's advice if you are worried that your child is seriously unwell.

- **Heat exhaustion or dehydration:** often a long drink of cool water and rest in a cool room is all that is required.

- **Poor vision:** if your child's headaches occur after watching television, arrange for an eye test.

- **Migraine:** if there is a family history of migraines and your child also complains of stomach aches, nausea and dislikes bright lights or loud noises, he could have a migraine. Treat with junior paracetamol and bed rest in a dark, quiet room.

- **Stress:** a headache caused by stress may sometimes be a plea for attention.

- **Cold or flu:** both can be accompanied by a headache. If combined with other symptoms, such as nausea, vomiting, a high temperature, a rash and obvious illness, call a doctor immediately.

Earache

Earache is a common problem for children, and sometimes it can persist.

- **Otitis media (ear infection):** young children and babies often suffer from this infection of the middle ear, usually after an upper respiratory tract infection. The child feels generally unwell, has a temperature and may pull her ears, or in the case of babies, move her head from side to side.

- **Glue ear:** if a child suffers from persistent otitis media, the ear becomes filled with a thick fluid that impairs hearing. The problem can be treated in hospital by inserting tiny tubes, called grommets, into the ear. This allows the fluid to drain out.

NOTE: earache can be treated with painkillers, decongestant drops and antibiotics if there is an infection. However, nothing – including warm olive oil – should be put into a child's ear unless under medical advice.

Otitis media is a common infection in children, causing pain in the ear and a raised temperature.

ALLERGIC REACTIONS

WHAT IS AN ALLERGIC REACTION?

An allergy is a condition in which the body reacts with unusual sensitivity to a substance or substances, which is then known as an allergen.

- The immune system is the body's natural defence against a harmful substance. Antibodies are programmed to recognise these, sticking to them and acting as markers for specialised defensive cells to destroy them.

- An allergic reaction occurs when the body reacts as if a harmless substance is, in fact, harmful. The severity of the reaction depends upon the number of markers. The more markers there are, the more histamine is released from the cells. Histamine is a substance that causes an inflammatory response and produces allergy symptoms.

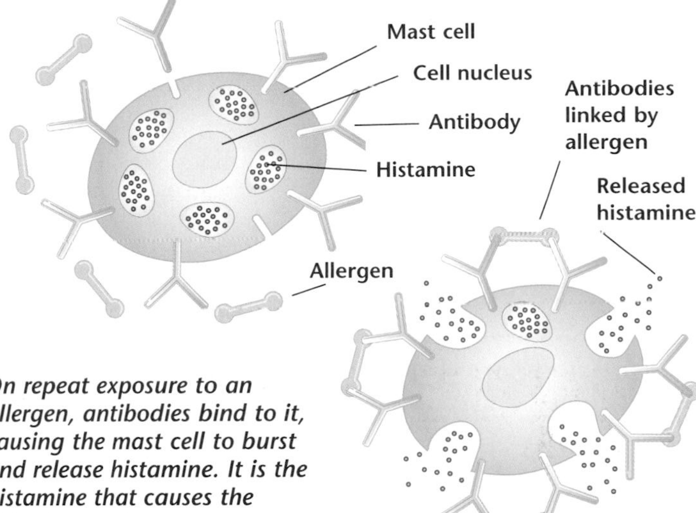

On repeat exposure to an allergen, antibodies bind to it, causing the mast cell to burst and release histamine. It is the histamine that causes the allergic reaction.

Most usual allergens

Severe allergic reactions can be triggered by:

- Nuts
- Eggs
- Seafood
- Grains
- Milk
- Wasp and bee stings
- Drugs, such as penicillin and aspirin
- Rubber products, such as latex

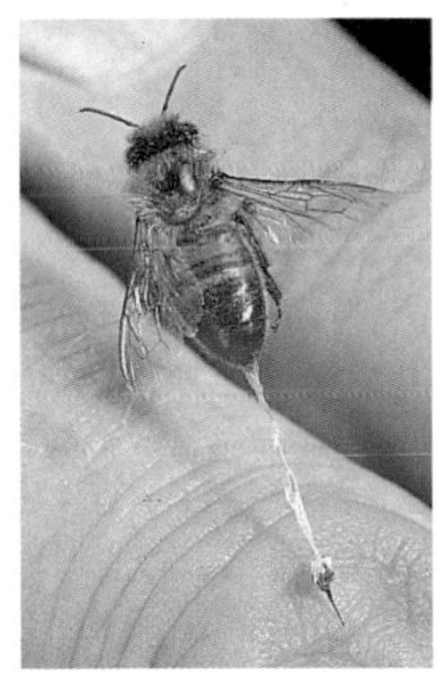

An allergic reaction to a bee sting is quite common.

Allergy facts

Allergies are increasingly common, with 25 per cent of children believed to have some sort of allergy.

1 The link between allergies and increased pollution has proved inconclusive.

2 Most children will outgrow allergies after puberty.

3 Someone who has inherited a tendency to allergies in general is referred to as 'atopic'.

4 Exposure of a three to six month old baby to a substance appears to heighten susceptibility, but only rarely will a child under one have a severe allergic reaction.

5 An allergy is different from a sensitivity or intolerance. In an allergy, the tiniest amount of a substance will cause a reaction.

ANAPHYLACTIC SHOCK

Generally, allergic reactions produce symptoms that require only basic treatment. Sometimes, though, the symptoms can be life-threatening.

- In some people, the body becomes 'sensitised' to a particular allergen. The first time that the person encounters the allergen, the reaction may be mild, but, subsequent attacks are more serious as a greater amount of histamine is released.

- The quick release of large quantities of histamine causes a life-threatening condition called anaphylactic shock, or anaphylaxis. Emergency measures must be taken.

- Those with a nut allergy are particularly prone to sensitisation, although the phenomenon can occur with any allergen.

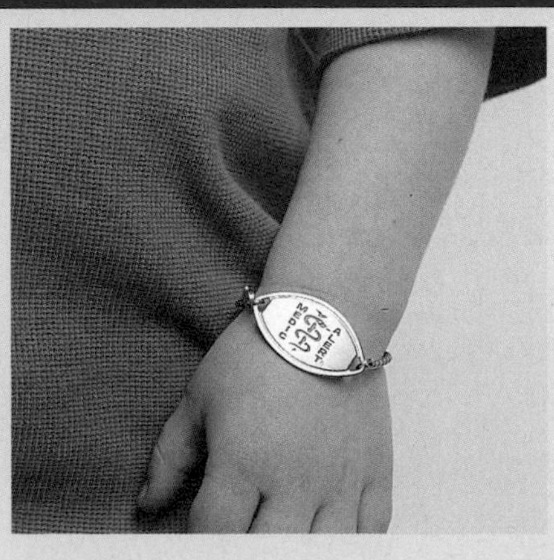

A child who is at risk of anaphylactic shock should wear a medic alert bracelet. This provides important information that could help to save his life.

Signs and symptoms

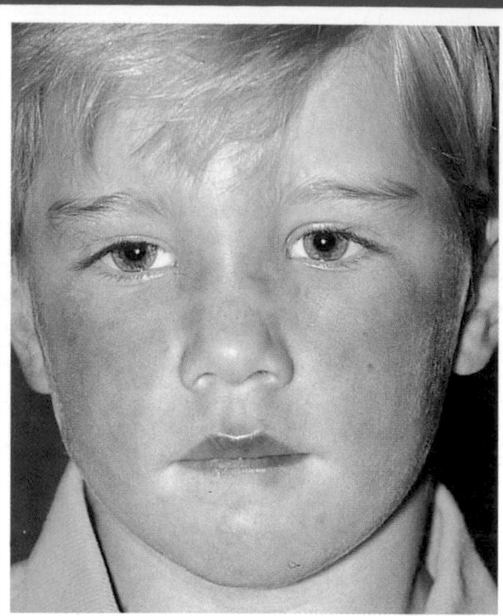

The effects will depend on the severity of the allergic reaction. Anaphylactic shock can develop within a few minutes of contact with the allergen, or after a couple of hours.

- The signs and symptoms of minor allergic reactions include redness and swelling around the site of the bite or sting, puffy eyes, rash, nausea, tummy ache, diarrhoea and, occasionally, joint pains.

- The very first signs of anaphylactic shock can be mild, such as a runny nose and a rash.

Most symptoms of an allergic reaction, such as an itchy rash and swelling, are not serious and soon disappear.

- The symptoms quickly worsen, with red blotchy skin, tightness of the throat and breathing difficulties (as the histamine causes the tissues of the throat to swell up). The lips, tongue and face swell, too, and some people experience vomiting and diarrhoea. There may be light-headedness and an irregular heartbeat.

- Children who also have asthma are at increased risk of a severe attack, because of their susceptibility to breathing difficulties.

First-aid treatment

1 Call the emergency services immediately if you suspect that your child is going into anaphylactic shock. Give any information you have about the cause of the condition.

2 If your child has an adrenaline (epinephrine) syringe for self-use (the hospital may have issued him with one if he has had anaphylactic shock before), help him to use it or give it yourself if you have been trained to do so.

3 Placing your child in a sitting position may help to relieve breathing difficulty, but don't do so if breathing is hindered. If he becomes unconcious and is breathing, put him into the recovery position.

4 Be prepared to give rescue breaths and chest compressions if necessary.

NOTE: antihistamine tablets or syrup can be given, but not if your child is having trouble breathing, because of the danger of choking.

Preventing allergic reactions

The only way to prevent anaphylactic shock is to avoid the allergen responsible. Treat any symptoms immediately.

- If there is a family history of an allergy, mothers are advised to breast-feed exclusively for four to six months and to avoid the allergen during pregnancy and while breast-feeding.

- A specific allergen cannot be identified other than by 'challenge testing' with it, and it would be unsafe to do this. Record any allergic reactions and avoid the allergens in the future.

- Children who are thought to be at risk from anaphylactic shock are given adrenaline syringes that can be used as soon as the symptoms appear – EpiPen and Anapen are both used in Britain. You, your child (if he's old enough) and any carers should know how to use the syringe.

- Buy your child a warning bracelet that states the nature of any allergy and the possibility of anaphylactic shock.

Medical treatment

Anaphylactic shock can be treated successfully so long as medical treatment starts without delay.

1 Adrenaline (epinephrine) is given by intramuscular injection, or, in special cases, directly into a vein, and usually symptoms start to abate fairly quickly. Further adrenaline injections may be needed over the next 24 hours.

2 An antihistamine is given either by injection or by intravenous drip, to combat the build-up of histamine.

3 Hydrocortisone may be given after an attack to prevent long-term consequences, especially for asthmatics.

4 A blood sample may be taken to confirm that the condition was, in fact, anaphylactic shock.

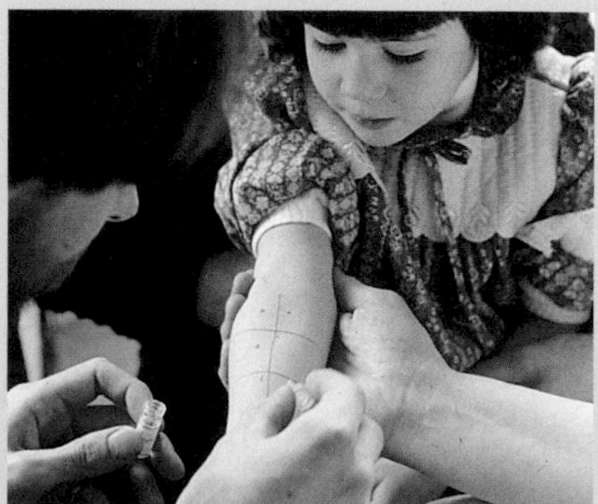

If your child is thought to be have an allergy, patch testing may be carried out to try to identify the substance that is causing the reaction.

ANIMAL BITES

WHY BITES HAPPEN

Children can benefit greatly from having a pet. But, if an animal is teased or harmed by a young child, it is likely to retaliate by biting.

- It is rare that children are bitten by animals, but when it does happen it can cause serious injury and be a frightening experience for the child concerned.

- For an animal to 'turn' on a child contradicts the impressions that pets are gentle, affectionate creatures – a confusing situation for a trusting young mind.

- Bites are usually from dogs or cats (and, in the toddler years, other children). However, with an ever-increasing range of pets available, a child may encounter hamsters, mice and even snakes.

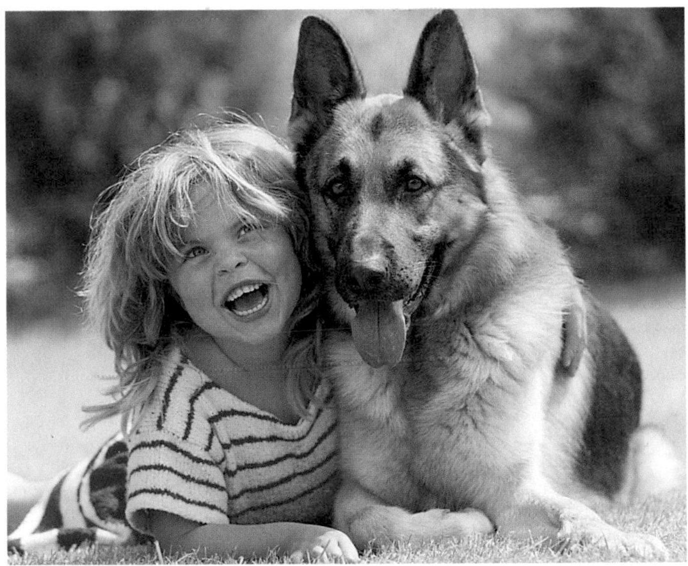

Children tend to trust animals, so it can be upsetting when a pet that was considered 'friendly' turns nasty.

The appearance of animal bites

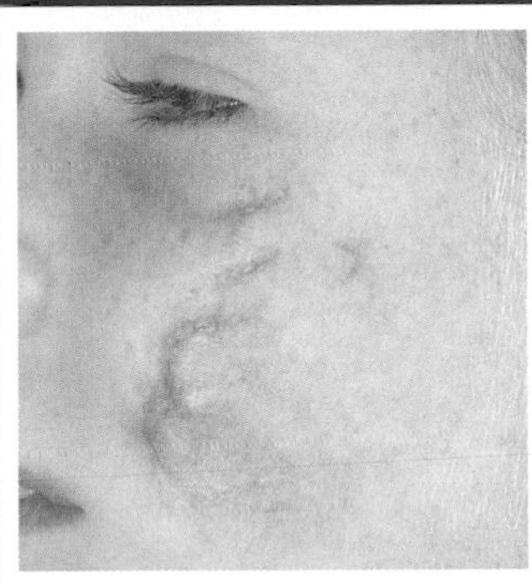

Animal bites are often superficial, requiring only minor treatment, but in some cases they may be serious enough to need stitches.

- An animal bite usually takes the form of puncture marks, tears, scratches or, at worst, ripped flesh or crush injuries.

An animal bite usually punctures the skin and is quite likely to leave a scar.

- The wound may bleed and rapidly become swollen and inflamed.

- The areas most often bitten tend to be the ones that are either at the level of the animal or those not covered by clothing. These include the face, hands, arms, feet and legs. Small children are at greater risk of a bite on the face because of their proximity to the animal.

When to seek help

A doctor should examine a child who has been bitten because of potential complications, such as:

- **Localised infection:** there are many varieties of bacteria in the mouth of any animal. If the skin is punctured, there is a possibility that the organisms could cause local infection, or enter the bloodstream and travel to other areas of the body.

- **Damage to underlying tissues:** if teeth pass through the skin, they can also penetrate tissues such as tendons and muscle.

- **The transmission of serious infections:** the child may be infected with tetanus or rabies.

First-aid treatment

Offer comfort and take steps to relieve pain and prevent infection.

1 Ensure the child is now safe and comfort and reassure him.

2 Wash minor bites with soap and water and cover with a plaster or dry dressing.

3 Serious bites or those that are bleeding should be treated by elevating the wounded area and covering with a sterile dry dressing, applying gentle but firm pressure.

4 If the skin has been broken or the child is in severe pain, seek medical attention.

5 It is advisable to seek a doctor's advice before giving junior paracetamol to a child who has been bitten. He may need further treatment.

NOTE: Do not to give any drugs to a child whom you are looking after, or who is visiting, without parental consent.

Medical treatment

The doctor will want to know about the animal that gave your child the bite, for example, whether it was known to you or whether it was domestic or wild. He will then assess the general condition of your child and examine the wound.

- If the wound is superficial, it will be cleaned and dressed. Antiseptic cream may be applied if appropriate.
- If the wound is deep or has caused damage to the underlying tissues, stitching may be necessary. But, if at all possible, the wound is left open to encourage healing and to lessen the risk of infection.
- The affected area may be X-rayed if the injury is close to bone or to a joint.
- If your child has not had a recent tetanus injection, a booster will be given.
- A course of antibiotics is often prescribed because of the risk of infection.

Tetanus is not easy to treat but it can be prevented by immunisation. Children usually have a booster injection for tetanus before starting school.

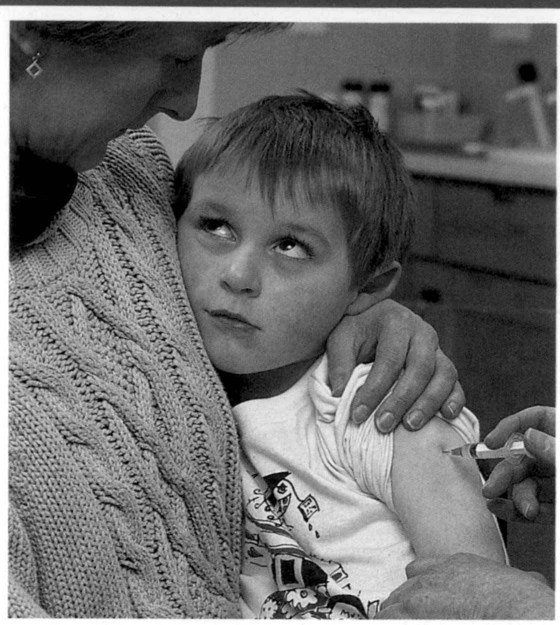

Rabies

Rabies is a virus that is spread through the saliva of an infected animal.

- The virus attacks the nervous system causing a potentially life-threatening condition.
- Rabid animals often behave strangely, foaming at the mouth and appearing agitated and aggressive. Others, such as monkeys, can appear perfectly normal so it is always wise when travelling to find out about the prevalence of rabies in that region.
- If your child is bitten by an animal that you think may be rabid, get medical help as soon as possible.

Rabies is extremely serious. However, there are, at present, no documented cases of rabies in Britain.

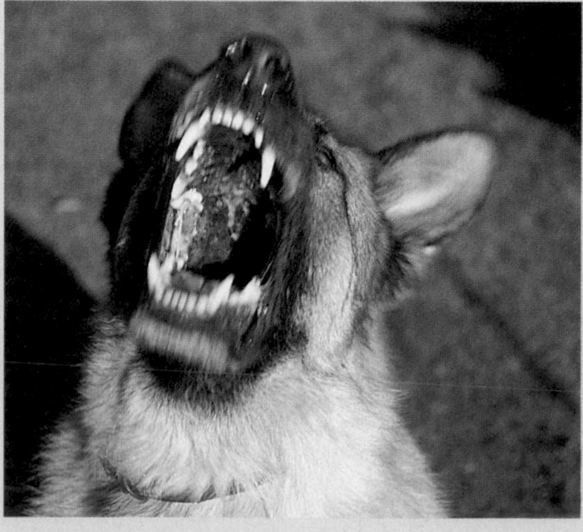

Snakebites

The adder is the only poisonous snake in the UK and its bite is very rarely fatal. However, it is conceivable, though not likely, that your child may be bitten during a holiday abroad. After calling for medical help, first aid to treat a snakebite centres on preventing the venom spreading around the body. Snakebites are usually received on the lower leg.

1. Lay your child down, keeping the heart higher than the wound, and keep him as still and calm as possible.
2. Gently wash and dry the wound. Do not attempt to rub the bite or to suck or cut out the venom.
3. Apply a compression bandage directly over the affected area. Loosen if toes become numb or cold.
4. Using a second bandage, work from the toes to the knee applying firm, even pressure.

Preventative measures

The most obvious advice to parents is to instil in their children an awareness that animals are not always as gentle and cuddly as they appear. Even the most patient animal could react aggressively if it is teased or inadvertently hurt, or if it is scared by sudden loud noises.

- Never leave a young child alone with an animal, even if the animal is thought to be harmless.
- If you have a caged pet, make sure that your child is unable to poke his fingers through the cage. Either keep the pet out of reach or use a fine wire mesh.
- Teach your child never to approach a strange animal, or to tease or hit animals.
- When travelling abroad with your child, take advice from your GP and make sure that your child has received appropriate vaccinations for that country.

APPLYING BANDAGES & DRESSINGS

DEALING WITH MINOR INJURIES

Cuts, grazes and sprains are a common occurrence in young children. Although a child may be distressed by a fall, injuries are often minor and can be dealt with at home.

- Always keep a well-stocked first-aid box at home so that you have everything that you need to hand.
- Play 'doctors and nurses' with your child, and apply bandages and plasters to her dolls and teddies. This will help her to feel more confident about being the patient.
- If a cut becomes infected, seek medical advice.

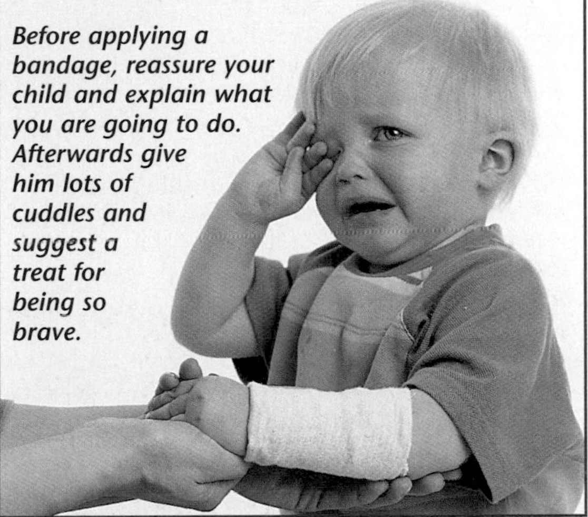

Before applying a bandage, reassure your child and explain what you are going to do. Afterwards give him lots of cuddles and suggest a treat for being so brave.

Dressings

Dressings can be used to cover minor wounds after they've been cleaned and dried. They help to control bleeding and keep the area clean. Always wear disposable gloves when applying a dressing to help prevent cross-infection.

- **Sterile dressings:** these consist of a dressing pad attached to a bandage in sterile packaging. Various sizes are available.
- **Non-adhesive sterile dressings:** some dressing pads are designed so that they do not stick to the damaged skin.
- **Gauze pads:** these can be used to clean around a wound. They can also be used for extra padding.
- **Skin closure tapes:** these sticky strips are used to hold the edges of a cut together before applying a dressing. Use them on your own child only.

Plasters

Plasters protect small cuts or grazes after they have been cleaned and dried. They stop germs getting into the cut, and protect against knocks.

- **Individual fabric plasters:** pre-cut plasters that are quick to apply and stick well.
- **Waterproof plasters:** these plasters stay on even in water, keeping the cut clean and dry

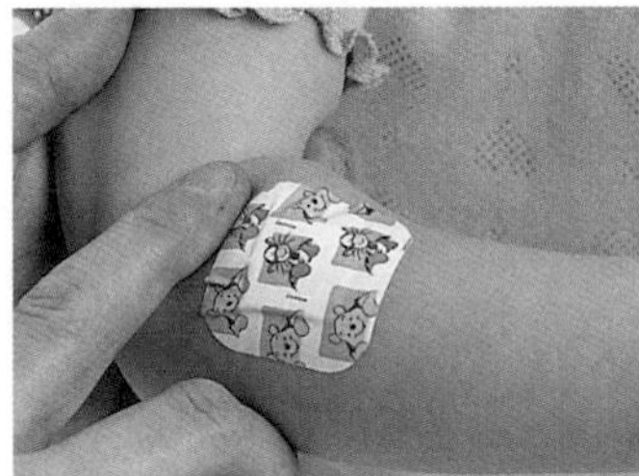

NOTE: some children are allergic to plasters and may develop a rash when they are applied. If this happens, remove the plaster immediately. Instead, use a dry dressing secured in place with micropore (a non-allergenic tape).

If your child is reluctant to wear an ordinary plaster, try letting him choose plasters featuring his favourite cartoon characters.

Bandages

Bandages are used to hold dressings in place, usually on limbs, or to help support a sprain.

- **Stretch bandage:** for holding dressings in place. The skin around a cut may swell so the bandage must be able to stretch.
- **Crêpe bandage:** a soft, stretchy bandage that holds dressings in place. It also provides support for a sprain.
- **Tubular bandage:** this sleeve-like bandage supports sprained joints.
- **Triangular bandage:** ideal as a 'sling' for a damaged arm.

NOTE: most bandages can be washed and reused.

Applying a rolled bandage:

If you are bandaging a limb, follow the steps below:

1 Wrap a clean, rolled bandage around the limb, starting at a point lower than the injury. Keep it taut as you move up the limb.

2 Finish wrapping at a point above the injured area. Secure the end with a safety pin or, in a young child, dressing tape.

3 Check that the bandage isn't too tight, both after putting it on and later. The fingers or toes should be their normal colour – if they are darker, reapply the bandage more loosely. If the bandage covers a wound, remove it daily and apply a clean dressing.

First aid for cuts and grazes

Dealing with a cut or graze is straightforward if you remember a few simple steps:

1 Wash your hands and put on disposable gloves, if available.

2 Wash the cut thoroughly using running water to remove any dirt and debris. Pat the area dry with kitchen roll or a clean cloth.

3 Cover the area, either with a plaster or a clean dressing-pad secured with dressing-tape. Elevate if possible.

4 Examine the wound daily. If the dressing gets wet, remove it immediately and apply a new one.

5 Check that the wound is healing properly. If the affected area becomes red, more swollen and painful, or if pus appears to be forming on the wound, seek medical advice.

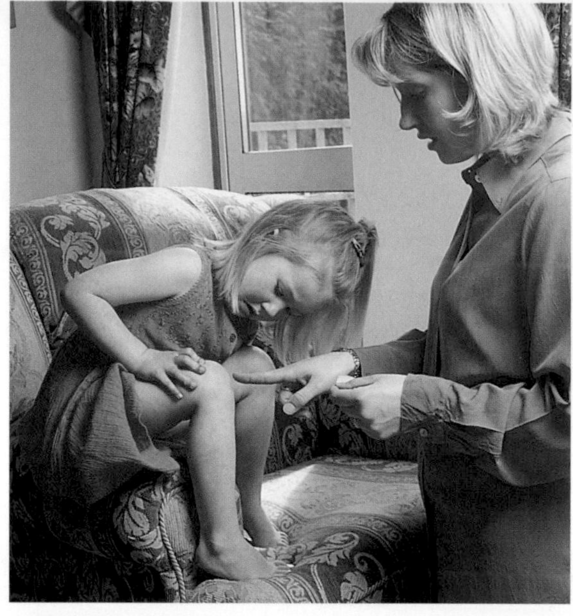

When treating your child's cuts and grazes, first make sure the wound is clean. Applying an antiseptic is not essential but may give extra reassurance.

When to call the doctor

Although you will be able to deal with most of your child's cuts and grazes, seek medical advice if:

- The cut is deep, gaping or has jagged edges.
- Your child has a deep face or head cut, especially if it follows a knock to the head.
- There is something embedded in the wound or it is very dirty.
- The bleeding does not stop after applying pressure.
- The wound was caused by an animal bite.
- There is pain or signs of infection, such as redness and pus.

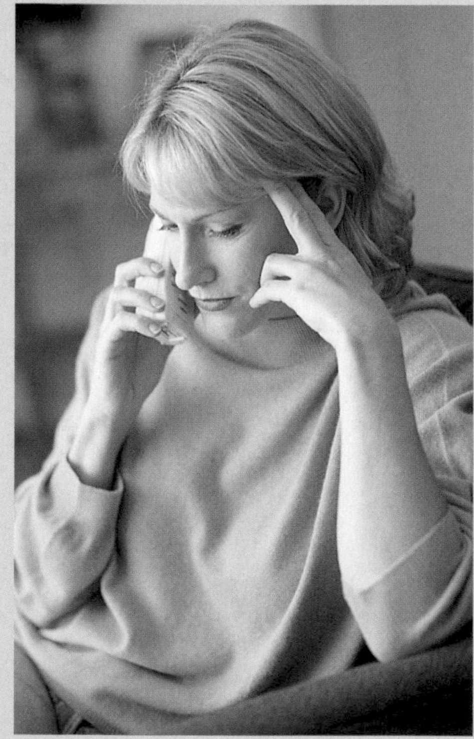

NOTE: normal childhood vaccinations will protect your child against tetanus.

Cuts and grazes are not difficult to treat at home, but seek medical advice if there are signs of infection. It is easier to treat problems in their early stages.

Antiseptics

Antiseptics may be used on your own child but not on another without parental permission. Antiseptics come in various forms:

- **Liquid antiseptic:** either in a bottle or in sachets. A bottle of antiseptic may be one of the cheapest options, but don't use it if it has passed the expiry date.
- **Cream or gel in a tube:** take care not to touch the wound with the tube as it may pick up germs. Put some of the cream on to a clean swab and then apply to the affected area.
- **Antiseptic wipes:** these can be very useful if you are away from home. Always clean the wound from the centre outwards. Discard each wipe after use.
- **Antiseptic sprays:** these are quick and convenient. Hold the spray upright and apply from about 7.5cm (3in) away.

NOTE: always read the instructions on the label. Do not use antiseptics on babies aged under three months. Store antiseptics in a cool place out of the reach of children. Check the expiry date regularly.

Keep antiseptic cream or wipes in your first-aid box along with a selection of plasters and bandages.

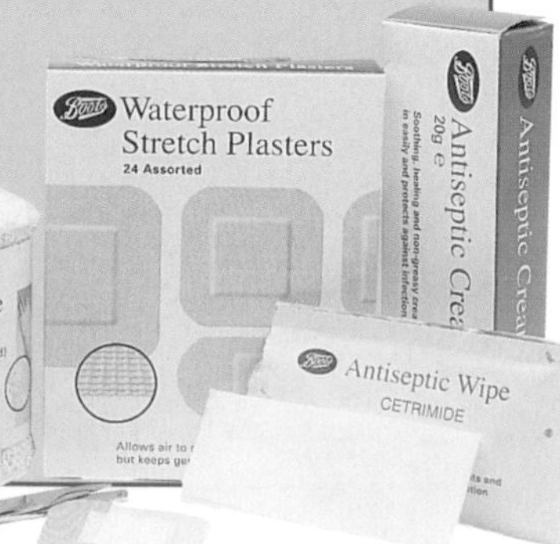

BITES & STINGS

An insect bite or sting is a painful experience for anyone, and will come as a nasty shock to your baby or toddler. While stings are more dangerous, bites from mosquitoes or horseflies can be a persistent problem in certain parts of the country. The following tips can help soothe your child during the spring and summer months.

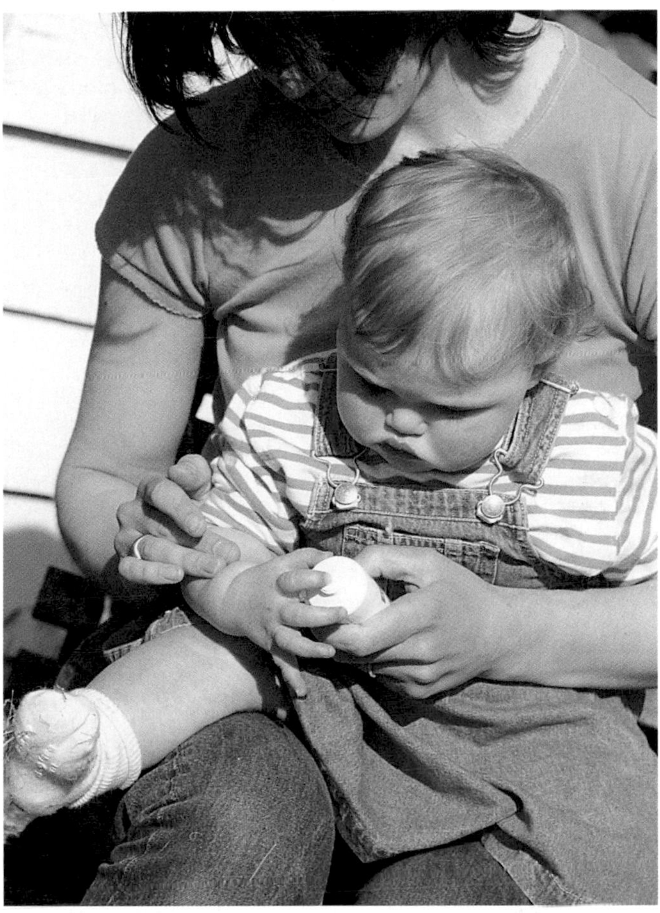

Bee and wasp stings

- If your child is stung by a bee, both the sting and its poison sac will remain embedded in her skin. Take care when removing the sting not to squeeze the sac, which will release more poison into the skin. Scrape the sting out with a clean fingernail or the edge of a credit card rather than using tweezers.

- A wasp sting is similar to that of a bee, but the sting and poison sac are rarely left behind. Wasps can sting repeatedly; bees sting once only.

Symptoms

- Bee and wasp stings are painful, but the effects are usually temporary and any swelling or tenderness, disappears within a few hours.

- Stings to the inside of the mouth need prompt medical attention, because any swelling could obstruct your child's airway. Call a doctor, and give your child cold drinks or, if she is aged two or over, an ice-cube to suck until she receives treatment.

Treating bee and wasp stings

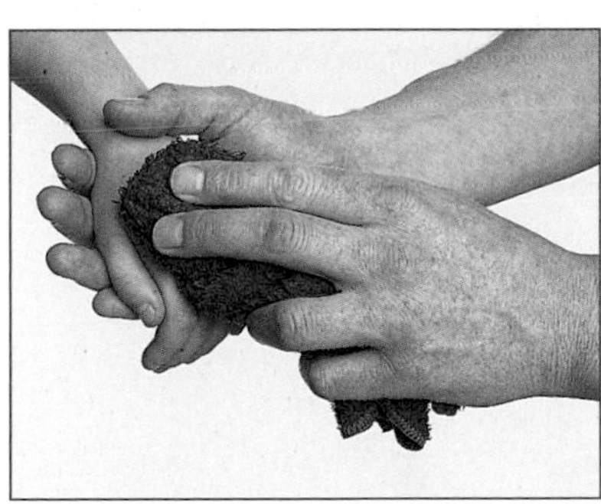

A cold compress can reduce swelling, but an antihistamine spray will help to minimise the skin's reaction to the sting.

- Apply a cold compress or an icepack wrapped in a tea-towel to reduce swelling.
- Apply an antihistamine cream to reduce the skin reaction, checking the instructions carefully.
- If necessary, give your child the appropriate dose of infant paracetamol (not suitable for babies under six months unless prescribed by your GP).

NOTE: do not use antihistamine cream or give paracetamol to a child other than your own without parental permission.

As well as soothing creams, a child over six months of age can be given infant paracetamol to ease the pain of a sting or bite.

Jellyfish stings

Jellyfish stings are relatively rare and most are not serious.

Symptoms

Red swelling with pain and irritation, with shards of jellyfish tentacles still stuck to the skin.

What to do

Ensure that there are no pieces of jellyfish left on the skin by washing with sea-water. Ideally, hold an icepack over the stung area for 10 minutes to ease the pain and swelling.

- A sting from a warm-water jellyfish, such as a Portuguese man-of-war, should be washed with vinegar or sea-water. Keep your child as still as possible and call the emergency services.

Bites

Mosquitoes and gnats

Bites from mosquitoes are most common in hot climates, but gnat bites are prevalent in the UK. Mosquitoes tend to congregate where there is shade and moisture; standing water is needed for them to reproduce. They become airborne at sunrise or sunset on calm and humid days. Fine mesh netting over a baby carrycot or pushchair can help deter them.

Symptoms
A red, itchy weal with a white centre and a small puncture mark.

What to do
Apply an appropriate after-bite milk or cream (seek advice from your pharmacist). Alternatively, apply an antihistamine cream. It is important to reduce the itching, as scratching can turn mosquito bites septic. If bites become infected, apply an appropriate antiseptic cream and consult your GP.

- If you are planning to visit a country where malaria is a risk, get advice from your GP about preventative treatment well before you travel. Malaria is carried and transmitted by mosquitoes.

Horseflies

Horseflies give particularly nasty bites and suck the blood of their victim.

Symptoms
A painful local reaction and swelling that lasts for a few hours.

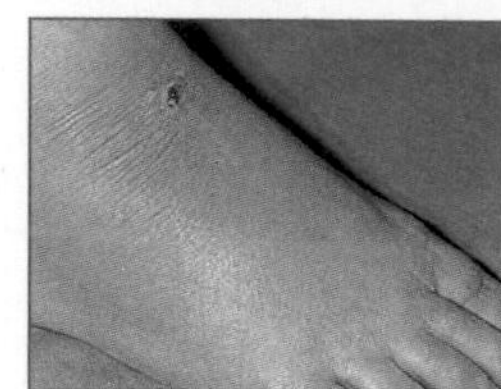

What to do
Apply a cold compress or an icepack wrapped in a tea-towel. Treat with an appropriate antihistamine cream (ask your pharmacist for advice).

Fleas

Flea bites are usually mild, and may occur when a household pet becomes infested.

Symptoms
Small itchy red spots or weals, usually on the arms or legs.

What to do
Apply calamine lotion or camomile cream (available in pharmacies and health-food shops). More importantly, treat your pets for fleas and spray any infested furniture and carpets. Wash pet bedding.

Bites and stings first aid

Insect bites and stings respond well to treatment. Here are some basic items to keep in your first-aid box to help prevent as well as treat bites and stings. Remember, you can use these products on your own children only:

- Insect repellent formulated for babies, available from high-street chemists
- Infant paracetamol
- Appropriate antihistamine cream (ask your pharmacist for advice)
- Appropriate after-bite milk or cream (again, seek advice from your pharmacist)
- Calamine lotion
- Aloe vera gel
- Camomile cream
- Antiseptic cream
- Local anaesthetic gel
- Adrenaline kit (if there is a family history of allergies, or if your child is already known to be allergic to stings)

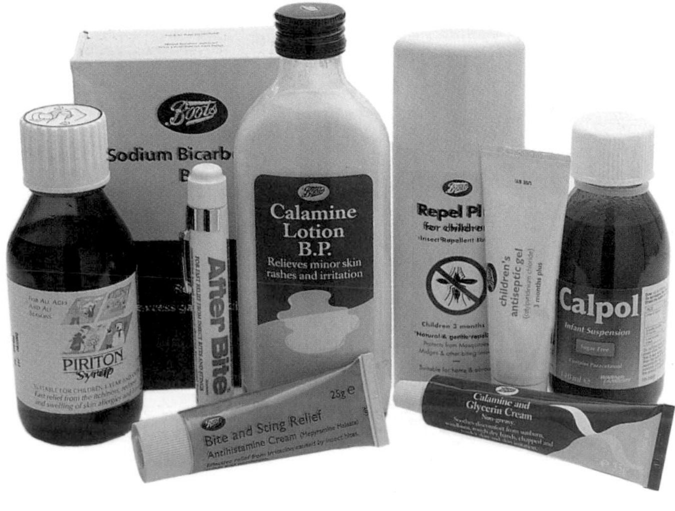

Beat the bugs

1 To prevent bites and stings, apply a repellent cream to any exposed areas of your child's skin before going outside.

2 Dress your child in loose-weave natural fabrics with long sleeves and long trousers whenever possible, but especially in the evenings if you are in a hot country. Pay attention to socks and hats but avoid brightly coloured clothes.

3 If you are travelling abroad, use a plug-in mosquito machine at night. These are available from chemists and come with sachets or tablets of repellent, which slot into the machine.

4 Avoid taking sweet foods and drinks out of doors where wasps are prevalent. Use clear drink containers rather than cans, so you can see if a wasp has got inside.

5 If a wasp approaches your child, wave it away calmly. Discourage her from running away from it, especially if she is brandishing sweet food: a wasp is more likely to sting if antagonised.

6 You can apply the cut side of an onion to a bee or wasp sting if you don't have a medical cream to hand.

BLEEDING

TYPES OF BLEEDING

Bleeding occurs when blood vessels are cut or damaged, allowing the blood to escape into the tissues or out on to the skin. There are three main types of blood vessel, each giving a different pattern of bleeding.

- **Arteries:** carry oxygen-rich blood away from the heart and towards the tissues under great pressure. Arterial bleeding will be bright red, the colour of oxygenated blood, and may spurt out of a wound.

- **Veins:** carry blood away from the tissues and back to the heart. Venous blood has had much of its oxygen removed and so is a darker red. It does not pump out of a cut, but there may still be a large quantity.

- **Capillaries:** the tiny vessels that carry blood through the tissues. Damage to these will cause oozing rather than profuse bleeding.

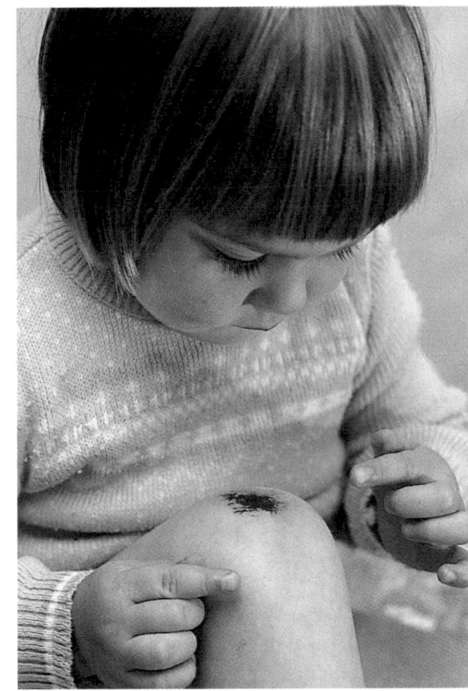

Most children's cuts and scrapes are superficial and will stop bleeding after a short while – mostly you'll just need common sense and a well-stocked first-aid kit.

First aid for minor bleeding

Minor cuts and scrapes are an inevitable part of childhood. Reassurance and simple first aid are usually enough to cope with the situation.

1 Wash your hands with soap and water before tending the wound.

2 Clean the wound with plenty of tepid water.

3 Dry the wound by patting with a clean swab and then place a fresh dressing over the damaged area.

4 Raise the wound up above the level of the heart if possible, supporting the affected limb.

5 Apply a plaster or a dressing pad secured by a bandage.

6 You may want to keep your child sitting quietly for a while before he goes back to play.

When giving first aid, always explain to your child beforehand what you are going to do – this will help her to remain calm.

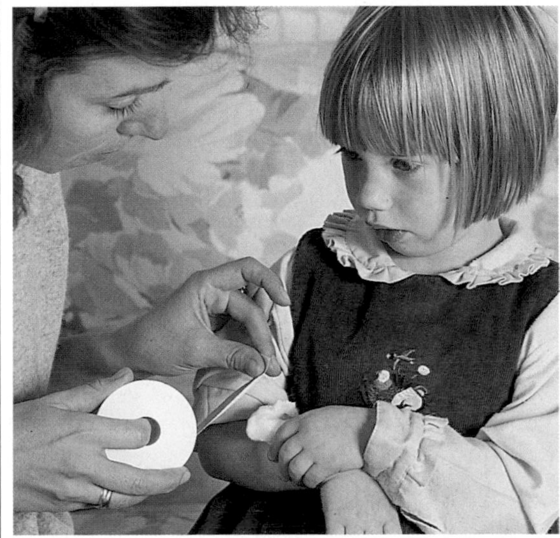

When to seek medical help

Most cases of minor bleeding can be treated at home. It is important, though, to recognise when further help is needed. Seek medical attention when:

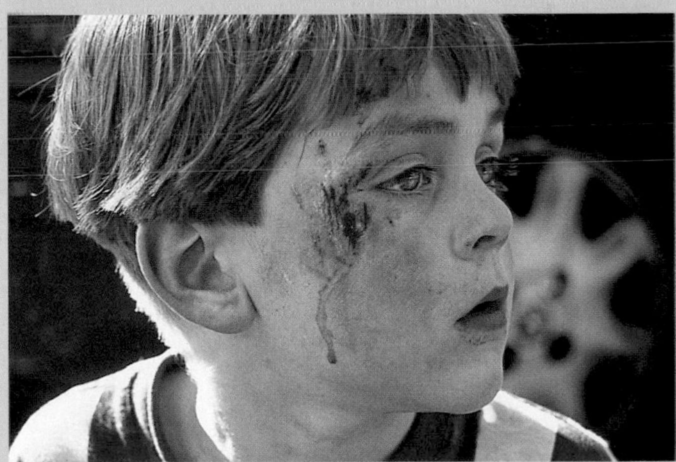

- Bleeding is severe, or there is a large wound.
- You suspect that there may be internal bleeding.
- There is bleeding of the scalp following a blow to the head.
- An object is sticking into or embedded in the wound.

If your child has a head injury, it is important that he is examined by a doctor whatever the extent of the bleeding.

- A minor wound or nose-bleed will not stop bleeding.
- The wound shows signs of infection, such as redness, swelling or pus formation.

First aid for serious bleeding

Serious bleeding can be very frightening, but try to remain calm as your child will be looking to you for the reassurance she needs. Your main aim should be to stop the bleeding before too much blood is lost, so you will need to act quickly.

1 Expose the wound by removing clothing and check whether foreign objects, such as glass, are embedded in it. If a foreign object is present, try pressing both sides of the wound. Raise the injured limb above your child's heart and apply pressure over the wound with your hand, using a clean dressing or cloth. This should stop the bleeding.

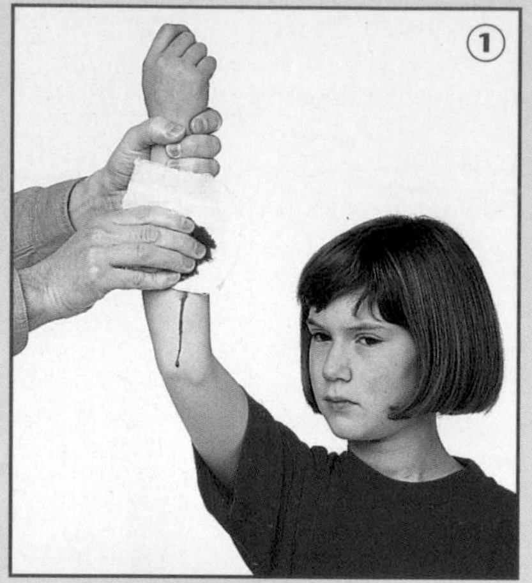

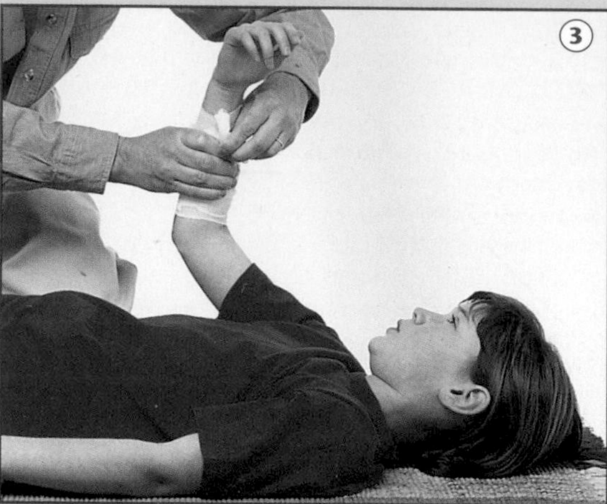

2 Continue to apply pressure while supporting the limb up above the heart, preferably with your child lying down. If there has been a lot of bleeding, you must lay your child down to minimise shock. Arterial bleeding (with bright red, spurting blood) will need at least 10 minutes of firm pressure.

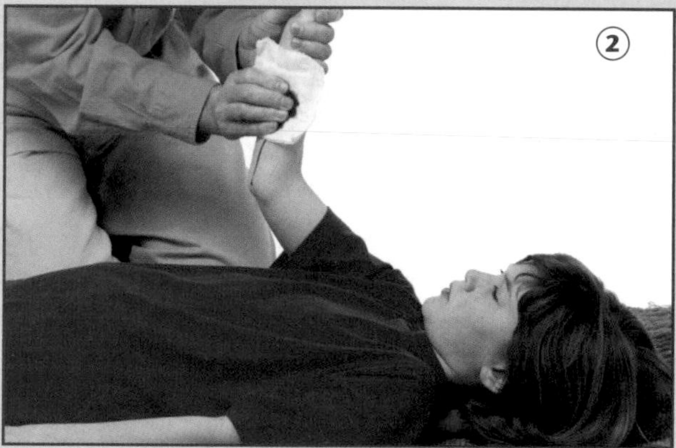

3 Apply a pressure bandage. Leaving the original pad where it is, cover it with a sterile dressing and secure it in place with a firm bandage. If the blood soaks through, apply another dressing and bandage on top.

4 While trying to control the bleeding, it is important to seek medical attention, calling 999 for an ambulance if necessary.

Aftercare

Looking after a wound means keeping it clean, dry and protected. To care for a wound:

- Change the dressing daily, using a clean or sterile dressing pad and a clean bandage if possible.
- Look for signs of infection, such as redness, swelling, pus or increased tenderness.
- Do not disturb any scab that is forming, as this is the body's way of healing.
- Protect wounds by limiting your child's activities.
- Take your child to the doctor if a wound shows any sign of infection.

Dealing with an infected wound

A wound should begin to heal in 48 hours but cannot do so if it is infected. Any break in the skin can lead to infection by micro-organisms, especially if the wound has dirt in it. An infected wound may become hot, red, painful and swollen and pus may form. To reduce the chances of infection:

- Clean the wound well with plenty of water when the injury first happens – antiseptic may help.
- Change the dressing regularly, being careful to wash your hands before and afterwards.
- Make sure your child completes the full course of any antibiotics that the doctor prescribes, even if the wound begins to heal well.
- Keep an infected wound well covered and do not allow your child or anyone else to touch it.
- Make sure your child is fully inoculated – if he is, he will be safe from tetanus, a serious infection that can spread from a dirty wound.

NOTE: check with your GP if you are not certain about your child's inoculations.

Antiseptic solutions can be useful on minor wounds. Do not apply to another person's child, because they might have an allergy to it.

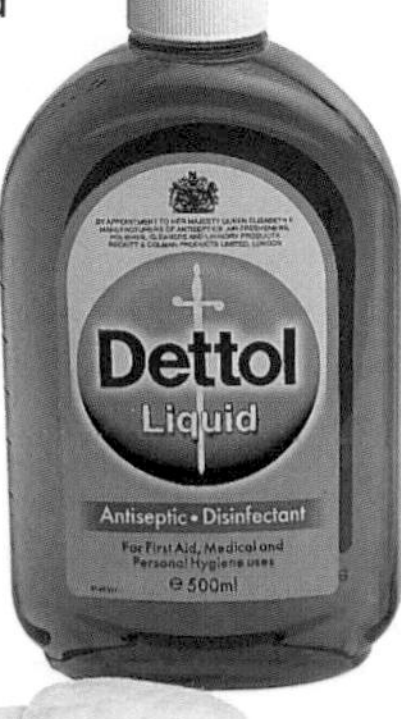

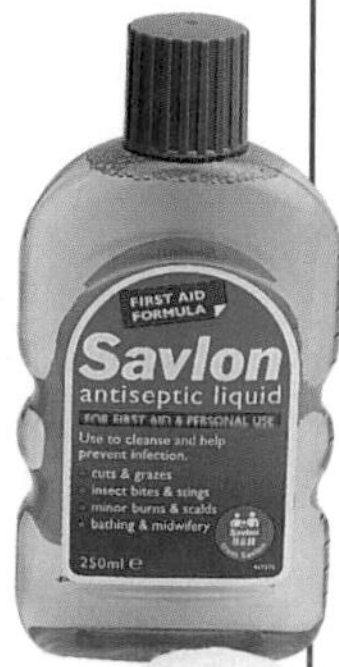

BURNS

THE RISK OF INJURY

Children under five are more likely to suffer from severe burns and scalds than any other age group.

- Every year, over 3000 pre-school children are taken to hospital suffering from burns and, sadly, many die or are disfigured for life. Burns are the second most common cause of accidental death in young children, after road traffic accidents.

- Children who are aged under five, especially toddlers, are active and inquisitive. They are too young to realise the danger posed by heat and certain objects and situations. Young children also have small bodies and delicate skin, factors that can intensify the damage caused by a burn.

- There are steps you can take that will reduce the risk to your child. The first is to have preventive safety measures in place at all times. Secondly, it is vital to know what to do, and what treatment to apply, if a burn occurs.

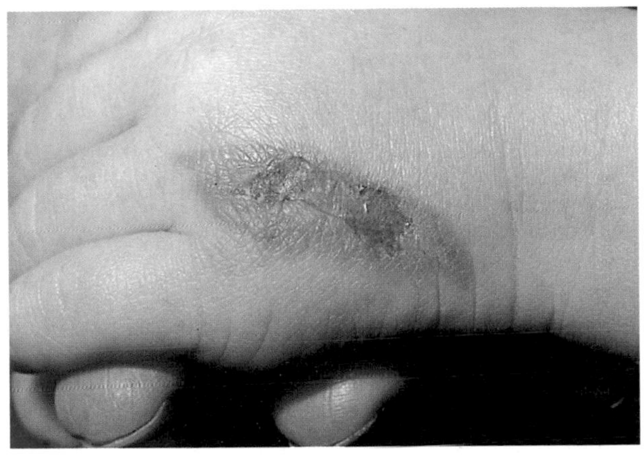

A partial thickness, or second degree burn, may be more painful than a full thickness, or third degree burn. This is because a third degree burn destroys the nerve endings that transmit pain.

Types of burn

Burns can be divided into three main types. Depending on the skin damage, they may be superficial, partial thickness or full thickness. They are also described as first, second or third degree.

1 **Superficial, or first degree burn:** this type of burn is the mildest and most common of the three groups. Only the outer layer of the skin is damaged. There will be some redness, swelling and tenderness before the area heals naturally. The scar will probably heal within a week.

2 **Partial thickness, or second degree burns:** this type of burn is more serious. The outer layer of the skin burns through but there is no damage to underlying tissues. It is usually painful and there may be raised blisters as well as redness and swelling.

3 **Full thickness, or third degree burns:** this type of burn is the most serious of all. All the layers of skin are burned through and there may be damage to the tissues beneath. Although these burns may be painful, there is sometimes little or no pain because of damage to the sensory nerve endings.

When to seek help

Always seek medical aid in the following circumstances:

- If the child is under two years old.
- If the burn involves the face – especially the nose or mouth, or is blocking the airways.
- If there has been smoke inhalation, which can block the airways.
- If the area affected is bigger than the palm of the child's hand.
- If the burn is located around the chest area, as this can constrict breathing movements.

Preventing burns

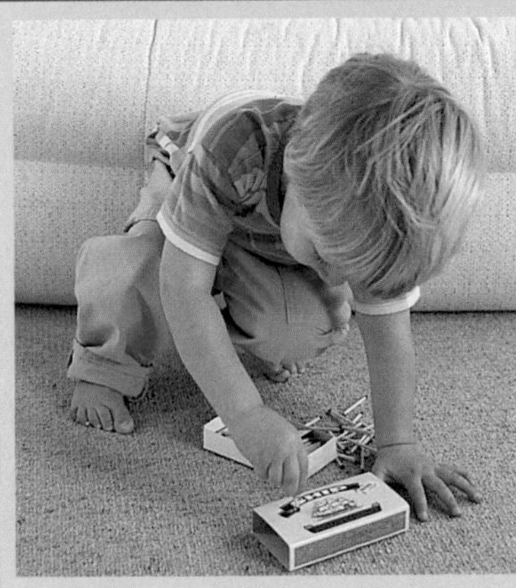

It is vital to keep flammable items, such as matches, out of the reach of young children.

Hazards in the home are one of the primary causes of burns in children.

- Half of all burns suffered by young children take place in the kitchen. Watch your child at all times, especially when you are cooking. Turn pan handles inwards and don't let electric cords dangle down. Use a playpen to keep a young child safe if you are busy.
- Keep matches and lighters well out of your child's reach and sight.
- Keep corrosive substances safely locked away.
- Fit smoke alarms on every floor of the house and test them regularly.
- Use a fireguard around any heater. Make sure it covers the whole heater and is attached securely to the wall.
- Put cold water in the bath before hot water to avoid scalding.

Home emergency treatment

All but the most superficial burns in young children require medical attention, but your actions in the first few minutes may make a big difference to the degree of injury your child sustains.

1 Cool the burned area immediately with lots of cold water for at least 10 minutes. If no water is available, use another safe and cold watery liquid such as milk. Keeping the burn immersed in water will help to ease the pain. Hold the burned area up off the ground to keep it clean, and try not to touch it.

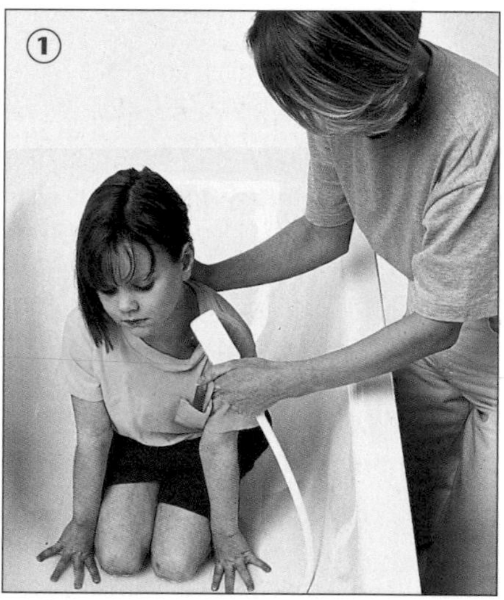
①

2 Remove any clothing or jewellery around the burned area, which might become tight as the burn swells. Cut around any clothing that is sticking to the skin – lifting such material away may remove the skin.

3 Cover the burned area with a clean, preferably sterile, dressing or cloth. Do not use anything fluffy, such as cotton wool, which would stick to the burn. Alternatively, once cooled with water for at least 10 minutes, cover the burned area with cling film or a clean plastic bag.

4 Do not give the child anything to eat or drink. Assess the child for signs of shock, such as pale, cold sweaty skin and rapid pulse and breathing. Remember to keep her warm.

5 If the burn is severe, especially if caused by fire with smoke, keep a check on your child's breathing. Be ready to resuscitate her if necessary.

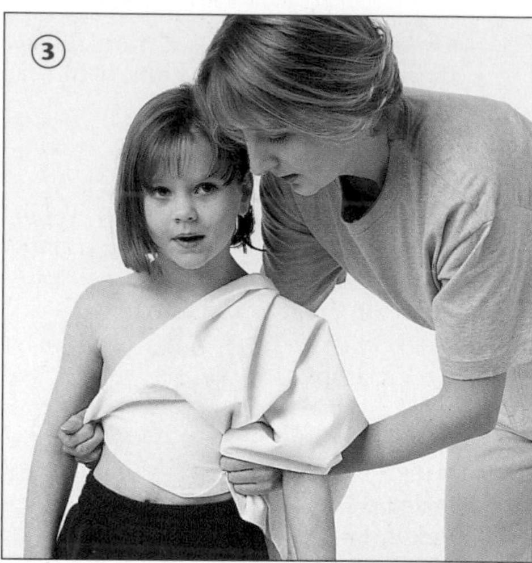
③

Precautions

✘ Do not put butter or other greasy substances on to a burn. These retain heat and stop the skin from cooling.

✘ Do not put ice directly on to a burn as it can damage the skin.

✘ Do not try to remove anything, such as clothing, that has stuck to the burned area.

✘ Do not burst blisters.

Chemical burns

Chemical burns are caused by corrosive substances that may irritate and damage the skin, or be absorbed into the body to cause further harm. A chemical burn always requires medical attention, but the immediate treatment is similar to that used when burns are caused by heat.

1 Remove your child from any spillage of chemicals. Wear rubber gloves if you have them.

2 Use large amounts of water to dilute the chemical and clean the area. Continue running fresh water over the burn for at least 20 minutes.

3 If there is a large amount of powder on the skin, brush it off carefully first.

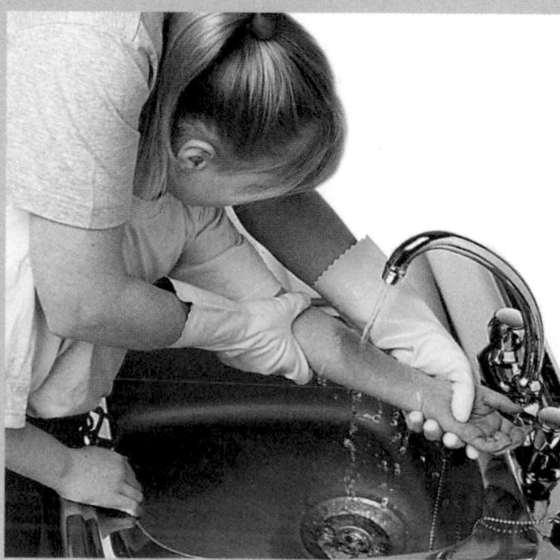

4 Remove clothing covering the burned area while you are flooding it with water, unless it sticks to the skin.

5 Seek medical help, letting the doctor know which substance caused the burn.

Wear rubber gloves for protection while running fresh water over the burn.

Hospital treatment

A child may need minor treatment, or may be taken to a specialist burns unit for expert attention. If your child is admitted to hospital with serious burns, he may receive:

- Fluids into a vein to make up for fluid lost at the burn site.
- A blood transfusion, if necessary.
- Pain relief, which will be adjusted if necessary to ensure that your child is not in great pain.
- Antibiotics, to treat infection.
- Skin grafting in serious, full thickness burns, to replace lost skin.
- Surgery at a later date, to help loosen any scars that form.

CHEST & ABDOMINAL INJURIES

WHAT CAN CAUSE INJURIES?

Although a child's body is more flexible than an adult's, it is also weaker, so the risk of suffering injuries to the chest and abdominal regions is just as high. The risk of injury is increased by the fact that children are often more active than adults and less aware of danger.

1 Injuries to the chest and abdomen commonly occur as the result of a fall, usually from some height. Injuries are even more likely if the torso makes contact with a hard or penetrating object on landing.

2 Injuries involving vehicles are common. They may occur when children are involved in road traffic or cycling accidents or when they are playing near vehicles, such as cars and tractors that are being used off the road.

3 Injuries sometimes occur as the result of physical abuse. Medical staff are always alert to this possibility and will therefore inquire closely about the circumstances of any serious injury or multiple injuries.

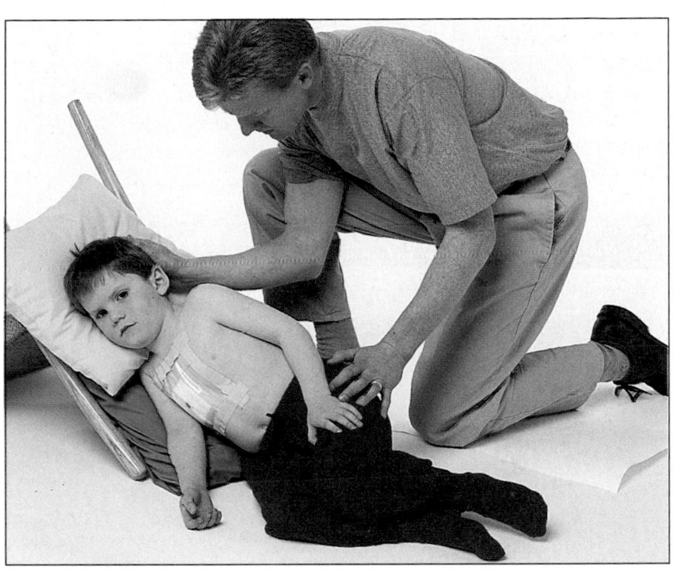

A chest injury can cause internal damage so It is important to act promptly. Place a dressing on the wound (as described overleaf), turn the child on his injured side and seek immediate medical help.

Types of injury

The type of injury and the damage that results will depend on the nature of the child's accident.

- **Fractured ribs:** the ribs protect the heart and lungs and are designed to absorb impact. However, fractured ribs may result from a severe blow to the chest. A fractured rib will cause pain when inhaling deeply. Rest is the only form of treatment. A fractured rib will normally repair itself within three to six weeks.

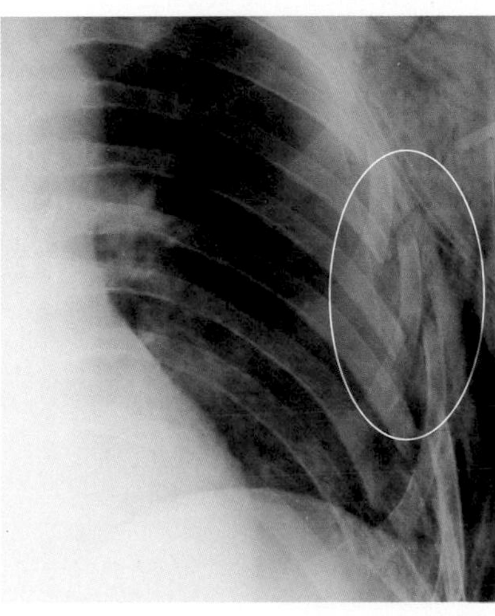

- **Crush injuries:** when the chest or abdomen are crushed, most of the damage is internal, but often the only obvious external sign of injury is bruising. A crushed chest usually involves one or more broken ribs, which may puncture the lungs. If several ribs are broken the result may be a condition known as flail chest. A section of the chest wall becomes detached, leading to the collapse of one or both lungs and possible damage to the heart. This condition requires urgent medical attention.

- **Penetrating injuries:** the damage that occurs when an object penetrates the skin depends on the depth of penetration. If it has only penetrated the surface layers of skin and muscle, it is unlikely to cause severe damage. A deeper wound may damage internal organs.

A serious blow to the chest may result in a rib fracture (circled). This may be confirmed by X-ray.

Symptoms

Even if there is no visible external evidence, there may be signs of internal damage.

- Internal injuries to the chest may cause breathing problems, particularly if a lung has been penetrated. If blood bubbles from a wound, this is a sign that air has entered the chest and that the child has a collapsed lung.

- Coughing up bright red frothy blood is a sign of a lung injury.

- Abdominal injuries may cause the abdomen to become tight and the child may complain of pain or tenderness. Muscular spasms may occur.

- The child is likely to show signs of shock. The skin becomes pale, cold and moist. Breathing becomes shallow, the pulse is weak and rapid, and the child may complain of dizziness, fainting, blurred vision and nausea. He may also become thirsty and restless.

Hospital treatment

In hospital, Accident and Emergency staff will carry out any necessary resuscitation. As soon as the child's condition is stable, they will assess the extent of any internal damage and begin appropriate treatment.

- Internal damage is assessed using imaging techniques, such as X-ray, CT scanning and MRI.
- If a pneumothorax is diagnosed, where air is trapped between the two layers of membrane covering the lungs, a tube will be inserted into the chest cavity to allow air to escape.
- If internal bleeding in the abdomen is suspected, medical staff may undertake a procedure known as a peritoneal lavage. A small tube is inserted into the abdomen to extract fluid. If the fluid contains blood, surgery may be necessary so that the damage can be investigated and repaired.
- Recovery from chest and abdominal wounds depends on the extent of the injury. After a minor injury the patient may be allowed home with instructions to rest. More serious injuries may require a stay in hospital.

First aid for chest injuries

In the event of a chest injury, take immediate action and telephone for an ambulance. Check the child's pulse and breathing regularly until help arrives.

1 If there is a penetrating wound, put on disposable gloves and cover the area with your hand.

2 Place the child in a comfortable position on the ground so that his head and chest are raised.

3 Cover the wound with a sterile dressing. Use adhesive tape to seal the dressing on three sides only, leaving one side free for air to escape .

4 Place the arm on the injured side diagonally across the child's chest. Hold the arm in place with a triangular sling. This will give added support to any fractured ribs.

5 Turn the child gently, ensuring that the head and torso remain raised, so that he is leaning towards his injured side. Make sure that he is comfortable and supported with cushions.

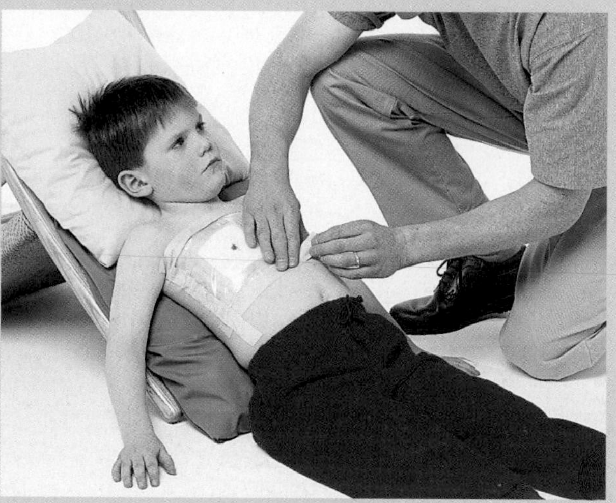

After suffering an injury to the chest, a child's lungs are particularly vulnerable to damage. It is important to cover the wound, leaving space for air to escape.

First aid for abdominal injuries

Take immediate action and call an ambulance. Check the child's pulse and breathing regularly. Do not remove any object that is protruding from a wound; removal may cause further damage and more bleeding.

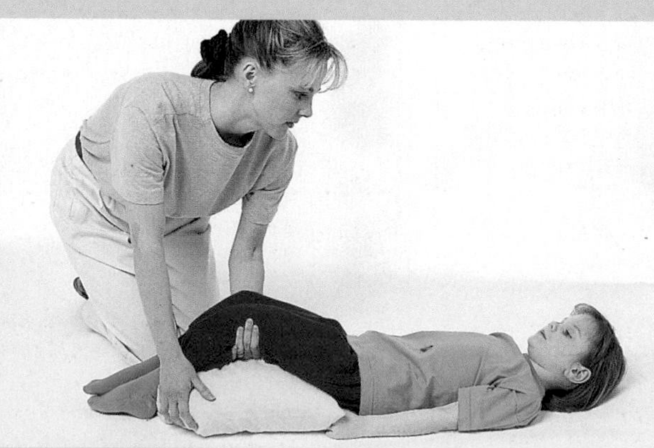

If a child has an abdominal injury, lie her on her back with a cushion under her knees. You should then cover the wound with a sterile dressing and tape it in place.

1 Expose the wound gently by removing clothing from around it.

2 If there are no organs protruding from the wound, place the child on her back, with a cushion under the knees to reduce the strain on the stomach muscles. This helps to keep the wound closed.

3 If there are organs protruding from the wound, raise the knees and place a blanket or coats under the child's shoulders. This position helps the natural action of the stomach muscles.

4 Cover the wound with a dressing and tape it into place. Do not attempt to push any protruding organs back through the wound.

5 If the child is about to cough or vomit, and there are no organs protruding, reduce the strain on the wound by pressing down on it with the flat of the hand.

CHILLS & HYPOTHERMIA

BODY TEMPERATURE

A child's normal body temperature is 36–37.2°C (97–99°F). A 'thermostat' in the brain helps the body to maintain a balance between heat gain and loss.

- The temperature-regulating mechanism in babies is underdeveloped so they are at risk of developing hypothermia if, for example, they are in a cold room.
- The difference between a chill and hypothermia is a matter of degree. While a chill is a mild, easily reversed condition, hypothermia is serious and requires immediate action to be taken.
- Exposure to cold environments causes heat to be lost faster than the body can generate it. For example, immersion in cold water can increase heat loss by up to 25 times.

If your baby has a chill, his temperature will drop slightly. However, if he has contracted hypothermia, his body temperature will drop dramatically.

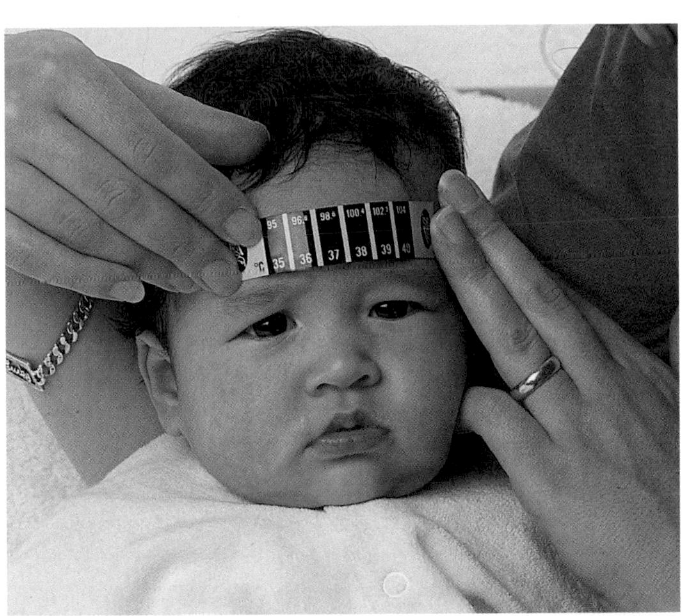

From a chill to hypothermia

A chill is a slight lowering of body temperature, which can result from being in a cold draught or not wearing enough warm clothing. Hypothermia is said to have occurred when the body's core temperature drops below 35°C (95°F).

- A chill affects the surface layers of the body only and, if appropriate action is taken, such as putting on warmer clothing, the cooling process is quickly reversed.
- If sufficient action is not taken to reverse the effects of cooling, the cold may penetrate deeper into the body, which may cause the body's core temperature to drop enough for hypothermia to set in.
- Small babies and the elderly are more prone to chills and hypothermia than adults. Infants have a lower volume to surface ratio than adults and thus their bodies cool more rapidly. Elderly people tend to cool down more easily because they often have a slower metabolism and are less active than younger adults.
- Contrary to popular belief, a chill is not the direct cause of a cold. But when body temperature is lowered, resistance to infection may be reduced, allowing the common cold virus to invade.

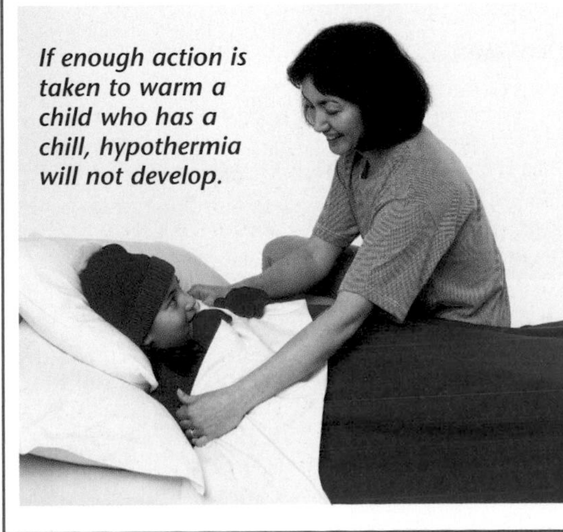

If enough action is taken to warm a child who has a chill, hypothermia will not develop.

Physical effects

Moderate hypothermia can be reversed, but a severe case can be fatal. The effects will depend on how far and at what speed the temperature drops.

1. Hypothermia depresses the central nervous system.
2. Below 33°C (91.5°F) the electrical activity of the brain becomes abnormal.
3. The hypothalamus in the brain, which normally controls body temperature, starts to malfunction.
4. Finally the whole body starts to slow down. The heart rate drops and breathing becomes slow and shallow.
5. As the blood supply to the brain is reduced, the child becomes unconscious.
6. If the body temperature falls too much, the heart becomes arrhythmic, kidney and lung failures occur, and the result is usually coma and death.

Signs in babies

The body goes through a series of stages before hypothermia sets in. Be aware of the signs that a baby is developing hypothermia.

- **Shivering:** this is a result of the involuntary rapid contraction and relaxation of muscles, as the body tries to use them to generate heat.
- **Curling up:** you may notice that an older baby or a toddler instinctively curls up in a ball to reduce the surface area exposed to cold air.
- **Cold skin:** the skin may look healthy but feel cold to the touch. This occurs as a result of the body attempting to maintain the temperature of the blood being sent to the brain, heart and other vital organs. The skin often becomes pale and cold to the touch due to the lack of blood being supplied to it, and may look red or blue.
- **Behavioural changes:** a baby may be drowsy and limp. He may be unusually quiet or cry, and may refuse to feed. Signs in an older child include being lethargic, feeling dizzy and nauseous, losing co-ordination and starting to stumble. A child with severe hypothermia may become confused and actually remove clothing.

Preventing chills and hypothermia

The obvious way to prevent the body from cooling down is to avoid exposure to cold. In cold conditions take precautions to keep your baby warm.

- For a baby sitting in a pram outside on a hot day, a single layer of clothing may be sufficient, but on a cold day in winter you will need to put your baby in several layers of clothing.
- In a cool room your baby will need more layers of clothing than in a warm, centrally heated room. At night make sure that your baby is covered with adequate bedding.
- Don't overdo clothing or bedding. Remember that a baby can be too hot as well as too cold. Keep room temperature at 18°C (64°F).

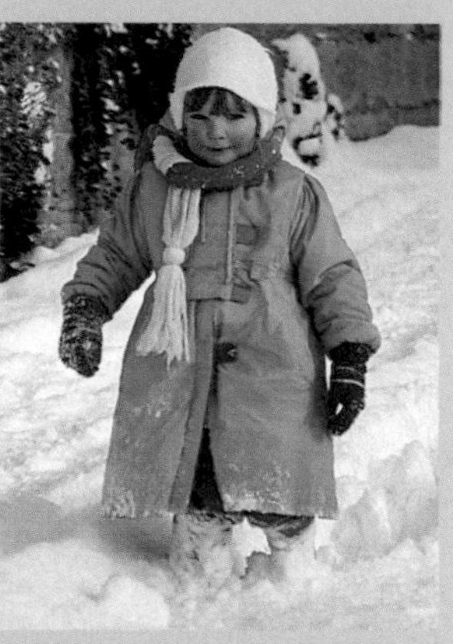

In cold conditions, make sure you dress your child in several warm layers of clothing and a hat.

Treating hypothermia in babies

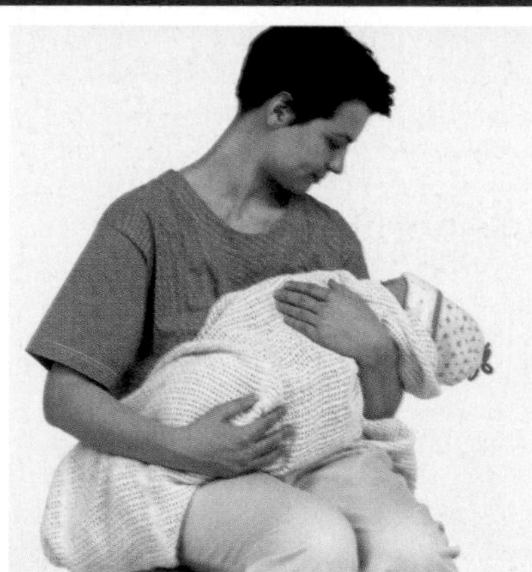

Wrap a baby with hypothermia in a blanket and hold him against you to warm him.

Hypothermia requires immediate treatment. The sooner a baby or child can be warmed, the greater their chances of survival.

1. Dial 999 and ask for an ambulance.
2. Wrap your baby in a blanket. Warm him gradually – warming him too quickly may place a strain on his heart.
3. Put a hat on him to prevent further heat loss through his head.
4. Hold him against you so that he can benefit from your body heat.
5. If possible, move your baby to a warm place. Stay with him.

NOTE: if your baby is not breathing, give artificial respiration immediately. If there is no pulse, give cardio-pulmonary resuscitation.

Treating hypothermia in children

As with a baby, a child with hypothermia must be treated immediately to increase her likelihood of survival.

1. Call a doctor immediately.
2. Give your child a warm bath and then wrap her in warm towels or a blanket.
3. Dress your child, including a hat, and put her to bed. Do not put a hot-water bottle next to her skin as it is essential that she warms up gradually.
4. Give her a warm drink and a high-energy food, such as chocolate.
5. Stay with your child so that you can monitor her condition.

NOTE: if your child is not breathing, give artificial respiration immediately. If there is no pulse, give cardio-pulmonary resuscitation.

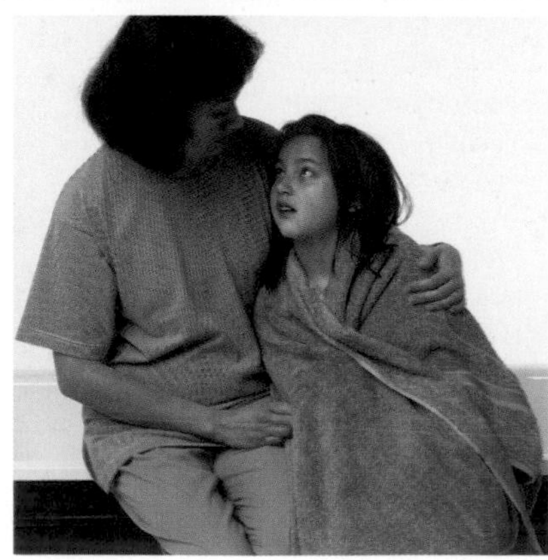

A child with hypothermia should be wrapped in a blanket and moved to a warm room.

CHOKING

WHY CHILDREN CHOKE

Each year, dozens of children die from choking. Babies and toddlers, especially, tend to put anything at all that will fit into their mouths. The item may be too big to swallow and get stuck in the airway.

Children are especially at risk because as they choke the back of their throat expands, and as they try to breathe by taking a deep breath the object is sucked further downwards.

When to take emergency action

When the following symptoms are present you need to act quickly:

- Your child cannot speak or make a sound
- His lips are blue
- His skin is a dusky colour
- He loses consciousness and collapses

If urgent action is not taken, death or brain damage will take place within four minutes. If your child is still breathing and has choked, staycalm, dial 999 and get first-aid emergency advice from the Ambulance Service.

Preventing choking

The sight of a choking child is every parent's worst nightmare yet, like many childhood accidents, by taking a few preventive measures the chances of your child choking can be reduced significantly.

- Do not leave small objects – such as toys, coins, marbles or half-deflated balloons – lying around for your curious toddler to find.
- Keep older children's toys separate from young children's toys.
- Avoid vending machine toys. These do not have to meet safety regulations and often contain small parts.
- If your child has no or few teeth, blend his food or cut it up very small.
- Never let your child run or play while eating.
- Never allow your child to run with pencils, lollipops or crayons in his mouth.
- Keep all adult snacks away from exploring toddler hands.
- Never let siblings feed younger children unsupervised. Infants tend to choke on food, especially peanuts. Older children are more likely to choke on other things, such as pen caps, paper clips and chewing gum.

AVOID giving children the following foods until they are at least four years old:

whole grapes
carrot/apple chunks
sweets
popcorn

Nuts A child should not eat nuts until they can open the packet. **Peanuts** are common culprits in choking. They will often not lead to complete airway blockage but will get stuck further down in the lungs and lead to chest infections and wheezing. Don't have peanuts near children, to avoid the risk of choking and/or a severe allergic reaction.

Beware balloons!
Balloons are an unsuspected hazard in many households. They can easily obstruct the airway. especially if they have almost but not quite fully deflated. Such balloons do a very effective job of completely blocking the airway and are extremely difficult to shift once stuck.

Emergency procedure for a choking infant under one year old

The management of a choking baby under one year old is different from that of a small child or an older child. You cannot use abdominal thrusts on a baby because these could cause damage to his organs.

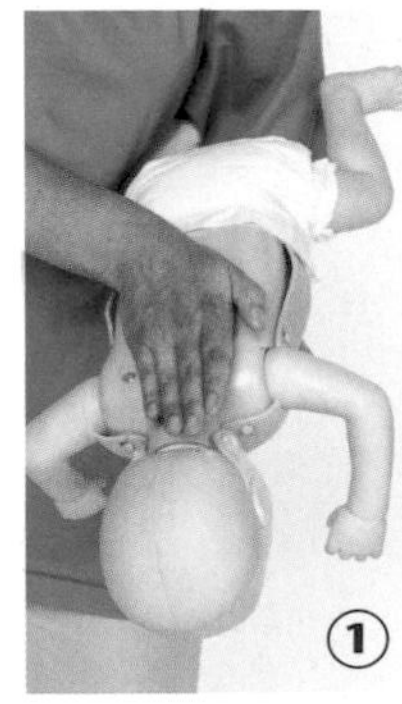

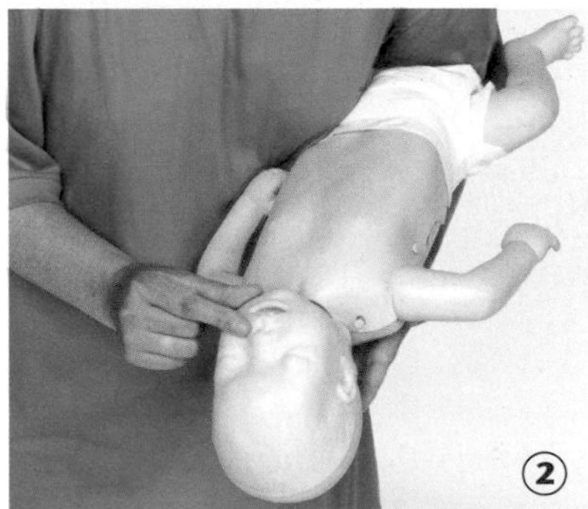

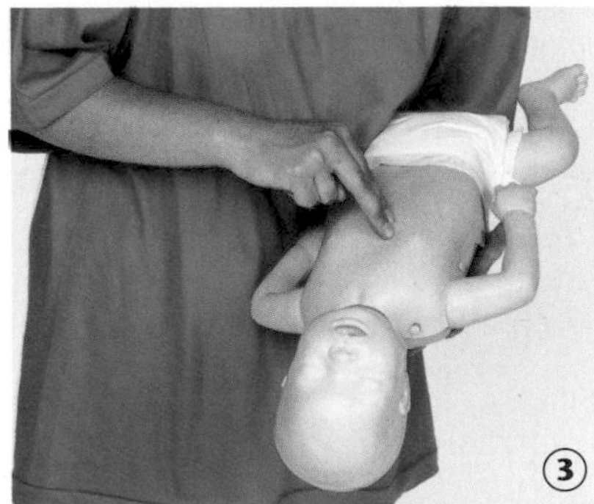

1 Place the baby face down against your forearm with his head lower than his trunk (demonstrated here with a dummy). If he is big, you can lie him face down across your lap. Slap firmly five times between his shoulder blades using the heel of your hand.

2 Check his mouth and remove any obvious obstruction with your finger.

3 If this does not work, turn him on to his back and rest him on a firm surface if you can. Using two fingers, push over the sternum five times in quick succession, at a rate of one push every three seconds. Then check the mouth.

Repeat steps 1–3 if necessary. If the obstruction still does not clear, take the infant with you and dial 999 for an ambulance.

Dealing with a choking child

The following procedure is recommended for children aged between one and seven years old. Children who cannot yet stand can be treated lying down on your lap, and older children can safely be treated while standing, seated or lying down.

1 First encourage the child to cough to bring up the obstruction. If he begins to weaken or stops coughing, bend him forwards and give up to five firm slaps between the shoulders using the heel of your hand. Check his mouth.

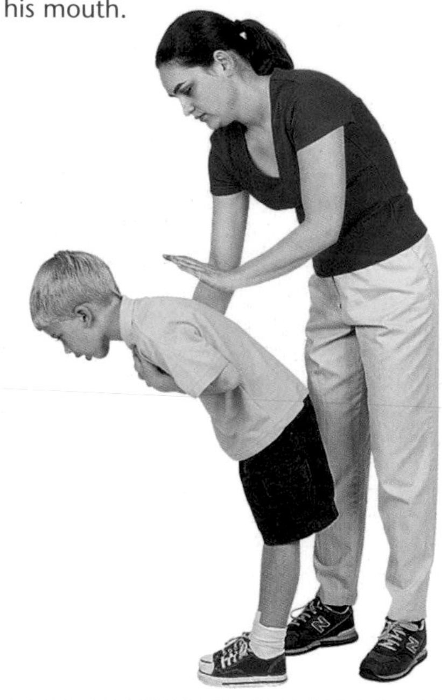

2 If this doesn't help, stand or kneel behind the child, make a fist and place it against the lower breastbone. Grasp your fist with your other hand and press into the chest with a sharp inward and upward thrust. Repeat up to five times once every three seconds. Stop if the obstruction clears.

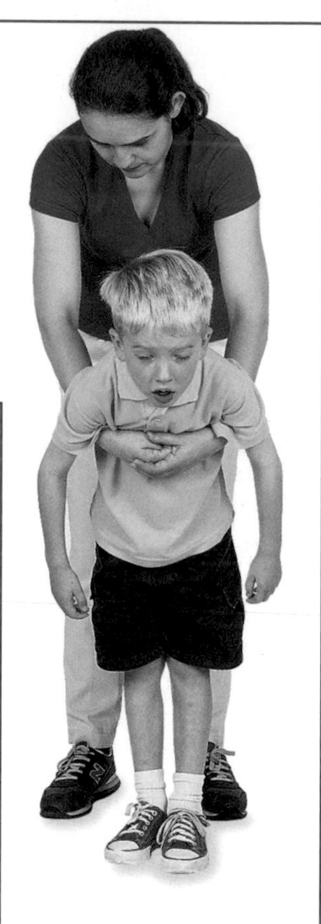

3 Check his mouth. If the obstruction has not cleared, try abdominal thrusts with your fist just above the child's navel. Give up to five thrusts. Check his mouth. If choking continues, dial 999 and repeat steps 1–3 until help arrives.

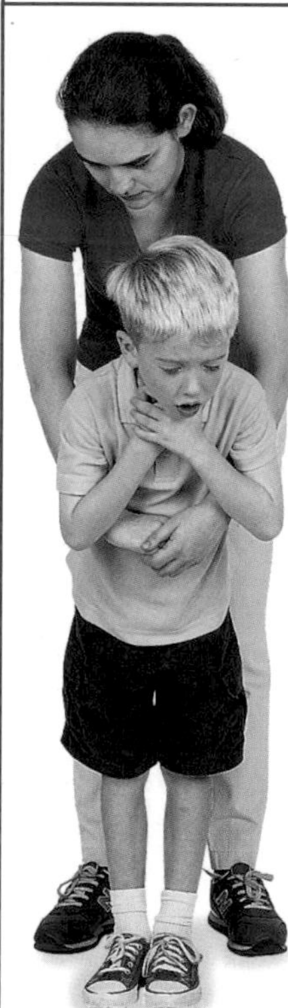

Swallowed objects

If you have seen an object in your child's mouth and then cannot find it, you must suspect that he has swallowed it. If he has not choked at all, the likelihood is that the object has passed into his stomach, but you cannot safely assume this. It may be stuck along the route to his stomach and could still result in choking.

You must call your local Accident and Emergency department and get their advice. What will happen then depends on what your child has swallowed. He will be X-rayed if it is something that shows up on an X-ray, such as a coin. If the X-ray shows that your child is not at risk of choking, you will be advised to look out for the object in his stools. If it is stuck in the upper gullet, it will have to be surgically removed.

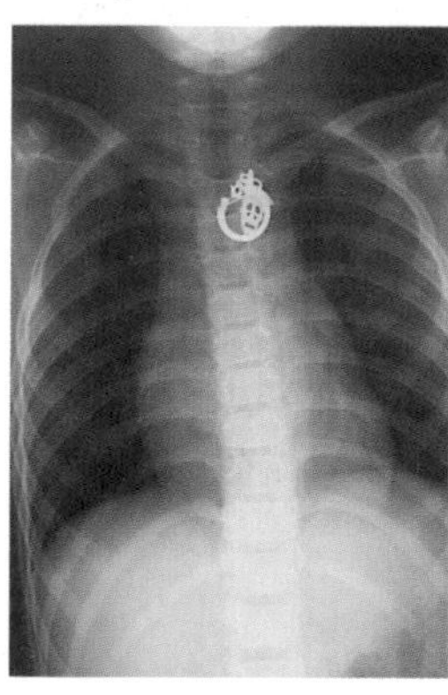

In some cases, X-rays can provide proof that a missing object, such as this keyring, has been swallowed.

Take care!

If your child has a sudden unexplained coughing fit you must assume that he has inhaled a foreign body, even though he may seem fine. If this is followed by wheezing, or raspy breathing, a foreign body is highly likely and this is a medical emergency. As your child is still able to breathe it is best not to try any actions yourself as this may lead to complete airway blockage. Call 999 immediately. As soon as you reach hospital, there will be a medical team ready to remove the foreign body under controlled conditions using a bronchoscope.

CUTS & GRAZES

DEALING WITH CUTS AND GRAZES

Toddlers and young children are naturally inquisitive and, in their eagerness to explore new surroundings, they are bound to experience many tumbles and falls.

Most accidents will result in minor cuts and grazes, but your child is also at risk of causing himself a serious injury. As a parent, you should know how to treat a minor cut at home and be aware of what action to take in case your child sustains a more serious injury.

IS YOUR CHILD IN SHOCK?

If your child has suffered a fairly serious cut and is bleeding profusely, he may go into shock. This happens when blood pressure falls abnormally low. Symptoms of shock include a rapid, weak pulse, shallow breathing, dizziness, grey-blue skin (especially on the lips), nausea and sweating.

What to do?

- Apply pressure to the wound to stop the bleeding.
- Make him comfortable and loosen his clothing. Reassure him.
- If possible, raise his legs so that the blood returns to his head.
- Keep your child warm with a blanket, but don't let him get too hot.
- Seek medical help immediately.

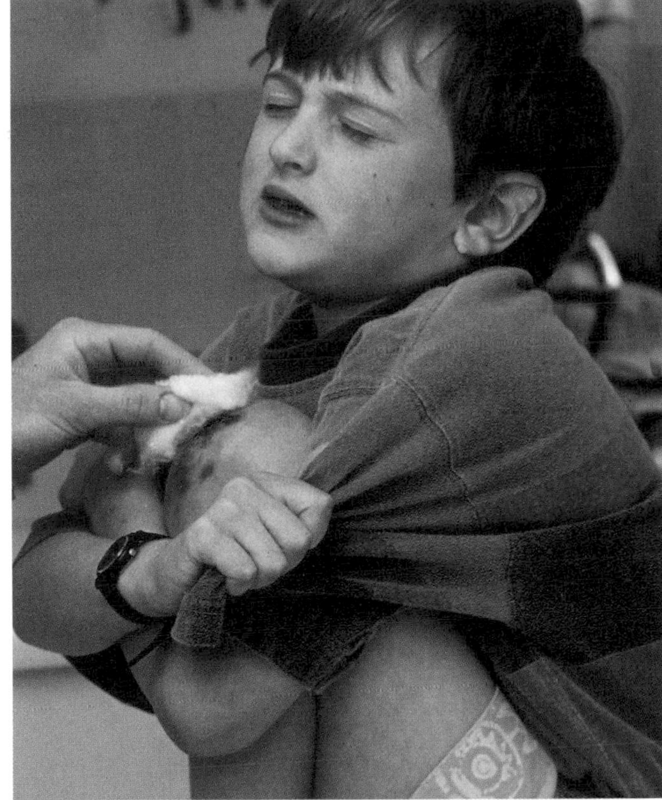

A minor cut can be treated at home by cleaning and covering it. If you are at all concerned, especially if you later suspect an infection, seek medical help.

When to seek medical help

There are some situations that require you to take your child to hospital immediately after you have given emergency first aid. These are when:

- Your child has cut his face badly.
- The wound is very dirty or has something embedded in it.
- The wound is gaping or has jagged edges.
- Bleeding is profuse, even after applying pressure.
- The cut is large or deep.
- You suspect a wound has been caused by a nail, broken glass or an animal.
- Your child has a puncture wound, i.e. a deep wound with only a small hole in the skin.
- Your child is in shock.

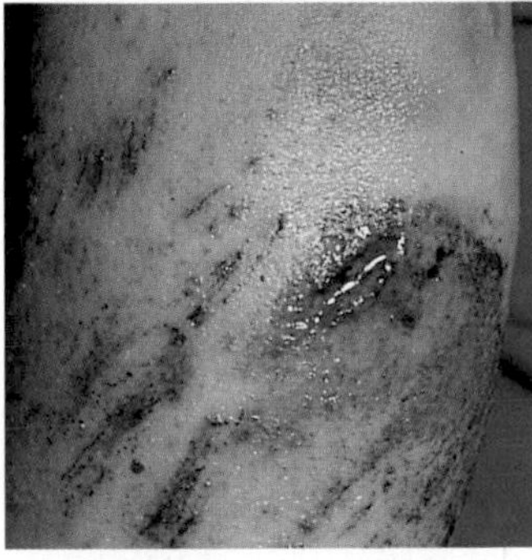

A wound caused by a rusty nail could become infected, so get hospital help. If infection sets in (left), your child will feel a burning sensation around the wound and it may ooze pus and become swollen. Seek medical help.

Dos and Don'ts

If your child hurts himself, it is often difficult to think clearly about what to do. It may be useful to have a check-list of dos and don'ts.

✔ Do seek medical help for your child if you are in any doubt about his condition.

✔ Do consult your GP if the area around your child's wound becomes red and tender after treatment. It could be infected.

✔ Do add a handful of salt to your child's bath each day, to keep the wound clean and promote healing.

✔ Do cover a wound if your child is prone to picking and scratching, which could lead to infection.

✔ Do take a course in first aid. Contact St John Ambulance on 0870 235 5231 for details of courses that are run in your area.

✘ Don't attempt to move your child if he is badly hurt but out of danger.

✘ Don't attempt to remove any object that is embedded in your child's wound.

✘ Don't elevate a limb which may be broken.

✘ Don't apply a tourniquet or tie a dressing in place so tightly that you cut off circulation.

✘ Don't fall behind with keeping up your child's tetanus injections. Check with your GP's surgery to find out if he is covered.

Treating minor cuts step by step

With some basic equipment, a calm approach and this simple guide, you can confidently treat your child's minor cut at home.

1 *Your child may be a little upset, so sit him down while he calms. Then wash your hands to prevent any infection getting into the wound.*

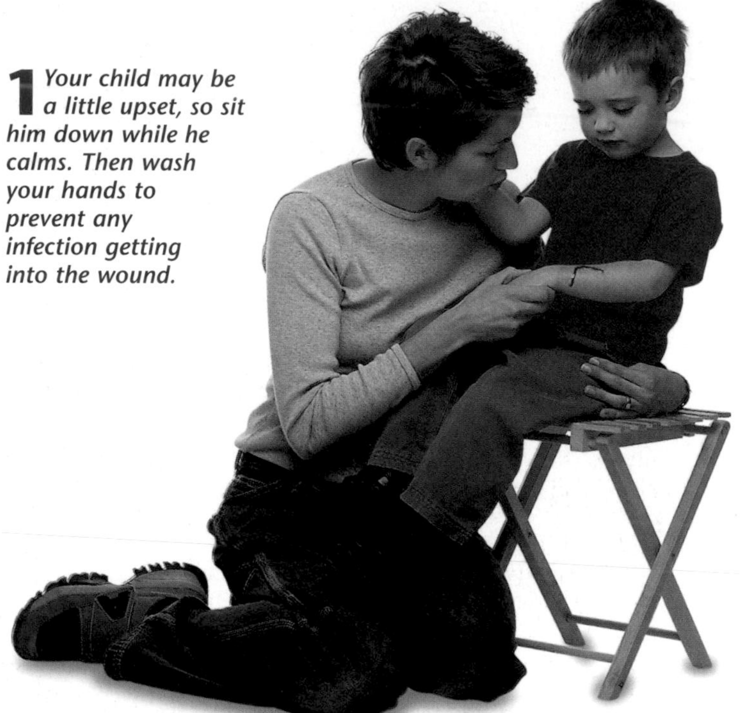

2 *Hold the wound under cold running water until it is clean and no grit or dirt are present. Gently pat the skin around the wound with kitchen roll or a clean cloth so that it is completely dry.*

3 *Apply a sterile dressing or sticking plaster. Some cuts benefit from being held together with skin closure tapes, which help to ensure that the wound heals neatly.*

First aid at home

Every home should have the basic equipment necessary to administer first aid. Make sure you always have a supply of the following:

- Bandages (crêpe, elastic, gauze and triangular)
- Antiseptic wipes or spray
- Sticking plaster or surgical tape
- Sterile gauze
- Adhesive dressings
- Packet of skin closures
- Tweezers
- Safety pins
- Blunt-tipped scissors

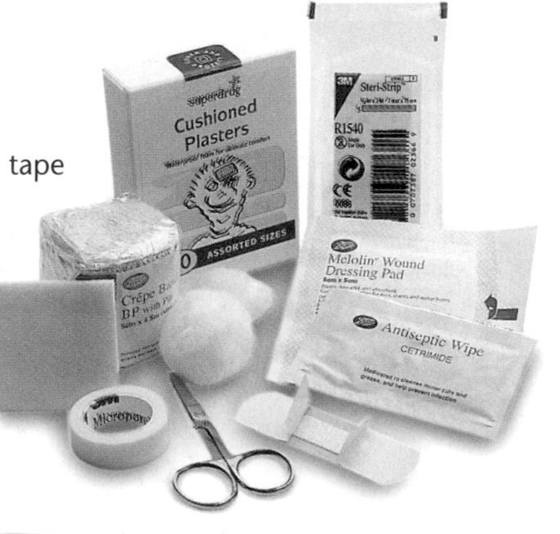

4 *Change the dressing daily until the wound has healed completely. This will keep it moist, which will help it to heal more quickly.*

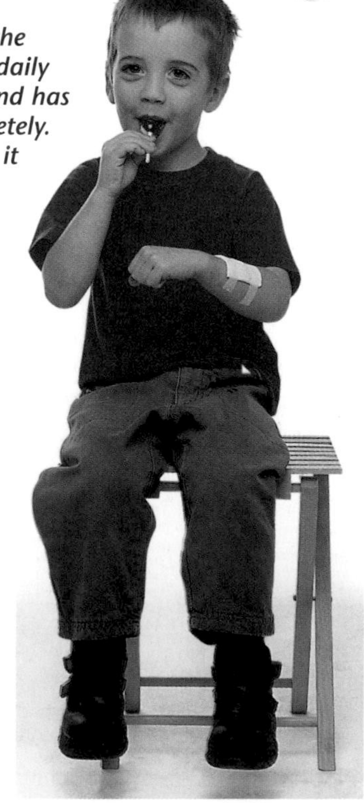

DEHYDRATION

WHAT IS DEHYDRATION?

Normally, the fluid taken in from food and drink is balanced by the fluid lost as urine, stools and perspiration. If your child loses more than he takes in, he will become dehydrated.

- A large proportion of body weight is water – approximately 80 per cent of a newborn baby's body weight and 60 per cent of a child's body weight.
- Dehydration involves a gradual loss of fluid from the body. In the early stages, the body is able to compensate for this loss and maintain normal functions.
- If the process of dehydration is allowed to continue, the kidneys will stop working, shock will follow and eventual collapse.
- Babies are at a greater risk of rapid dehydration than older children.

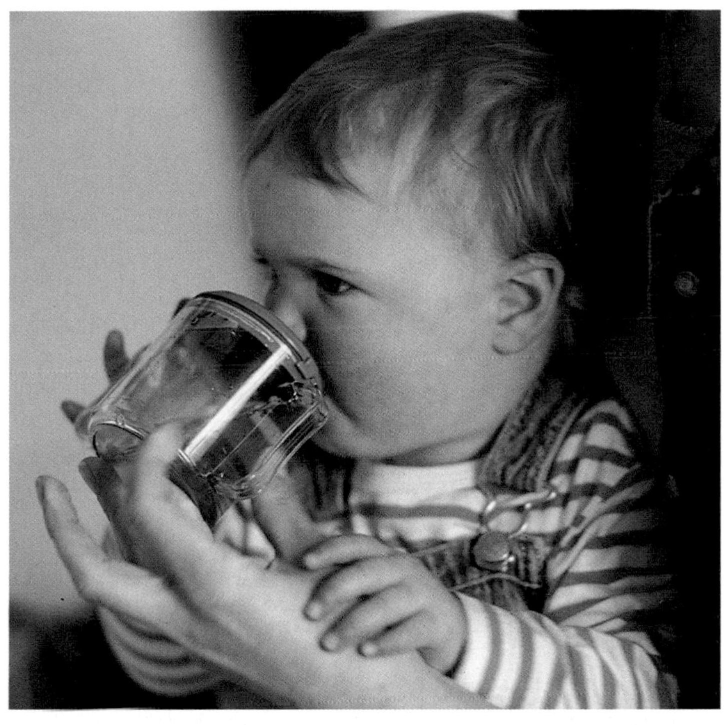

Dehydration can be extremely serious in young children, so you should make sure your child has sufficient fluid intake, especially if he is unwell.

Causes

There are many possible causes of dehydration. The most common are:

- **Diarrhoea:** with or without vomiting (gastroenteritis).
- **Vomiting:** loss of fluids through vomiting can cause dehydration.
- **Heat exposure:** a baby or child can become dehydrated outside on a hot day, even if he is kept in the shade; similarly, a very warm indoor environment can cause dehydration.
- **Strenuous activity or exercise:** children will often be so absorbed in a game or activity, that they will either not notice that they are thirsty or they will choose to ignore it.
- **Fever:** a child with a fever can easily become dehydrated through sweating.
- **Certain medical conditions:** for example, kidney disorders and diabetes; some drugs, such as diuretics, can cause dehydration.

Symptoms

Dehydration is classified into stages according to the amount of body weight lost as water at each stage.

Mild dehydration

- Slightly dry mouth and lips.
- Urine is concentrated – a little darker than usual and reduced in volume; a baby's nappy will be less wet than usual.
- Your child is thirsty.

Moderate dehydration

The signs for mild dehydration, plus the following:

- Darker, more concentrated urine.
- A baby not producing a wet nappy for several hours.
- Dry, inelastic skin.
- Sunken eyes and no tears when crying.
- Sunken fontanelle – the 'soft spot' on top of your baby's head, which is usually flat.
- Your child is lethargic (drowsy) or irritable.
- Increased thirst.

Severe dehydration

The signs for mild and moderate dehydration, plus the following:

- Very pale or mottled skin, cool to the touch.
- Your child is increasingly lethargic or irritable.
- Eventual collapse.

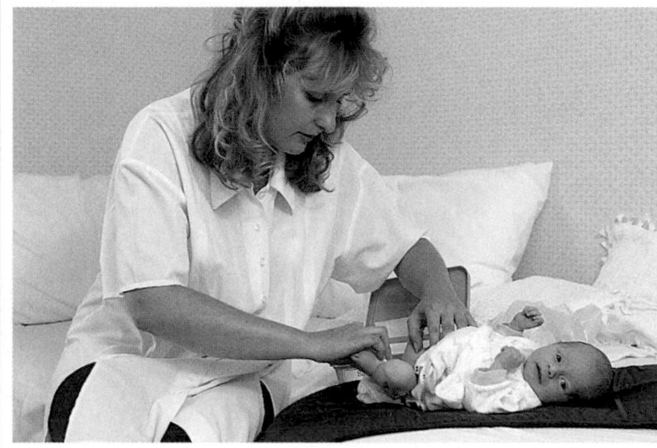

Be alert for signs of dehydration, such as the frequency of your baby's wet nappy and the colour of his urine.

What to do if your baby is dehydrated

Young babies can become dehydrated within the space of a few hours. A baby with any signs of dehydration, even if mild, must be taken to a GP immediately. If there is to be a delay in seeing a GP, the baby should be taken to a hospital emergency department instead.

1 Offer a feed immediately. A breast-fed baby should be offered a breast-feed. Your doctor may recommend you continue to offer breast-feeds, but more frequently than usual, even if your baby is vomiting or has diarrhoea.

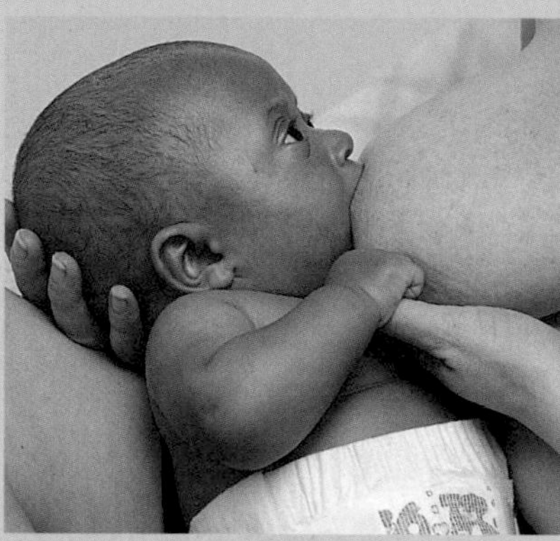

If you suspect that your baby may be dehydrated, offer a feed immediately and seek medical advice.

2 A bottle-fed baby should be offered his usual formula but, if he also has diarrhoea and/or is vomiting, in smaller amounts and more frequently than usual. Alternatively, you can give oral rehydration solution (ORS) – seek advice from your health visitor or GP about preparing these solutions correctly for your baby.

3 If your baby refuses to take a bottle, try feeding with a spoon or from a small cup.

NOTE: never give anti-diarrhoea medicine to a baby unless instructed by your doctor.

What to do if your child is dehydrated

Mild dehydration can usually be treated at home, but if you are unsure, always call your doctor.

- A child should drink approximately 1.5 litres of fluid a day at least, but when dehydrated, additional fluids are needed to replace those lost.

- The exact amount of fluid needed depends on your child's weight, but as an approximate guide, aim to give at least 60–90mls of fluid every hour.

- The way the fluids are given depends on the cause of the dehydration, but you should aim for your child to have no remaining signs of dehydration after four hours. His urine should be straw coloured and he should no longer feel thirsty. If after four hours your child's dehydration is getting worse, call a doctor.

When to talk to the doctor

- A baby with any signs of dehydration must be taken to the doctor immediately. A child should be taken to a doctor if he shows signs of moderate or severe dehydration.

- A baby or child with moderate or severe dehydration will need to be admitted to hospital for treatment and is likely to need intravenous replacement of fluids to replace fluids lost.

- A baby or child must also be seen by a doctor under the following circumstances: if he has severe watery diarrhoea for more than six hours; if he has severe vomiting for six hours or more; if he is showing other signs and symptoms in addition to mild dehydration, such as blood in the stools, or fever.

How to prevent dehydration

Diarrhoea and vomiting:
- If bottle-fed, offer small, frequent amounts of your baby's formula milk.
- If breast-fed, continue to breast-feed as usual, offering more frequently.
- If not vomiting, a baby who has been weaned should also continue to be given his usual diet.
- If your older child is vomiting, offer small amounts of oral rehydration solutions frequently.

Hot weather:
- Give your baby or child extra fluids.
- Bottle-fed babies can be given cool boiled water in hot weather; breast-fed babies can be offered more frequent feeds.
- If travelling, take plenty of drinks with you.
- NEVER leave a baby or young child unattended in a car on a hot day.

Exercise:
- Encourage your child to take a break for a drink during strenuous exercise or very active play.

Fever:
- More fluid than usual is needed to replace that lost through sweating.
- Offer small amounts of your child's usual drinks frequently, or give oral rehydration solutions; breast-feed your baby or offer him his formula milk more often than usual.

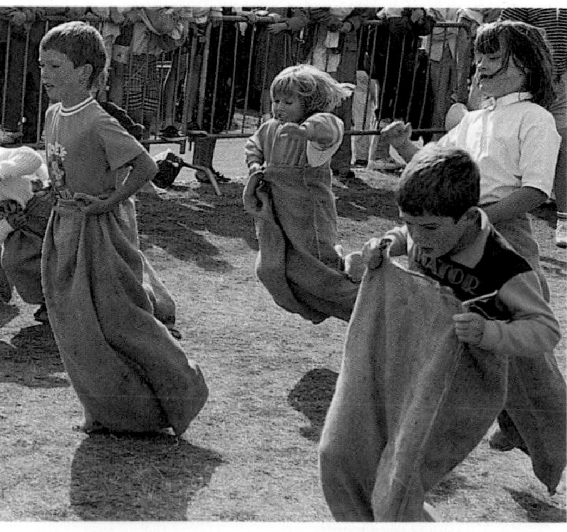

When your child is involved in active play, give him plenty of drinks, or fresh, juicy fruit, which provides fluids.

DISLOCATIONS

WHAT IS A JOINT DISLOCATION?

Joint dislocation is the complete displacement of the two bones in a joint so that they are no longer in contact, usually as a result of injury. There may be recurrent dislocations and a strengthening operation may be needed.

- Dislocation is usually accompanied by tearing of the joint ligaments and damage to the joint capsule (the membrane that surrounds the joint). It is the tearing that makes the injury so painful.

- It most often occurs to the shoulder, thumb, finger, jaw and hip. Injury severe enough to cause dislocation can also cause one or both of the bones involved to break.

- Joint dislocation is rare in children because they are very resilient. It takes a great deal of force, such as that caused by a road traffic accident, landing hard on concrete or a fall down the stairs, to remove a joint from its socket.

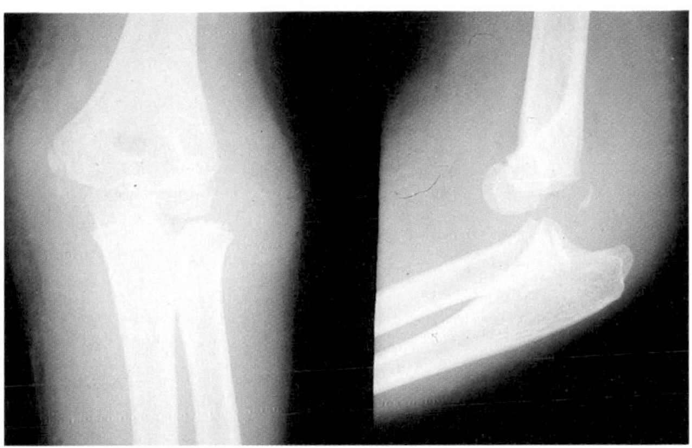

Joint dislocation, such as the one shown in this X-ray, occurs when the two bones in a joint are no longer in contact. This is usually caused by a severe fall or accident and is extremely painful.

Symptoms

Children are resilient, so your child will usually have had a nasty fall and normally hit the ground (or hard surface) with some force. Dislocation restricts or prevents the movement of the joint and is usually accompanied by severe pain.

1 If a joint has dislocated, you will probably hear it click out of place.

2 The joint will look misshapen and swollen.

Precautions

The most important thing is not to move the injured child unless it is absolutely necessary.

✘ Do not give your child anything to eat or drink because a general anaesthetic will probably be required.

✘ Do not move your child until the injured part is secured and supported, especially if your child may have other injuries. He should be moved by trained rescue workers. You should move your child only if his life is in immediate danger.

✘ Do not try to replace a dislocated bone into its socket.

Assessing the injury

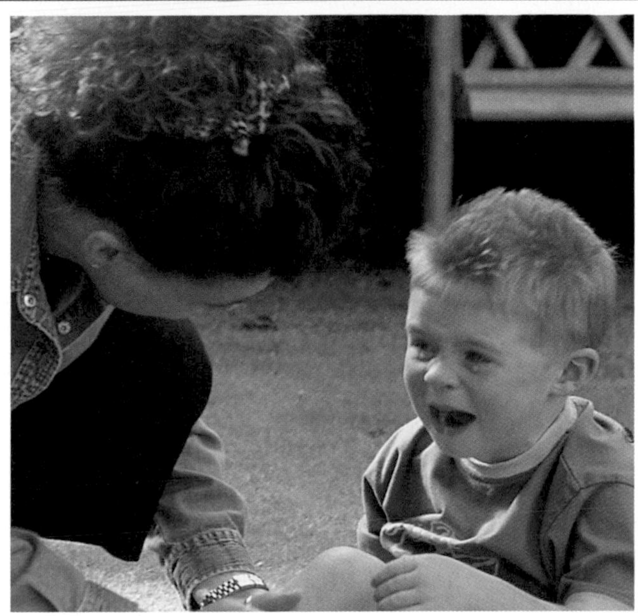

A baby or toddler may be unable to tell you where it hurts so you will need to assess the injury. Look for the following signs:

- Difficulty in moving the limb normally or at all. For example, your child may not be able to stand or walk, or he may leave an arm dangling by his side.

- Pain at or near the site of injury. This is made worse by movement. Sickening and severe pain often indicates dislocation (tenderness over a bone if it is slightly touched is a sign that the bone may be fractured).

- A shortening, bending or twisting of the limb.

- A 'grating' sensation of bones rubbing together, pain, tenderness and a swelling of the injured part are signs and symptoms of both fractures and dislocations. If in any doubt, treat as a fracture.

If your child has dislocated a bone he will be in immense pain and is unlikely to be able to move the injured limb at all. Seek urgent medical help.

First aid for dislocations

Fractures, sprains, strains and dislocations may be hard to diagnose. For this reason, first-aid treatment of any of these conditions is handled as though the injury is a fracture.

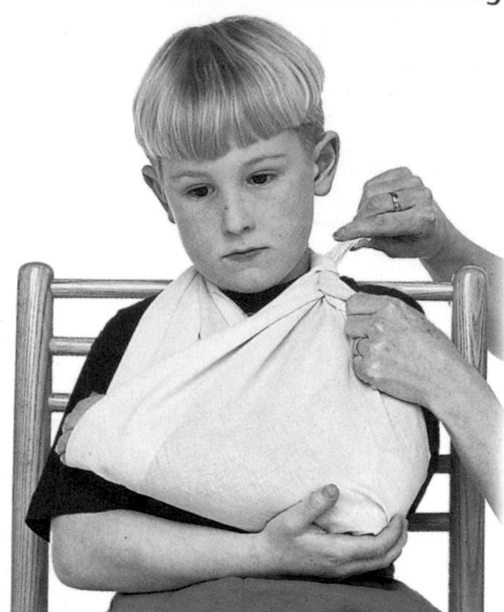

To steady and support an injured arm, the shoulder needs to be stabilised. Applying a sling or wrapping a sheet around the body and arm can help to hold it in place.

1 Assess the situation. Check your child's airway, breathing and circulation. If there is any blood loss, you must stop the flow of blood and treat him for shock.

2 Try your best to calm him down and keep him still. Stay close to him. The calmer he is, the less likely he is to move and cause further damage.

3 Steady and support the injured part. For a shoulder dislocation, apply a sling or wrap a sheet around the body and arm to stabilise it. For the lower limbs, roll blankets and lay them around the leg.

4 Bandage the injured leg to the sound one. This is very important for babies and young children because thrashing about can cause further damage to the joint. Applying a cold pack to the affected area may reduce pain and swelling.

5 Talk to your child throughout to keep him calm.

6 Dial 999 for an ambulance and stay with your child.

IMPORTANT

- A person without medical qualifications should not attempt to put the joint back in place because of the risk of seriously damaging the nerves or worsening any fracture.
- You should aim to prevent movement at the injury site and arrange immediate removal of your child to hospital.

Complications

In some cases, a dislocation is followed by potentially serious complications, but this is rare.

1 Dislocation of the spinal vertebrae resulting from a severe back injury can damage the spinal cord, which can sometimes result in paralysis below the point of injury.

2 Dislocation of the shoulder or hip joint can sometimes damage nerves in the arm or the leg, which can again, in some cases, result in paralysis.

3 Occasionally, the tissue around a dislocated joint (usually the shoulder, although sometimes this can occur in the hip in children) becomes so weakened that it cannot support the bone any more. Even after the joint has mended, minimal pressure can cause another dislocation.

Congenital dislocation of the hip

Congenital dislocation of the hip (CHD) is a disorder present at birth in which the ball-like head of the femur (thigh bone) fails to fit into the cup-like socket of the pelvis to form a joint.

- The cause of congenital hip dislocation is unknown. However, it is usual for babies to move about freely in the uterus, which helps to mould their joints into shape. If the baby is in an awkward position, such as a breech, there may not be enough room for this process to take place properly.

- Babies are checked at birth for CHD, but the condition is not always picked up at that time. They are then checked at intervals until they can walk. This is a routine physical examination of the hip to check for instability and the range of motion.

- If the condition is found in early infancy, a special harness is usually used to manoeuvre the ball of the joint into the socket and keep it in position. Hip stabilisation can take place in as little as a month, but sometimes harnesses need to be worn for longer. Most babies grow out of these problems and their hips develop normally.

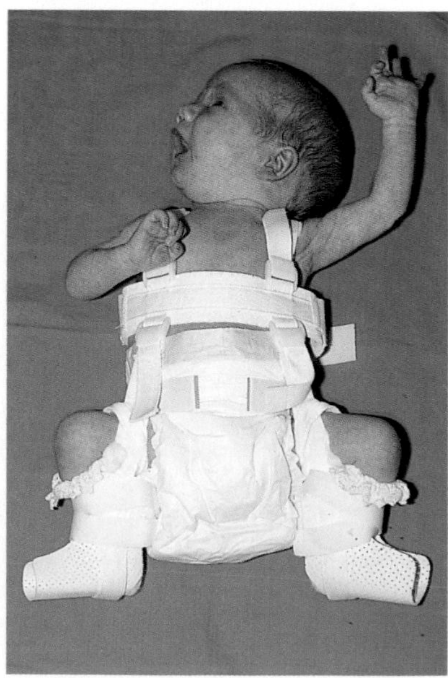

To cure a congenital dislocation of the hip, a special harness may be used to move the ball of the joint back into the socket.

ELECTRIC SHOCK

WHY IT HAPPENS

Babies and young children are in danger of getting electric shocks because they love poking their fingers or objects into holes or playing with wires.

- Electric shocks can be fatal, so it is very important to try to eliminate all risks of them happening in the first place. Check in all the rooms of your house that you have taken every possible precaution to guard your child from the dangers of electric shock.
- Effects of electric shock vary and depend on the type of current that passes through the body, how much current there is and how long it lasts. The mains electricity supply in Britain is of low voltage but has a 50Hz frequency, which can disrupt the body's electrical control systems.

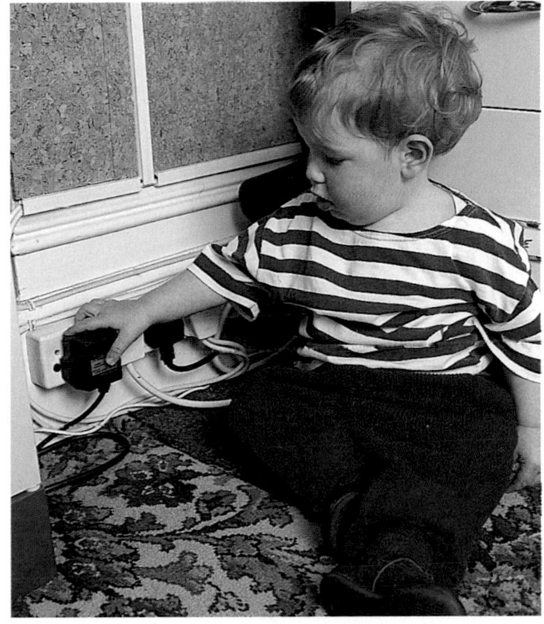

Plugs and wires are temptations that most toddlers simply can't resist, so never allow your child the opportunity to play near sockets.

The effects

The effects of an electric shock range from a mild tingling sensation to a heart attack.

- The electrical frequency can cause rapid, irregular heartbeat, leading to cardiac and respiratory failure.
- The muscles may go into spasm and contract rigidly.
- The current can cause a deep burn. There may be internal damage.
- The victim may turn pale, sweaty, listless; feel nauseous and cold; and have a rapid pulse and respiratory rate.
- High-voltage shocks are very dangerous and occur near power lines, overhead cables or live electric rails. If the electric shock is not fatal, the victim may be knocked unconscious, stop breathing and suffer severe burns and possibly internal injuries.
- Lightning can stun the victim, set clothing on fire and cause death instantly.

Seeking medical help

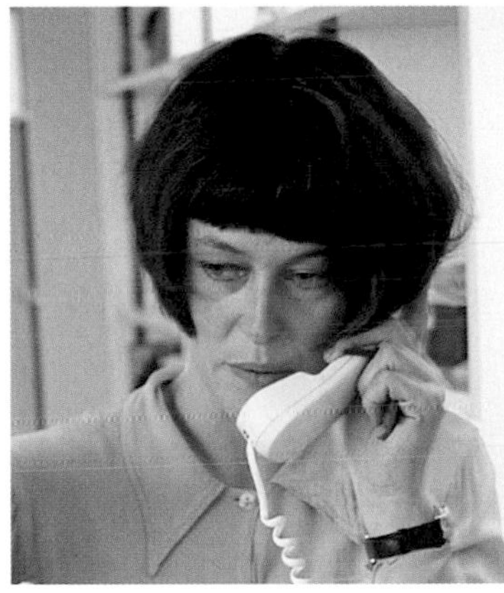

Even if the effects of the electric shock are minor, seek medical advice and arrange for your child to be examined by a doctor.

Call an ambulance for your child if he:

- Stayed connected to the live current.
- Required resuscitation.
- Was unconscious for any length of time.
- Suffered burns of over an inch in diameter at the contact sites.
- Is suffering from shock.

NOTE: Take your child to a doctor even if he has suffered just a mild shock. Any child under five who's had a shock should be seen by a doctor to ensure there is no internal damage.

First steps to dealing with an electric shock

Follow the guidelines below, taking care not to give yourself an electric shock.

1 In the case of a high-voltage shock outside the home, there is little that you can do. Never attempt to approach closer than 18 metres (20 yards), even if the casualty has been thrown clear of the electrical contact by the force of the shock. Electricity can 'arc' (jump long distances) until the authorities have turned off the mains supply.

2 To safeguard yourself indoors, put on rubber boots or stand on a pile of papers or a telephone directory – this is absolutely vital if the area concerned is wet. Then use a wooden object, such as a broom handle or a chair, to push the child away from the current and break the circuit.

3 Alternatively, turn off electricity at the mains.

4 If you can't turn off the electricity and don't have a wooden object, hold on to the child's clothing. Don't touch the child or anything wet.

Giving first aid

Once your child is clear of the danger, you can start to assess and treat her condition.

If your child is unconscious but breathing, place her in the recovery position, as shown here, while awaiting medical help. Tilt her head to keep her airways clear.

1 Your child may be unconscious. Once it is safe to do so, open her airways and check the breathing.

2 If breathing has stopped, give rescue breaths, and give chest compressions if necessary.

3 If your child is breathing but unconscious, place her in the recovery position and call 999. Keep checking her breathing while you wait for the ambulance.

4 If your child is conscious, look for signs of burns. Immerse any burns in cool water for 10 minutes, or hold them under running cold water. Immerse the damaged area only. Cover the burn loosely with a dry dressing or clingfilm and seek medical advice if the affected area is bigger than the palm of a child's hand.

5 Do not remove clothes that are stuck to the skin in case you cause further damage, but you can take off anything constricting, such as a belt.

6 Keep a close eye on her in case she goes into delayed shock.

Treating shock

'Shock' describes any condition that causes blood pressure to drop rapidly. Ultimately, it can lead to unconsciousness.

1 Lie your child down with his legs and feet raised on pillows above the level of his head.

2 Cover him with blankets.

3 Do not give him food or drink.

4 Seek medical advice and, if your child becomes unconscious at any time, place him in the recovery position and call an ambulance.

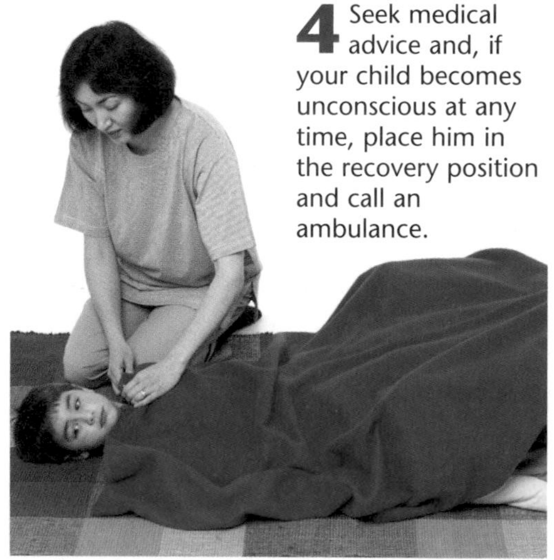

The basic treatment for shock is to lay the casualty down with legs raised and cover with a warm blanket.

Prevention

An electric shock can be extremely serious for adults and children, but the risks of it occurring can be reduced by taking a few preventive measures in the home.

- Use dummy covers for all spare electric sockets.
- Use dummy covers when you unplug an appliance – at night or when it is not in use.
- Keep all switches in the 'off' position unless in use.
- Teach your child that he should never play near to electrical apparatus or plugs.
- Get a qualified electrician to check the electrical circuits in your home and to install trip switches if they're not already there.
- Do not let a small child have an electric blanket – a wet bed or spilt drink can be dangerous.
- Ensure that all wires are well insulated. Bind up excess wire out of reach with a twist-tie.
- Christmas tree lights can be hazardous. Make it clear that they can be switched on when an adult is present only.

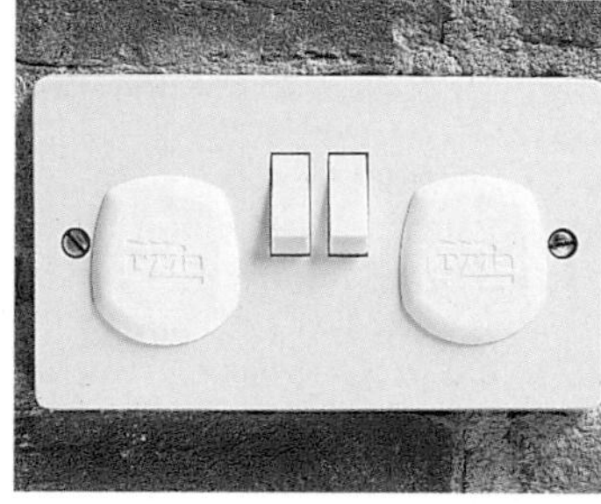

Dummy covers for sockets are available from shops such as Mothercare – these covers are absolutely essential if there is a young child in the house.

- Check all electronic toys and transformers at regular intervals for signs of wear and tear.
- Learn how to wire a plug or change a fuse or light bulb.
- Find out where your mains power switch is and know how to turn it off.
- Make sure your children are taught not to touch wires and to keep away from railway lines and pylons.

FAINTING

WHAT IS FAINTING?

Fainting is a temporary loss of consciousness due to an insufficient supply of blood to the brain. The medical term for fainting is syncope.

- Fainting usually affects children over 10, especially pubescent girls. If your child is under 10 years old and faints more than twice, you should seek medical advice.
- Fainting is often a reflex action. Overactivity of the vagal nerve slows the heart, reducing the blood supply to the head.
- As soon as the child falls to the ground, blood flows back to the head and consciousness returns.
- Fainting may occur without warning, but it is usually preceded by a feeling of dizziness or light-headedness.
- A child who is about to faint may also appear pale, yawn, feel cold or clammy, feel nauseous and have a slow heartbeat.

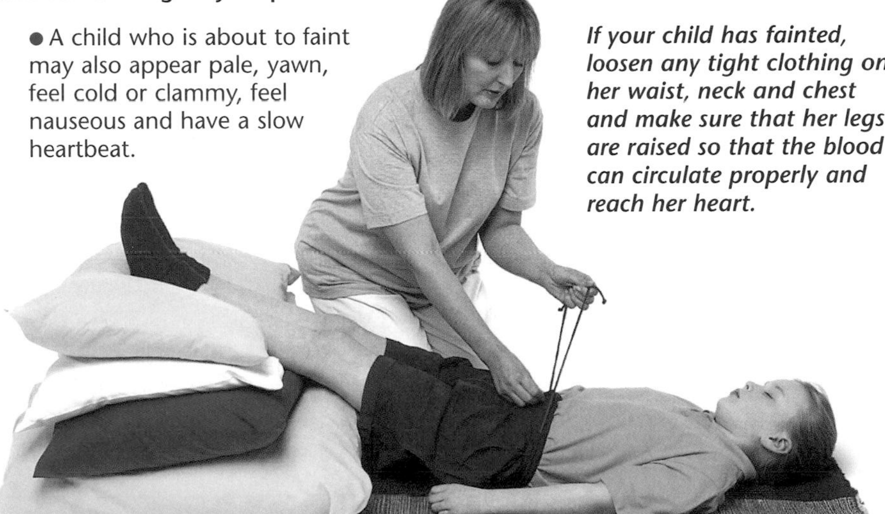

If your child has fainted, loosen any tight clothing on her waist, neck and chest and make sure that her legs are raised so that the blood can circulate properly and reach her heart.

Common causes of fainting

A variety of events may lead to a reduced blood flow to the brain. Fainting is more common in children and teenagers than in adults.

1 Lack of movement: movement helps to keep blood circulating around the body. Standing still for a long period of time may cause a pooling of blood in the legs, and the resulting lack of blood supply to the head can cause fainting.

2 Hyperventilation: abnormally rapid breathing, caused by conditions such as anxiety, can lead to dizziness and fainting.

3 Muscular relaxation: fainting can occur as a result of a general muscle relaxation, e.g. when having a hot bath.

4 Powerful emotional reaction: some people faint on receiving bad news and others faint at the sight of blood. Fear and pain can cause fainting.

5 Other extreme situations: hunger, dehydration, anaemia, fatigue and exhaustion can all cause fainting.

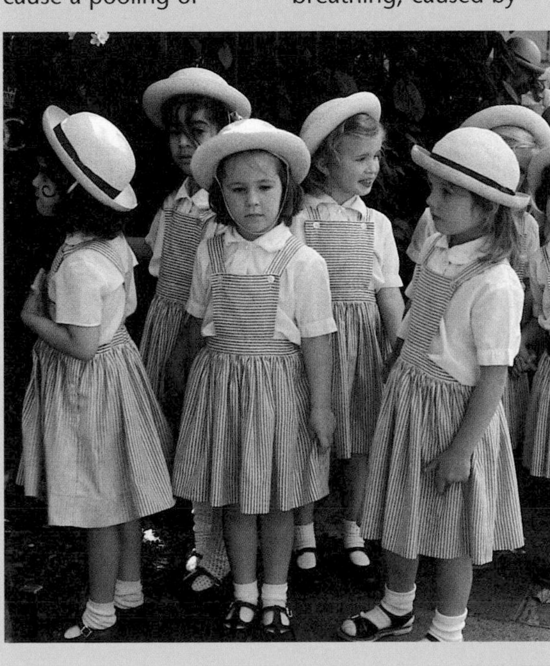

Standing to attention, or just standing still, and being in a crowd can cause a young child to faint.

Less common causes

Most cases of fainting have a simple cause and are a one-off occurrence. However, there are more serious causes that should be investigated by a doctor.

1 Shock: this involves reduced circulation, which can lead to fainting and a complete loss of consciousness.

2 A reduction in the supply of blood to the head: heart disease, pregnancy and a heavy menstrual period can all cause a person to faint.

3 An epileptic fit: this may cause loss of consciousness, and be confused with fainting.

4 Carotid sinus syndrome: in some people, stimulation to the carotid sinus in the neck causes the vagal nerve to send impulses to the heart, slowing it down and causing faintness.

What to do when a child faints

If your child has fainted, certain measures should be taken to bring her back to consciousness and make her comfortable once she has come round.

1 Check that your child is breathing, then position her with her head low and her legs raised above heart level. This will help the blood flow to the brain and circulate to the heart.

2 Make sure that your child has a supply of fresh air. Loosen any tight clothing.

3 Once conscious, your child should continue to lie down for at least 10 minutes and when she feels better, get up very slowly.

- **If your child feels faint:** position her with her head low and legs raised.

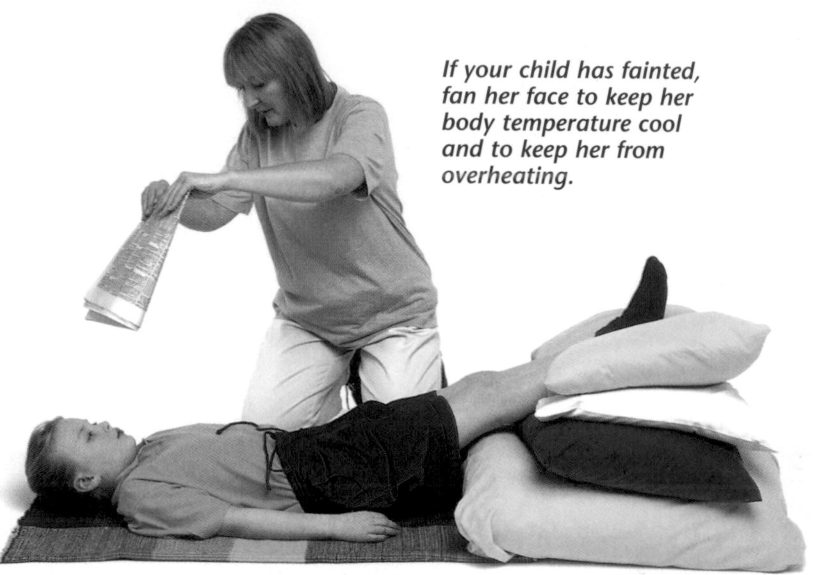

If your child has fainted, fan her face to keep her body temperature cool and to keep her from overheating.

When to seek help

Fainting attacks usually last for one or two minutes. If someone who has fainted remains unconscious for longer than this, additional first aid may be needed. Medical help should be sought under certain circumstances.

- Any fainting episode in a child should be reported to a doctor, particularly if fainting episodes occur more than twice.
- If there is a loss of consciousness for more than two minutes.
- If the head has been injured either before or as a result of fainting and collapse.
- If other symptoms are apparent, such as shaking, tongue-biting or urinary or faecal incontinence. These symptoms can indicate convulsions.
- If medication, alcohol or drugs are suspected as the cause.
- If the lips go blue – this could indicate choking, severe asthma or severe allergy-anaphylaxis.
- If a feeling of light-headedness persists.
- If blood or fluid loss occurs (through, for example, a severe nose-bleed, a heavy period, diarrhoea or vomiting). The child could be in shock, which can lead to fainting. Seek immediate medical help.

What to do when a child is unconscious

If your child is already unconscious when you find her, she may or may not have fainted. Until you know otherwise, assume that her unconscious state has a more serious cause.

1 Check that your child's airway is clear and that she is breathing. If your child is not breathing, begin mouth-to-mouth resuscitation immediately.

2 Check your child's pulse to make sure that blood is circulating properly. If there is no pulse, carry out chest compressions immediately.

3 As soon as your child is breathing comfortably, place her in the recovery position and call an ambulance. Make sure that someone stays with her at all times.

If your child is slow to regain consciousness but is breathing and has a pulse, place her in the recovery position and then call an ambulance.

FEBRILE CONVULSIONS

WHAT ARE FEBRILE CONVULSIONS?

Febrile convulsions are fits experienced by babies and young children. Affected infants may turn blue, stiffen, clench their fists, twitch uncontrollably and lose consciousness for anything from a few seconds to five minutes. Short convulsions are more usual. Although febrile convulsions are extremely alarming, in the majority of cases they are harmless.

Febrile fits are not the same as epileptic fits. Their cause is usually a sudden rise in body temperature (the word febrile means fever) as a result of a minor childhood illness – a middle ear infection, for example. The child's immature brain reacts to this sudden change in temperature by firing off abnormal electrical impulses, although it is not known why this happens. Only 2 per cent of children who suffer from febrile fits go on to develop epilepsy.

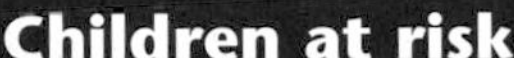

Children at risk

- Around 5 per cent of children suffer from febrile convulsions at some time and the condition has a tendency to run in the family.

- The risk is higher in children who suffer frequently from illnesses that involve a raised temperature and in those who have already had a febrile convulsion.

- Febrile convulsions are most common in children aged six months to three years, but can occur up to the age of five. Most children do grow out of them. This may be because their temperature control mechanisms and brains have matured sufficiently to cope with a rise in temperature.

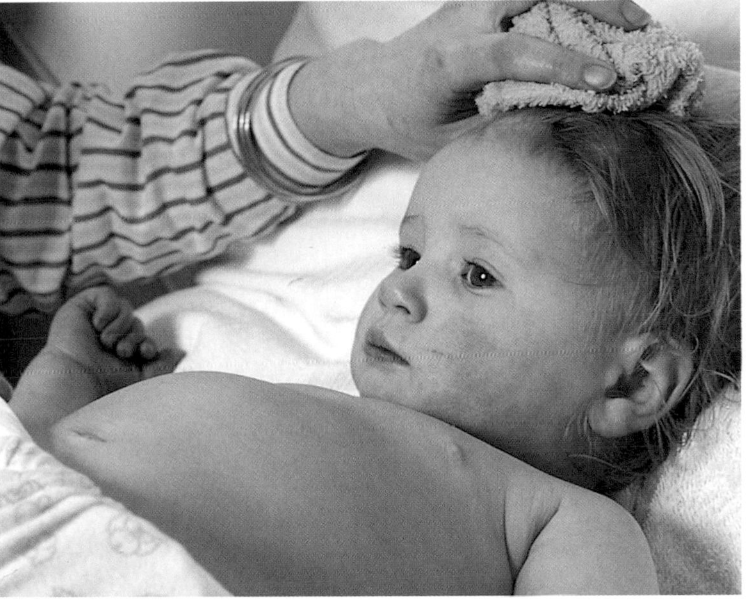

Febrile convulsions (fits) usually affect children between the ages of six months and three years. The condition occurs when a child's temperature rises too quickly. Lowering the fever reduces the risk of a fit.

What happens

- The first sign that a child may be at risk of having a convulsion is if his temperature rises rapidly.
- He may then start to look vacant and his muscles may begin to twitch.
- The child's head will be thrown back, his eyes will roll up and his whole body will jerk uncontrollably; his skin will look blue. In a short time, the child will lose consciousness.
- Depending on the severity of the convulsion, this state can last from a few seconds to a few minutes.
- Afterwards, the child will go limp and then gradually regain consciousness, before falling into a natural sleep.

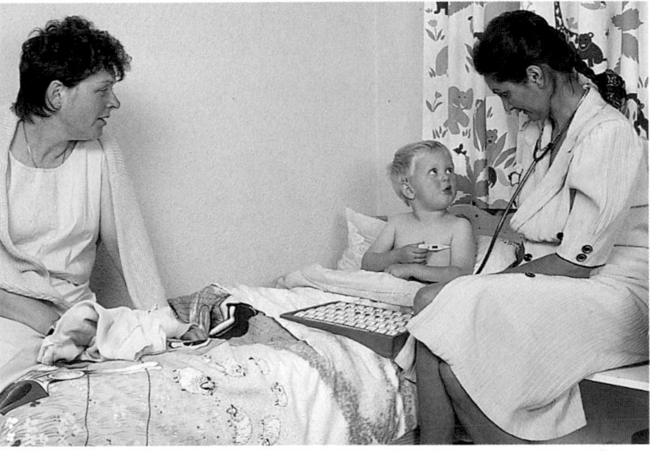

You should call your GP the first time that your child has a febrile convulsion. The doctor will want to ensure that the cause of the fit was nothing more serious than a viral infection.

When to call the doctor

- The first time a febrile convulsion occurs, call your GP immediately. Your child may need to go to hospital so that a proper evaluation can be made and causes other than a rise in temperature can be excluded.

  This evaluation is not normally repeated if your child has another convulsion. However, you should notify your GP so he can make sure that your child's fit was caused by a minor infection.

- If the convulsion lasts for more than five minutes or your child has repeated convulsions, you must seek urgent medical attention.

- After the convulsion, make an emergency call to your GP if your child has acute nausea, tremors, a rash, poor coordination, a dislike of bright lights, a severe headache or a stiff neck. Your GP will want to rule out the possibility of any serious illness, such as meningitis.

What you can do

If you realise that your child is having a febrile convulsion, you need to take immediate steps to lower his temperature. This is because the convulsions are usually triggered by a fever.

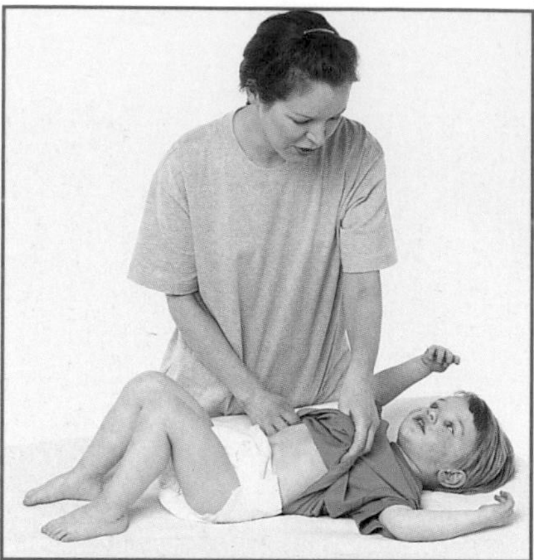

1 Lower the room temperature and strip your child down to his nappy or underwear. Put pillows or soft padding around him to prevent injury.

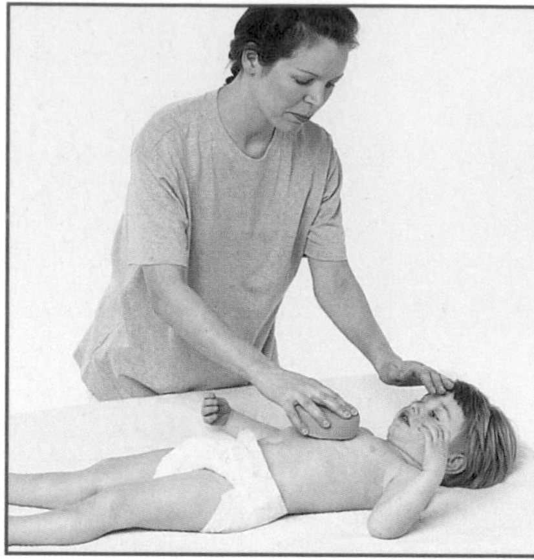

2 Sponge your child down, using tepid water. Do not let his temperature drop so low that he becomes cold.

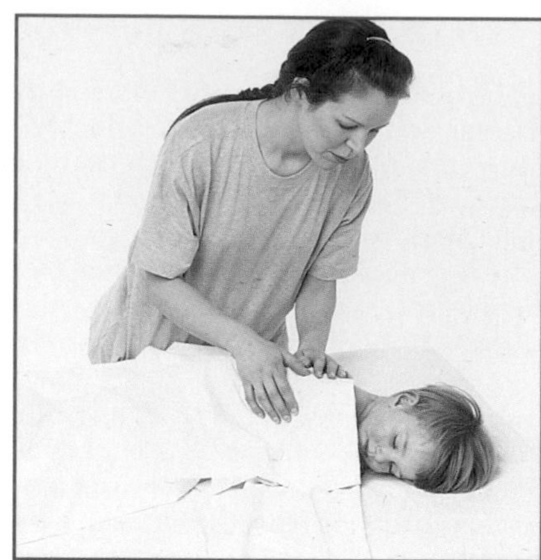

3 Once your child's temperature is controlled, his convulsions will stop. Place him on his side and make him comfortable. Keep checking his level of response and breathing until he recovers.

Guidelines

It can be extremely frightening the first time you see your child have a fit. Try to keep calm and follow these simple rules:

- Remove any hard or sharp objects nearby, such as a chair or a table that has sharp corners, so that your child does not hurt himself while he is thrashing about.
- Do not attempt to restrain your child in any way.
- Do not try to put anything in your child's mouth to stop him biting his tongue or lips – this rarely happens and, if it does, having something in his mouth is more dangerous.
- Once the fit has passed, place your child on his side (or into the recovery position, if possible) so that any secretions or vomit can drain out of his mouth.

Other causes of convulsions

On rare occasions, a convulsion may have a more serious cause than a mild childhood infection, such as:

- **Birth injury:** damage to brain tissue, usually caused by a difficult labour.
- **Infection of the brain:** such as meningitis and encephalitis.
- **Damage to the brain:** a brain haemorrhage, tumour or a skull fracture.
- **Epilepsy:** recurring seizures without fever.
- **Asphyxia:** may occur after a severe attack of whooping cough.
- **Immunisation:** the measles vaccine in the MMR injection can cause a febrile convulsion 8–10 days afterwards. However, it is more likely that your child will have a fit while suffering from measles than he will if he receives the vaccination.
- **Rickets:** a severe lack of vitamin D can irritate the membranes of the brain, so triggering a convulsion. This is rare in the UK.

Treatment and investigation

- To prevent further fits, give regular doses of paracetamol or ibuprofen when his temperature rises, or for the first 12 hours after a vaccination. If he is still hot, sponge him down with tepid water.
- If a convulsion lasts for more than five minutes, or if your child experiences a succession of fits in the same hour, a diazepam (Valium) suppository may be administered by the hospital or doctor.
- Your child may have to stay in hospital for tests. Blood and urine samples will be analysed to rule out a more serious cause.
- Other tests include a lumbar puncture to check the spinal fluid for signs of infection, and a brain scan (CAT scan) to eliminate the possibility of a brain disorder.

If the convulsions are unusual in some way, a CAT scan may be used to investigate the cause.

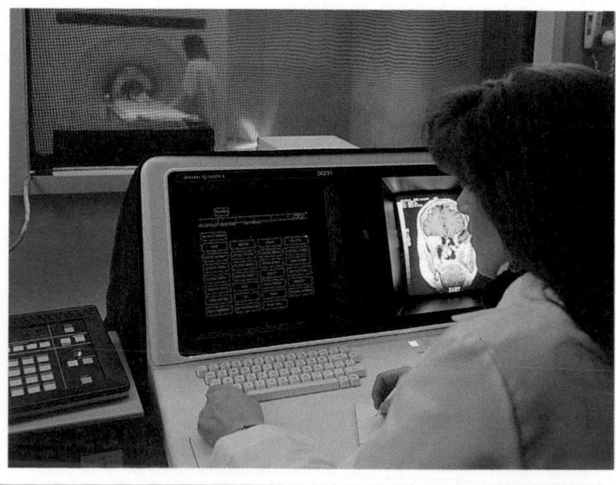

FOOT COMPLAINTS & INJURIES

FOOT PROBLEMS

Most foot complaints and injuries are minor, but they may cause your child a great deal of discomfort.

- Always ensure that your child's shoes fit properly. This will help to prevent general discomfort, and complications such as blisters will be less likely to occur. Have your child's feet measured regularly and budget for new shoes.
- Although your child may enjoy wandering around barefoot in the house, make sure she wears adequate footwear outside to prevent injury. Also ensure that there is nothing on your floor at home that could damage your child's feet.
- If your child has an infection, such as a verruca, seek advice from a pharmacist on the best way to treat it.
- If your child has a sprained ankle, take measures to reduce the swelling and seek medical advice if necessary.

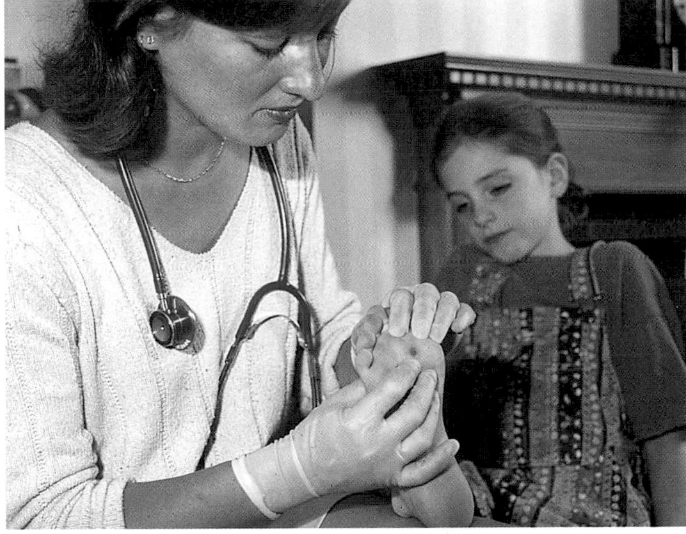

Minor foot complaints, such as veruccas, will usually clear up without treatment being necessary. If a verucca does not disappear naturally, seek medical advice.

Ingrowing toenail

An ingrowing toenail is a condition of the toe in which one or both edges of the nail press into the adjacent skin, leading to inflammation and infection.

- Causes of an ingrowing toenail include ill-fitting socks and shoes, the nail being cut incorrectly and poor personal hygiene.
- Temporary relief from pain can be given by bathing your child's foot in a strong warm salt solution. After bathing, the nail should be covered by a dry gauze dressing. If there is any infection, you will need to consult your GP for antibiotics.

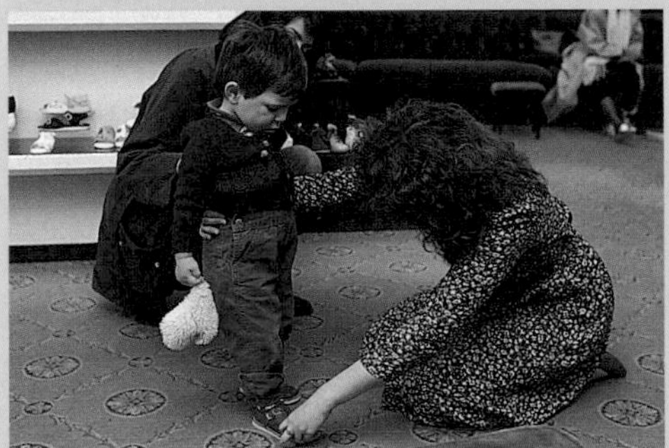

Ensure your child's shoes fit properly. Until he is three, have his feet checked every six to eight weeks.

Blisters

A blister is a collection of fluid under the outer layer of the skin, which forms a raised area usually oval or circular in shape.

- The fluid in a blister is serum that has leaked from blood vessels in the underlying skin layers after minor damage has occurred. It is usually caused by friction (such as a shoe that rubs) or a scald or sunburn. The fluid is usually sterile and it protects the damaged tissue.
- A blister is best left to heal itself. Do not burst the blister as the damaged tissue could become infected. Ensure your child always wears well-fitting shoes and socks.
- In the case of large, troublesome or unexplained blisters, seek medical advice.

Cramp

Cramp is a sudden, involuntary and painful muscle spasm. It occurs commonly during sleep, but can also happen after exercise. In children, it can be caused by excessive loss of salt and fluid from the body if the child has a fever and is sweating.

To relieve cramp in the foot:

1. Help your child to stand with her weight on the front of her foot.
2. When the first spasm has passed, gently massage the foot to relax the muscles.
3. If your child has a fever, ensure she has an adequate fluid intake and give junior paracetamol or ibuprofen to reduce her temperature. Consider giving rehydration sachets mixed with water – this will help to replenish the salts lost due to sweating.

Veruccas

These are known medically as plantar warts. A verucca is a hard, horny, rough-surfaced area on the sole of the foot caused by a virus called the papillomavirus.

- The infection is often acquired from contaminated floors at swimming pools.
- The wart is flattened and forced into the sole of the foot due to the pressure of the weight of the body. This can cause discomfort or pain when walking.
- Many verrucas disappear without treatment, but some persist for years or may recur.
- To relieve discomfort, a foam pad may be worn in the shoe.
- Verrucas can successfully be removed by crysurgery (freezing the verruca) or cautery (burning it), for which you will need to take your child to see a GP.
- You may wish to try to treat the verruca yourself using one of the over-the-counter preparations from your pharmacist. Always follow the instructions carefully and take particular care not to get the preparation on to the surrounding healthy skin as this can cause blistering and pain, which will further impede walking.

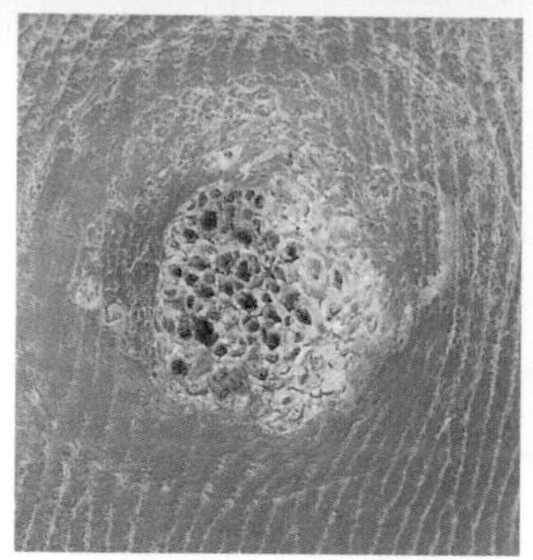

A verucca is a contagious lump found on the sole of the foot. It may cause a child discomfort and pain.

Strains and sprains of the ankle

If your child experiences pain when she puts weight on her foot or her ankle is swollen, it may be sprained. If you suspect that the ankle may be broken, secure and support it and take your child to hospital immediately. A sprain (usually caused by a wrench or twist of the ankle) can be treated with the RICE procedure: Rest the injured part; apply Ice or a cold compress; Compress the injury by wrapping it firmly; Elevate the injured part.

1. Steady and support the ankle in the most comfortable position.
2. Apply an icepack or cold compress to a recent injury to reduce swelling.
3. Wrap the ankle in a thick layer of padding and then bandage firmly.
4. Raise and support the injured limb to reduce the swelling.
5. Try to get your child to rest her ankle and seek medical advice if the pain persists.
6. You can give your child an anti-inflammatory medication, such as ibuprofen, to help with the pain and also reduce the swelling. If you are unsure what to give and at what dose, ask your doctor or pharmacist for advice.

Puncture wounds

Puncture wounds can occur as a result of standing on a nail or piece of glass, for example. There is usually a small entry site, but a deep track of internal damage. As germs and dirt can be carried far into the body, the risk of infection is high. Prompt action is needed to reduce blood loss, shock and infection.

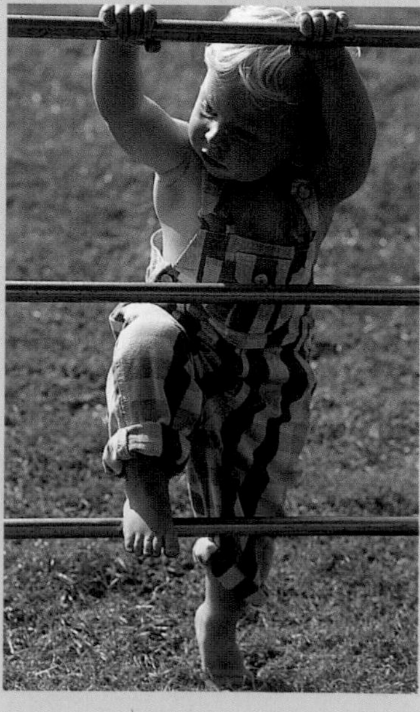

1. Control blood loss by applying pressure over the wound and raising the injured part. For a foot injury where, for example, your child has stepped on a nail, lay her down on the floor and raise her leg, resting it on your knee, while you treat the blood loss.
2. If you cannot apply direct pressure to the wound, for example, if an object or bone is protruding, press down firmly on either side. Do not attempt to remove the object.
3. Take steps to minimise shock, which can result from severe blood loss. Lay your child down with the injured part elevated, if you have not already done so.
4. Cover any open wound with a dressing, to protect it from infection and promote natural healing. Apply a sterile dressing and bandage it firmly.
5. Secure and support the injured part.
6. Wash your hands well with soap and water before and after treatment so that there is no spread of infection between you and your child.
7. If a foreign object is still in the wound, take your child to hospital for it to be removed and for treatment. She may need an X-ray.

Puncture wounds can have serious consequences – to prevent any injury, make sure your child always wears adequate footwear.

FOREIGN BODIES

DEALING WITH FOREIGN BODIES

Dirt, dust or other specks commonly become lodged in children's eyes, ears and noses, and babies especially may get something stuck in their throats. These sensitive organs need to be handled carefully.

Your child will become distressed if a foreign body becomes lodged in her eye, ear or nose, so reassure her and try to keep her calm.

If she has something in her eye it may be possible to remove it using the first-aid treatment shown overleaf, but do not attempt to remove an object from her nose or from her ear.

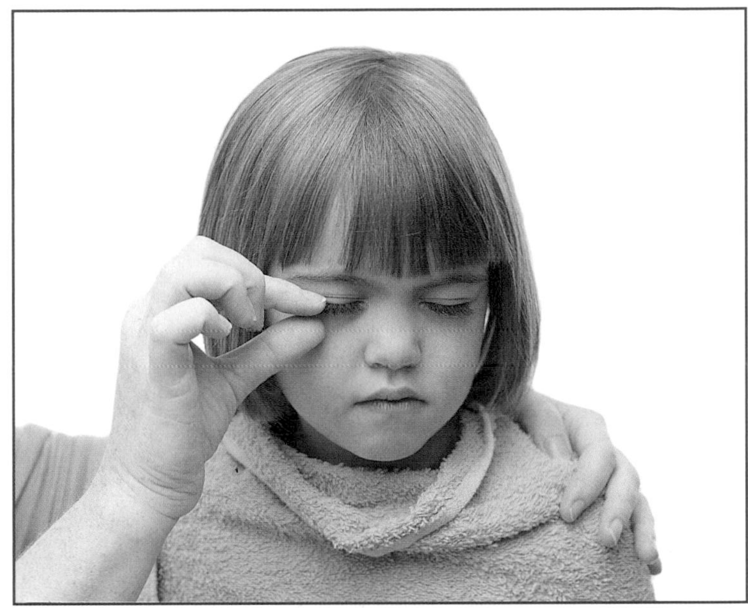

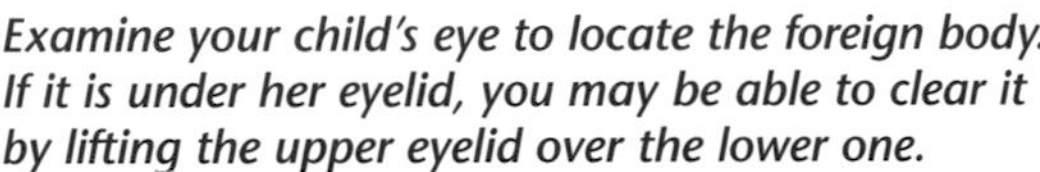

Examine your child's eye to locate the foreign body. If it is under her eyelid, you may be able to clear it by lifting the upper eyelid over the lower one.

What not to do

Eye	Ear	Nose
Don't attempt to:	**Don't attempt to:**	**Don't attempt to:**
● Remove anything that is embedded in the eyeball itself. ● Disturb or touch any piece of metal in the eye. ● Remove a foreign body that is in the iris and pupil – the coloured area of the eye.	● Remove any object from inside the ear. ● Try to dislodge an object or probe inside the ear, because you may pierce the eardrum.	● Remove any object that is stuck up the nose. If it is pushed further up, it can block the throat and damage the delicate nasal lining.

Seeking medical help

Take your child to hospital if she:

- Has an object embedded in the white of her eye or in the iris or pupil.
- Has a foreign body stuck in her nose or ear.

Call an ambulance if she:

- Is unconscious.
- Is choking, turning blue and becoming floppy.

Swallowing an object

Babies and young children often put small objects into their mouths or talk while they are eating. There is a risk that they could accidentally swallow something that becomes stuck in their windpipe (trachea).

- When an object has been swallowed, the signs that the windpipe is blocked include difficulty in breathing, gurgling and blueness around the lips and face. Your child may also be clutching her throat (a baby may wave her limbs around), be unable to speak or cry and, possibly, become unconscious.

- If your child is choking, give emergency first aid and call an ambulance.

- If your child has swallowed an object but is not choking, don't make her vomit. Bringing the object back up could cause further damage. Seek medical help.

Many incidents of choking are caused by babies being given toys that contain small parts. Always ensure that all toys are suitable for your child's age and conform to safety standards.

A foreign body in the eye

Position your baby or child so that you can see into her eye. You may need to hold her head still while you examine her.

First-aid tips

- Keep an eye irrigator and sterile eye solution in your first-aid kit.
- Make sure that your child does not rub the affected eye.
- Before giving first-aid treatment, ask your child to blink rapidly as this may be enough to dislodge the foreign body. Moistening the eye with eyewash may help.
- If the eye is still sore after removing the foreign body, seek medical help.
- When it is not possible to remove the foreign object, bandage lightly over both eyes and take your child to hospital. It is important to cover both eyes because movement of the good eye can cause movement of the injured eye.

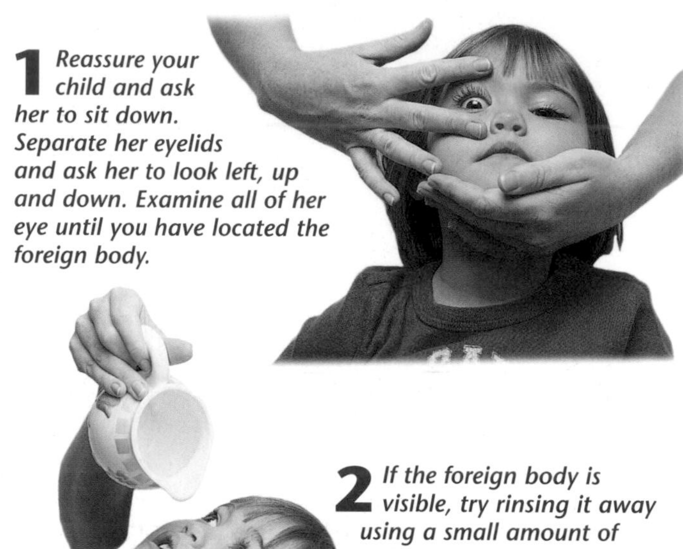

1 *Reassure your child and ask her to sit down. Separate her eyelids and ask her to look left, up and down. Examine all of her eye until you have located the foreign body.*

2 *If the foreign body is visible, try rinsing it away using a small amount of clean tepid water. Tilt your child's head back and gently trickle water into her eye to wash away the debris.*

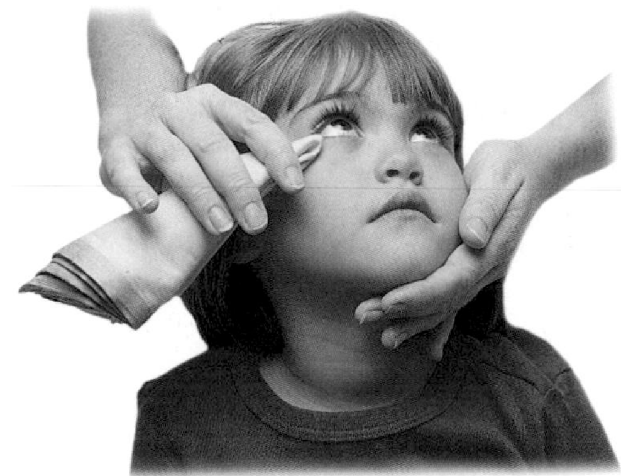

3 *If it is not possible to remove the foreign body from the eye with water, try using a handkerchief or cloth. Dampen the corner of the handkerchief, then gently use it to wipe the offending object off the eye.*

A foreign body in the ear

If your child complains of feeling pain or vibrations inside her ear, she may have something stuck in it. Hearing may be impaired on the affected side.

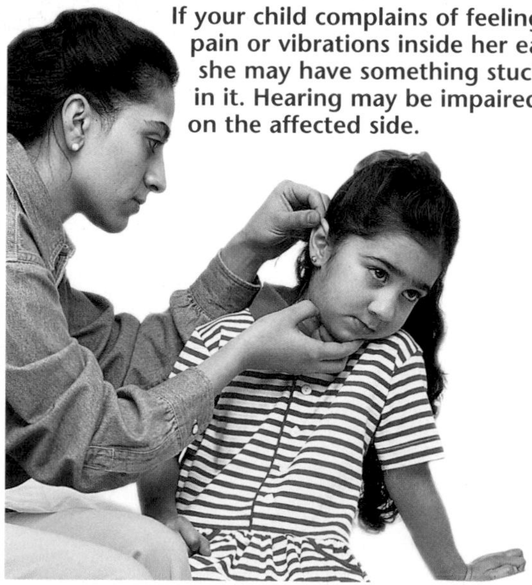

- Reassure your child.
- Take her to hospital.

NOTE: if an insect has crawled into your child's ear, it may be possible to rinse it out with tepid water.

A foreign body in the nose

It's all too common for a young child to try to push small objects, such as pebbles, marbles or sweets, up one or both nostrils. As a result, the nostrils may become blocked and swollen and sometimes start to bleed.

- Reassure your child.
- Take him to hospital.

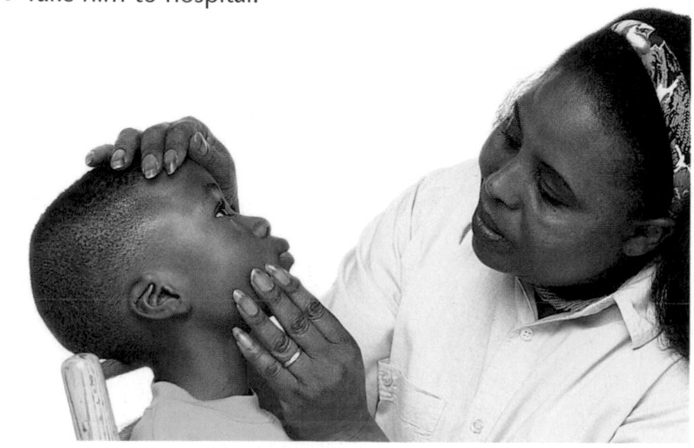

FRACTURES IN TODDLERS

WHAT IS A FRACTURE?

A fracture is a crack or break in a bone. Fractures can be serious, with the bone broken in several places or pushing through the skin. This is known as a compound fracture, and can be complicated by injury to adjoining nerves, muscles and blood vessels.

However, children's bones are so flexible and resilient that fractures are not usually that serious. Often, children's bones do not snap like an adult's, but bow or break the outer lining of the bone only, rather like new wood. Such breaks are called greenstick fractures. Complications, such as infection or failed healing, are much less common than with adults, and children's bones heal a lot quicker.

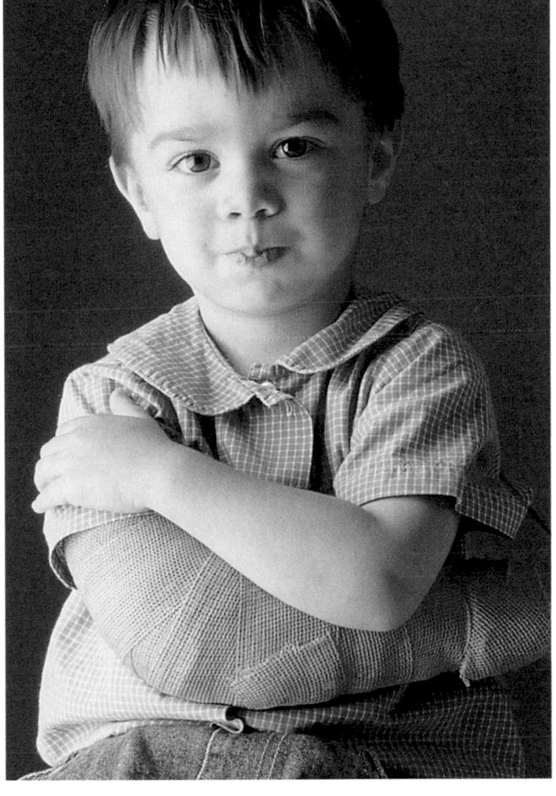

With their boundless energy, insatiable curiosity, early unsteadiness and total lack of any sense of danger, toddlers and young children are susceptible to fractures.

Signs of a fracture

A toddler may be unable to communicate where he is hurting, so it is possible for parents to be unaware of a fracture. Look out for the following signs:

- Swelling or bruising of a limb. (A toddler's healthy chubbiness at this age may mask any obvious outward signs of a fracture.)
- Limping or refusing to walk.
- Not using an arm or leaving the arm hanging by his side as if it is paralysed.
- Crying whenever the limb is used or touched.

What to do for a suspected fracture

Basic first aid is to support the broken bone – for example, strap a wounded finger to the finger next to it. However, this may cause further upset and pain.

1 The best thing to do is to take your child to an accident and emergency department or doctor's surgery as quickly as you can. Certain bones, such as the thigh bone (femur) and pelvis, can bleed profusely internally – any suspicion of such a fracture should be treated as an emergency.

2 Don't let your child have anything to eat or drink until he has seen a doctor because he might need a general anaesthetic.

After treatment, the doctor may give your child liquid paracetamol. This should help to ease the pain.

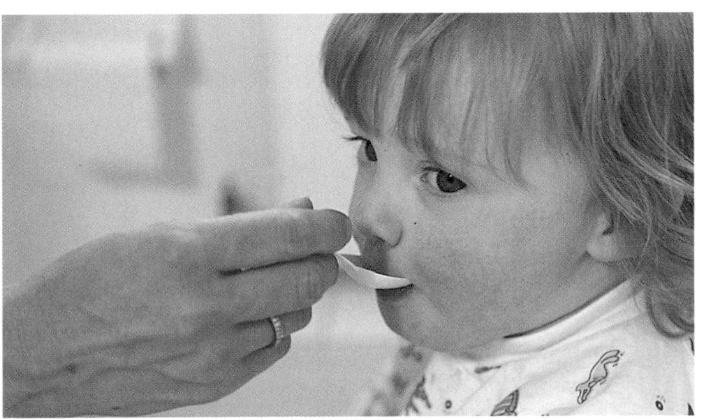

How are fractures treated?

Deciding on the best way to treat a fracture is often straightforward and a casualty doctor makes the decision.

- **Splint:** plaster of Paris is used most commonly. Initially, a half plaster is put on because of the swelling around the fracture. Once the swelling has reduced, a full plaster will probably be put on.
- **Manipulation:** the broken bone is pulled back into line and then plastered, under a general anaesthetic.
- **External fixation:** pins are inserted into the bone through the skin, and then fixed to hold the bones in place while they heal.
- **Traction:** for a bone that is badly out of line, the best way to ensure proper healing is to fix the limb, usually a leg, using a traction system, with the child bedbound.
- **Surgery:** if the fracture is too great to heal naturally, the surgeon will fix the two broken ends, using temporary metal plates and pins.

How does bone heal?

Fractures are like any other wound – if they are not protected, they will not heal properly. However, most bones will have healed in four to six weeks in the toddler age group. A broken bone goes through several stages as it heals:

1 Initially, there is bleeding, with swelling and pain around the fracture. Cells, called osteoclasts, get rid of the old, dead bone.

2 After a few days, chondroblast cells form new bone called soft callus. Callus is made of blood vessels, fibrous tissue, cartilage and bone.

3 Hard callus appears after two to three weeks. This may form a lump that can be felt under the skin. On an X-ray, the fracture line will no longer be visible, but a cloud of new bone will have appeared around the fracture site.

4 Remodelling is the final stage of healing. If the bone has healed out of shape, it is now restored to its original shape. This remodelling takes around three months for toddlers, while it may take several years for older children and adults.

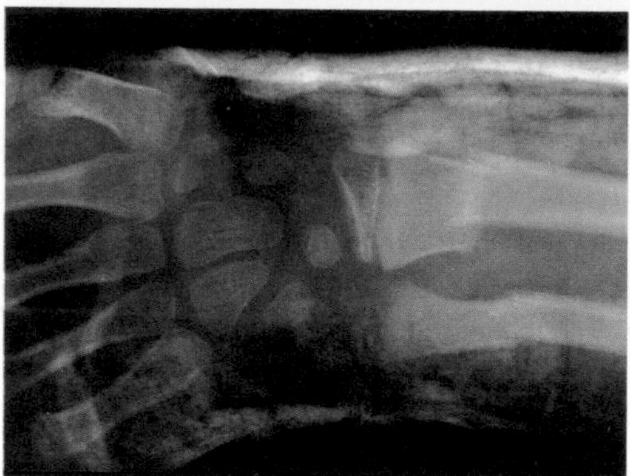

The above X-ray of a broken arm in plaster has been taken to assess how well the fracture is healing. The plaster cast protects the broken bone, preventing movement of the aligned ends until healing has progressed sufficiently.

Learning to walk

When toddlers are learning to walk, they may fall in such a way as to cause a particular type of fracture.

Toddlers will often keep one leg still when they fall, while the other twists underneath them. This twisting leads to a spiral-shaped fracture of the tibia, one of the two bones in the lower leg. A fracture of this kind can sometimes be missed because it's difficult to see on an X-ray.

Your child's mobility will be checked by your health visitor at the developmental checks.

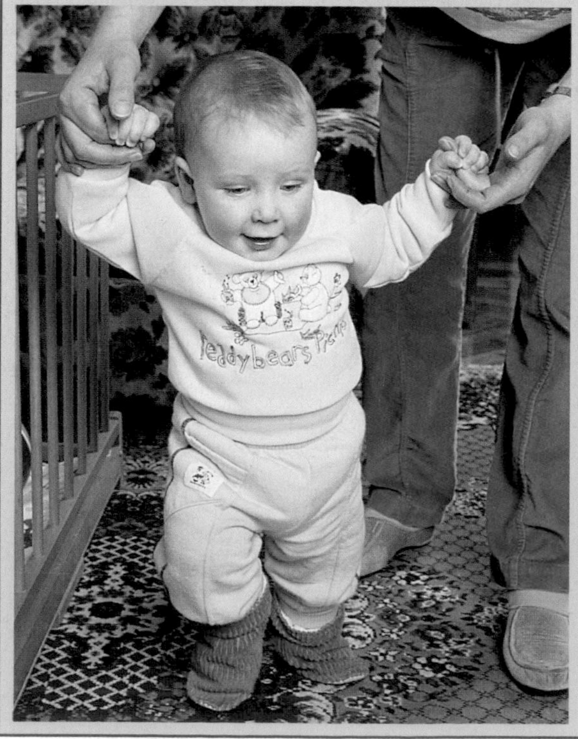

When your child is in plaster

Check his circulation and make sure that he doesn't develop an infection. Seek medical advice if you think there is a problem. Look out for the following signs:

- Toes (or arms) turn blue or white, are cold and not moving, or are swollen.
- There is redness, swelling or pus.
- Your child has a fever and/or is in pain, having been settled beforehand.
- The plaster seems soggy, broken or loose.

Long-term effects

Most fractures heal and cause no further problems. However, a fracture that involves a child's growth plate may have a lasting result.

- The growth plates (epiphyses) lie at each end of the long bones, and those most commonly affected are located in the fingers and the wrist.
- Any interference with these, such as a break, may stop the bone growing. The fractured bone may therefore be shorter than it would have been with normal development.
- This kind of fracture will be monitored closely by the orthopaedic doctors to ensure that growth is not affected.

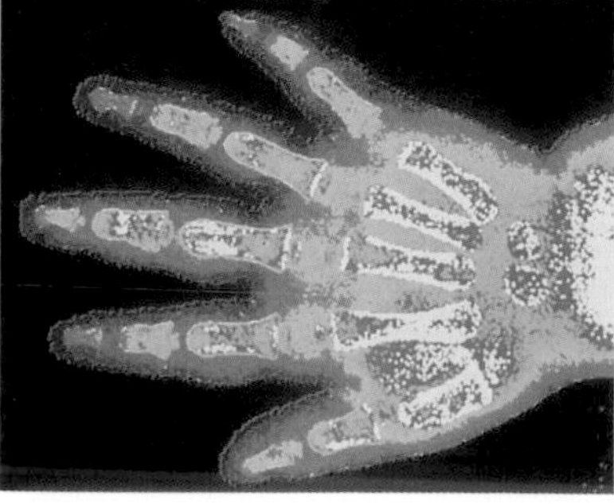

A child's hand, wrist, ankle and foot bones develop gradually in the first four to five years. In normal growth, a one-year-old child has three wrist bones, with the remaining six developing during early childhood.

HEAD INJURIES & CONCUSSION

HEAD INJURIES IN CHILDREN

Young children often get knocks on the head. These are seldom serious but parents need to be able to assess the severity of the injury and act accordingly.

Most children recover quickly from what is usually a minor bump that causes a few tears but does not need medical attention. However, you should check for signs of concussion and keep a careful eye on your child for several days.

If your child has had a head injury that led to him losing consciousness, he must not play any contact sport for three weeks.

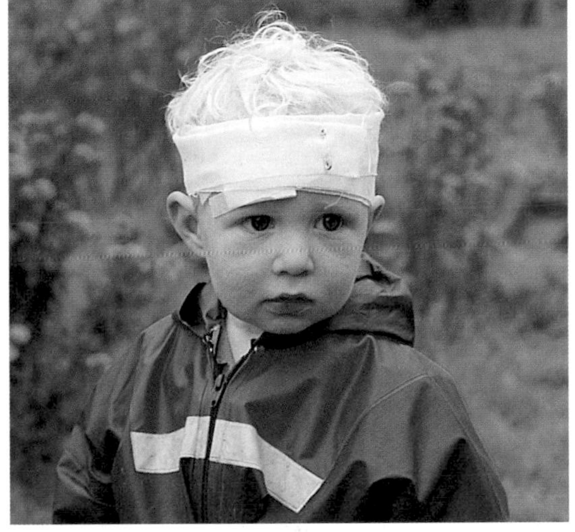

Even a minor cut can bleed for a long time. Pressure should be applied and a bandage wrapped fairly tightly round your child's head.

Types of head injury

Head injuries range in severity from a minor cut to, at the other end of the scale, damage to the brain.

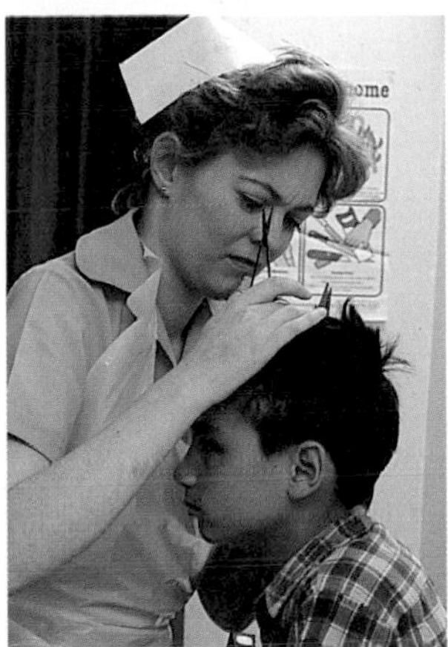

If your child has been involved in a head collision and you are unsure of the severity of the injury, seek medical advice.

- **Bruising/swelling to the scalp:** this will appear within minutes of a blow to the head.
- **Scalp wound:** even a tiny scratch can bleed profusely because the scalp is well supplied with blood vessels. Some may need stitching.
- **Concussion:** a blow to the head can 'shake' the brain, causing symptoms such as temporary loss of consciousness, nausea, dizziness, loss of memory and headache.
- **Fractured skull:** a fall from a height or a traffic accident may result in a fracture to the skull.
- **Penetrating injury to the brain:** occasionally, a splinter of bone from a fractured skull, or a sharp object can pierce the brain tissue.

Danger signs

If any of the following symptoms develop after a head injury, call for an ambulance:

- Loss of consciousness, however brief
- Visible severe wound or an abnormal dent in the scalp
- Vomiting
- Convulsions
- Dazed appearance, drowsiness
- No response when spoken to or touched
- Clear fluid leaking from ear or nose
- Blood in the white of the eye

When to seek medical help

Answering these questions should enable you to make the decision about whether to seek medical help. If in doubt, always call a doctor.

1 Is your child conscious? Feel the scalp for bumps and look for cuts, bruises or dents.

2 How distressed is he? Persistent crying, despite being comforted, will mean he's still in distress.

3 How is he behaving? Unusual behaviour may indicate concussion. A baby may be floppy; a toddler, irritable.

4 What is he telling you? An older child may be able to tell you that he is not feeling well and may complain of feeling sick or dizzy, or tell you that he is in pain.

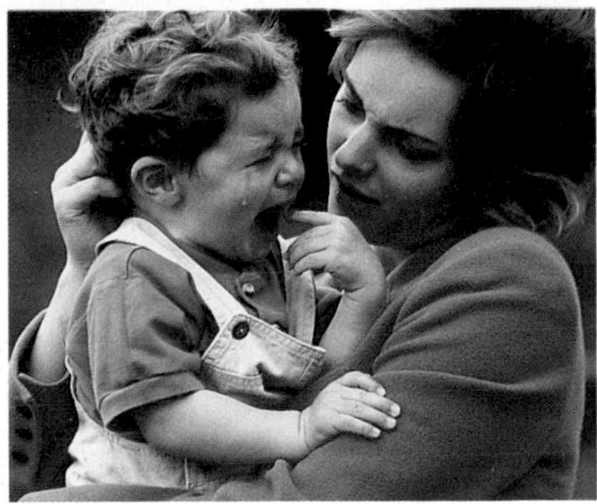

If your child continues to scream for a long time after a fall or bump, seek medical advice.

Delayed reaction

Some head injuries that initially appear to be minor can develop into serious cases. It is important to monitor your child's wellbeing closely in the days following an injury.

- In infants, the bones of the skull are not fused together, allowing brain tissue to swell without causing specific symptoms.

- In older children, the skull bones have fused together so that if the brain swells due to damage, signs of increased pressure inside the skull will gradually appear.

- Signs of increased pressure within the skull, which may lead to unconsciousness, include headache, unequally sized pupils, weakness in one side of the body or face, fever and drowsiness.

First aid at home

If your child seems to have no ill effects and the head injury is minor, basic first-aid measures are usually very effective.

- **Bruising and swelling:** you can use an icepack to reduce swelling. A bag of frozen peas is excellent for this, but remember to wrap it in a tea-towel first so that it doesn't damage the skin.

- **Bleeding:** the priority with a scalp wound is to stop the bleeding. Sit or lie the child down and place a clean dressing or kitchen paper over the wound (a clean handkerchief will do if you don't have a first-aid kit) and gently press for a few minutes. Once the bleeding has stopped, secure the dressing in place, using tape or a light bandage.

NOTE: you may want to apply a herbal remedy, such as arnica for swelling and calendula for cuts.

- **Serious injury:** if the injury is not minor and you are concerned about your child's condition, there are measures you can take while waiting for the ambulance. Keep the child still in a quiet room. If he is unconscious, check his breathing and pulse regularly and make sure that if he is sick, there is no vomit blocking his airway. Keep your child lying on his side, either on your lap or in your arms, to help keep his airway clear.

Hospital treatment

Once in the hospital, treatment very much depends on the severity of the injury, but a few basic principles will be followed.

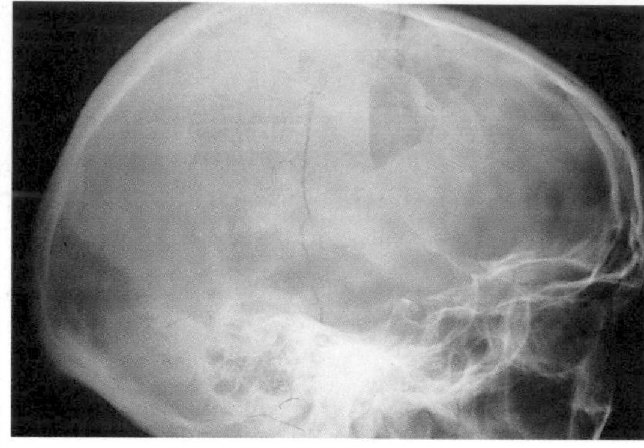

A skull fracture can occur if there is a serious blow to the head. An X-ray may be taken as part of the overall assessment.

1 A detailed neurological assessment of a child's condition helps to decide the extent of the injury, including the level of consciousness and symptoms that need monitoring.

2 The head injury is examined, cleaned, stitched if necessary, and covered with a clean dressing.

3 Skull X-rays may be taken to check for a fracture.

4 If there is any concern, an overnight stay in hospital will probably be recommended in order to monitor your child's condition.

5 More serious head injuries may involve intensive care and possibly even surgery.

6 CT scanning of the brain is sometimes carried out to check for signs of damage – whether temporary or permanent.

Preventing head injuries

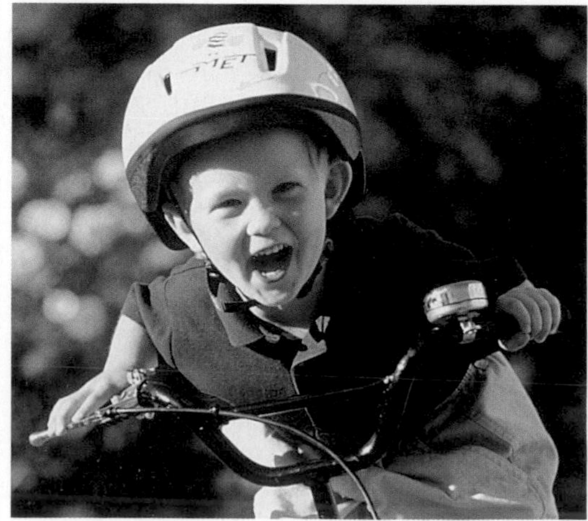

Although the occasional bump and bruise are all part of growing up and learning about the hazards in life, there are several steps you can take to prevent head injuries occurring:

- Think about where the 'toddler-level' sharp corners are in your house and fit protective safety guards.

- Fit all windows with safety catches and use window bars if appropriate.

Wearing a helmet has been proved to save lives. Insist that your child wears one when he is cycling or rollerskating.

- Install stairgates.

- Teach your child road safety from an early age.

- When travelling, strap your child safely into an age-appropriate car seat.

- Make sure your child wears a crash-helmet when riding a tricycle or bicycle.

HEAT EXHAUSTION & HEATSTROKE

OVERHEATING

Children, like adults, can suffer from the effects of heat in the warmer weather. Extreme heat may cause heat exhaustion and heatstroke, especially when it is combined with physical activity.

- **Heat exhaustion:** this is due to dehydration and is usually caused by a combination of heat, humidity and physical activity. It may develop very gradually. Your child may show symptoms such as headache, confusion and sickness and he may have cramping pains in his stomach and leg muscles. Although he will feel hot to the touch, his body temperature will not be significantly raised.

- **Heatstroke:** this is uncommon in the UK, but is a medical emergency. When heatstroke occurs, the body cannot maintain its normal temperature and so it starts to overheat. Heatstroke can be fatal if it is not treated quickly.

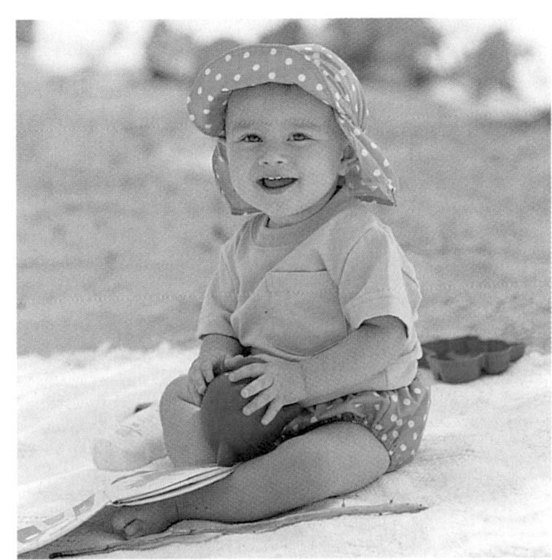

It's vital to protect your baby from the effects of heat by ensuring that he wears a hat in the sunshine and has plenty of cool drinks.

Causes

The body gets rid of excess heat by sending more blood to the skin to be cooled and by increased sweating.

1 On a very hot day the body cannot lose heat easily; the blood sent to the skin to be cooled will meet warm air.

2 In addition, if the atmosphere is very humid, sweat cannot evaporate well and so cannot cool the body effectively. More sweat is produced to try to bring the temperature down. If it's not replaced with fluids, this leads to dehydration.

3 Heatstroke may follow from untreated heat exhaustion. It occurs when the body's 'thermostat' stops working and cooling mechanisms, such as sweating, cease. The body's temperature rises to dangerous levels.

Symptoms

The symptoms and signs of simple heat exhaustion differ a little from those of the more serious condition of heatstroke.

Heat exhaustion:
- Pale, clammy skin
- Headache
- Thirst, nausea and vomiting
- Hot dry skin
- Rapid pulse and breathing
- Normal or only slightly raised temperature
- Cramps in the stomach or limbs
- Usually comes on gradually

Heatstroke:
- Headache and dizziness
- Confusion or strange behaviour
- Rapid pulse
- High temperature
- Less urine
- Unconsciousness
- May happen suddenly

When your child is at risk

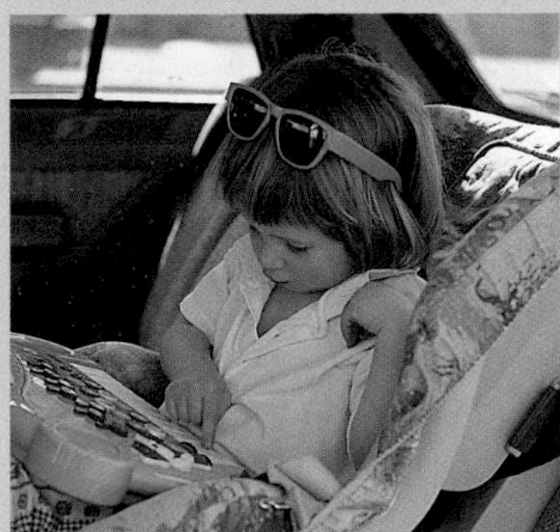

It is extremely important not to leave your child for any length of time in a car. Even if it doesn't feel very hot outside, a child can overheat quickly inside a vehicle.

Your child can suffer from the effects of heat in any situation where she is producing more heat than can be lost by her body.

- **At home:** playing in the garden, or in the park, on a hot sunny day may cause problems unless your child has frequent drinks and rests in the shade.
- **Overseas holidays:** summer holidays in the sun bring increased risks for your child, especially if he is not used to the heat.
- **In the car:** even if the weather is not particularly hot, the car can become very warm in bright sunshine. Your child may overheat, particularly if she is dressed warmly and strapped in a car seat.
- **Warm clothing:** many layers of warm clothing on a relatively mild day can cause overheating.

First aid for heat exhaustion

If you believe your child is suffering from heat exhaustion, you need to cool her down and give her drinks to replace the fluids she has lost. With a few simple steps she should soon be feeling much better.

1 Take your child to a cool place and lay her down.

2 Remove her outer layers of clothing.

3 Give your child tepid water or fruit juice to drink; or you can give her a rehydration solution, available from a pharmacist. Do not give her ice-cold drinks.

4 Sponge your child with tepid water.

5 Make sure your child rests in the shade until she is feeling better.

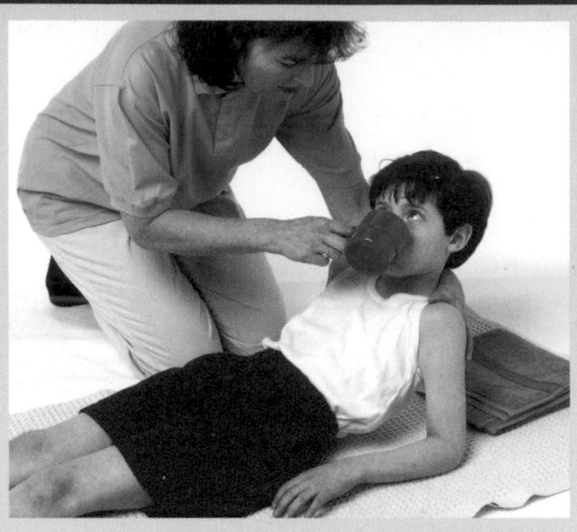

If you suspect that your child is suffering from heat exhaustion, lay her down straightaway and give her sips of tepid water or fruit juice to drink.

First aid for heatstroke

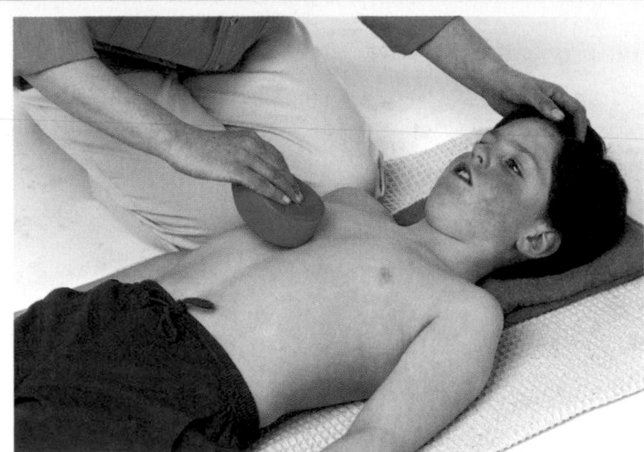

Once you have called for medical help, take measures to cool your child down. Remove his outer clothing, sponge him down repeatedly with cool water and fan him.

Heatstroke is a medical emergency and an ambulance should be called immediately. While you are waiting for help to arrive, take steps to cool your child down.

1 Quickly take your child to a cool place and lay him down.

2 Remove his outer clothing.

3 Sponge your child down with cool water.

4 If he becomes unconscious, put him into the recovery position.

Hospital treatment: in the rare event of heatstroke your child will need expert medical treatment. This will include an intravenous drip of a water and salt solution, which will help to replace the fluid he has lost through sweating. He may have to stay in hospital while the doctors check to see whether any of the body's organs have been affected by the high temperature.

Preventing overheating

Most cases of heat exhaustion and heatstroke are preventable if you follow a few simple guidelines.

- Give regular cool drinks in hot weather and encourage your child to drink them even if he does not feel thirsty. Ice lollies with a high water content also provide fluid and usually appeal to young children.

- Make sure your child takes regular 'breathers' where he sits quietly in the shade to cool off. Always keep babies in the shade.

- Dress your child in lightweight, loose-fitting clothing. Light colours reflect the sun's heat. Be very careful with babies, who are unable to tell you they are hot.

- Ideally, keep your child out of the sun between midday and 4 p.m., especially if you are abroad. Always protect your child with sunscreen in warm weather.

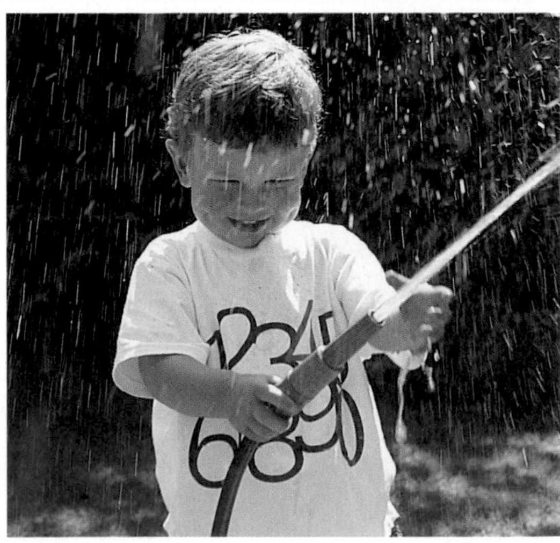

Allow your child to play with water outside. He will love to get wet and it will keep him cool.

MOUTH INJURIES

MINOR AND MAJOR INJURIES

Mouth injuries are common in toddlers and young children, and often occur when a child trips over or falls.

- Mouth injuries in children can range from a cut lip caused by a fall to a serious burn from drinking poisonous fluids.

- Although they may look unsightly and be distressing, most mouth injuries are minor and can be treated at home.

- More serious mouth injuries can result in blocking or partial blocking of the airway as a result of swelling or excessive bleeding. These types of injuries need urgent medical attention at a hospital to avoid potential suffocation.

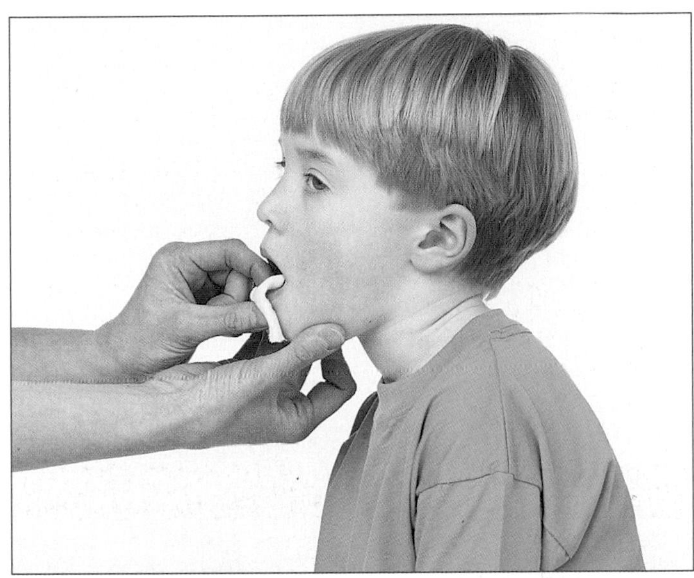

Mouth injuries are often very painful and children can find them distressing. However, most of these injuries are short-lived and can be treated at home.

Bleeding from the mouth or lip

Most children will sustain a cut to the mouth or lip at least once in their life as a result of a fall, or running into a solid object, such as furniture. Sometimes the piece of skin joining the top lip to the top gum (the frenulum) tears and this, like the rest of the mouth, will bleed a lot.

1 Sit your child upright with her head tilted forward. This will ensure that the blood doesn't run down her throat.

2 If you can see the site of the bleeding, place a clean pad of gauze, cotton or even folded paper tissue over it and tell her to hold it firmly in place with a finger, or do this yourself, making sure she can't choke on the pad. Hold this in place until the bleeding has stopped.

3 Don't give your child anything to drink as this may dislodge any clot that is forming. However, for small cuts, an ice lolly can act as a distraction and constrict the blood vessel, thereby reducing bleeding.

4 If the injury involves your child's tongue, it's important to look for swelling. This is a serious condition because a swollen tongue can obstruct the child's airway, and therefore result in suffocation.

Foreign objects

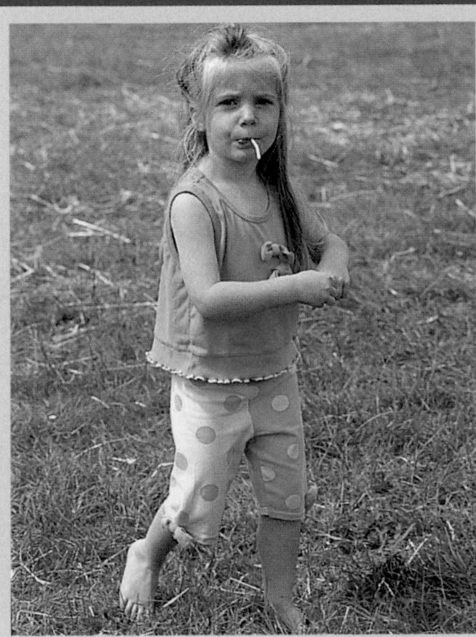

Serious injuries can be sustained if a child falls or runs into something, with an object, such as a lollipop or pencil, sticking out of her mouth. This can cause the airway or the base of the skull to be pierced, resulting in a life-threatening injury.

1 Do not allow your child to run around with something in her mouth.

2 In the event of choking, don't attempt to remove the object, unless the child cannot breathe.

3 Ask someone to call an ambulance.

Do not let your child run around with an object such as a lollipop in her mouth. If she falls, it could choke her or pierce her airway.

4 Try to maintain your child's airway, and don't let it become obstructed with blood. Sit your child upright with her head forward to allow blood to drain out of the mouth. Alternatively, place your child in the recovery position.

5 Stay with her and keep her calm until the ambulance arrives.

6 Once your child is at the hospital, the foreign object may have to be removed under general anaesthetic.

A knocked-out tooth

A milk tooth should not be put back into its socket because it may cause damage to the permanent tooth underneath. However, it is sometimes possible to save a permanent tooth if you can get rapid dental treatment.

- Either put the permanent tooth back into the socket and hold it there – make sure you put it in the correct way round. Then take your child to a dentist, dental hospital or an accident and emergency unit.

- Or put the tooth straight into milk and take your child and her tooth to the dentist, dental hospital or accident and emergency unit, where the tooth will be repositioned.

- The tooth (or teeth) will need to be held in place with a splint for approximately four weeks.

Abscess or infection in the mouth

If your child complains of a painful spot in the mouth, it may well be a mouth ulcer. An abscess under a tooth will usually cause toothache. If you notice a bad smell on your child's breath, it may indicate infection.

Mouth ulcers

- These appear as painful small, white craters.

- They are not serious but can indicate that your child is run down or stressed, has poor oral hygiene or has bitten the inside of her cheek.

- Mouth ulcers usually clear up quickly on their own. Ensure your child gets plenty of rest and supervise her toothbrushing. However, if they recur take her to the GP to check for underlying illness.

Abscess

- A painful, swollen gum, jaw or facial swelling can indicate an abscess.

- An abscess is usually the result of decay, or a crack in the tooth, through which bacteria set up an infection.

- Give your child liquid paracetamol for the pain and take her to see a dentist urgently.

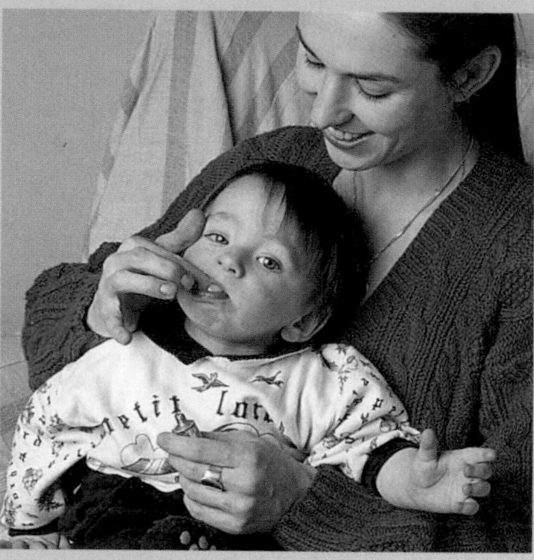

If your child is suffering from a mouth ulcer, a soothing mouth gel will help to numb the pain.

Burns to the mouth and throat

Burns to the mouth and throat arise from taking in hot food or drinks. They can also occur if a child swallows a poisonous substance.

Poisonous liquids

- If your child has drunk a corrosive liquid, such as bleach, weedkiller or dishwasher liquid, she may have red burn marks in and around her mouth and lips.

- Her breathing may sound harsh and high-pitched as a result of the swelling of damaged throat tissue.

1. Call an ambulance. Your child will require urgent hospital treatment.
2. Ask your child to tell you or point to what she has drunk and take the bottle to the hospital.
3. Don't make her vomit as the liquid will burn her gullet again as it comes back up.
4. Give sips of milk or water to help neutralise the acidity of the poison.
5. Wipe away any of the remaining liquid from your child's mouth with a cloth.
6. Stay with your child. If she becomes unconscious, put her in the recovery position.
7. Keep checking your child's breathing and give mouth-to-mouth resuscitation if necessary while you are waiting for the ambulance.

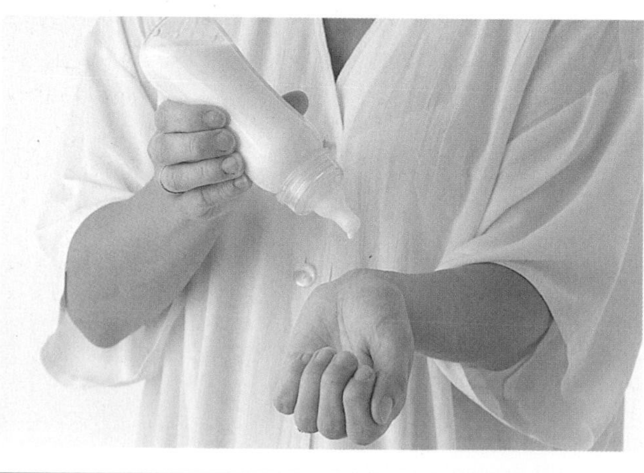

It's important to test the temperature of a liquid before giving it to a baby – if a drink is too hot it will burn the mouth. Test a few drops on the back of your hand.

Hot food or drinks

- Before giving warm drinks to a baby, always test the temperature by sprinkling a little on to the back of your hand. Be careful with food or drinks that have been heated in a microwave – they can feel cool on the outside but be hot inside, so ensure they are stirred and test the temperature yourself first.

- If your child does burn her mouth, give her cold water to drink immediately. Avoid giving warm liquids or ice as the mouth will be very sensitive to hot and cold temperatures at first.

- Watch for swelling in the mouth that could obstruct the airway. If the mouth blisters, take your child to your GP. An antiseptic mouthwash may be prescribed.

NECK INJURIES

THE ANATOMY OF THE NECK

As part of the spinal column, the neck consists of a series of intricately arranged bony vertebrae, interspersed with flexible discs of cartilage.

- The spinal cord, which is responsible for nervous control of the body's every move, runs through the centre of the spinal column. This is designed to protect the spinal cord while enabling the head and neck to move freely.

- The neck is vulnerable to a number of injuries, particularly in children. Any neck injury, no matter how mild, should be treated with great caution, because damage to the spinal cord can result in paralysis and even death.

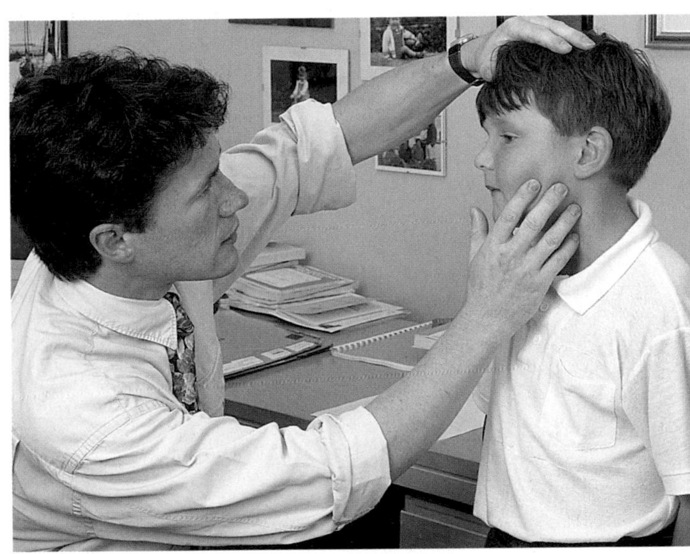

Any injury to the neck should be examined by a medical professional. A series of checks will be carried out to eliminate the possibility of serious damage to the area.

Causes of neck injuries

Children are particularly accident-prone, making their necks very susceptible to injury.

- **Falls:** any fall can result in neck injury due to landing awkwardly on the neck, possibly leading to a strain or fracture.

- **Sprains:** the muscles of the neck may become sprained during vigorous play.

- **Road traffic accidents:** even a mild car collision can cause whiplash to occur, whereby the head is thrown forward and back very quickly. This causes the muscles in the neck to be seriously sprained, and the vertebrae to be compressed or misaligned. Road traffic accidents are the main cause of neck fractures in children, which can be life-threatening.

- **Sleeping awkwardly:** children tend to wriggle around when they are asleep and may lie oddly so that they wake with a painful neck.

- **Torticollis:** this condition causes the muscles of the neck to undergo painful spasms and contract, pulling the head to one side. It may develop in newborn babies after damage to the neck muscles during a difficult birth. In children, torticollis may be caused by swollen glands in the neck due to infection.

- **Infection:** infections of the throat or ear can result in neck pain, due to the swelling of lymph glands in the neck in response to the infection. A sore neck may therefore be a symptom of an underlying infection. In rare cases, a stiff neck may be caused by meningitis, a life-threatening infection of the membrane surrounding the brain.

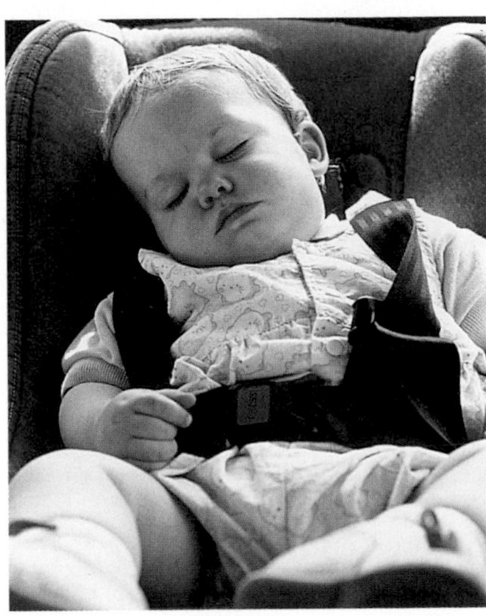

Make sure your child is securely strapped in during car travel. This will help to prevent a neck injury in the event of an accident.

Recognising a neck injury

Your child may be unable to tell you that he has a sore neck, but may appear generally unwell. Watch him closely for signs of the following:

- Swelling around the neck.

- Uncharacteristic behaviour – your child may become very quiet, for example, or appear extremely distressed.

- Your child may describe a numb feeling in his arms or legs or other parts of his body.

- He may hold his head awkwardly or lose his balance.

- If your child has a neck fracture, he may be unable to move.

- Any injury can cause the body to go into shock – your child may appear pale and clammy, and have irregular, shallow breathing and an erratic pulse.

- If the injury is severe, he may even lose consciousness.

Meningitis

Meningitis is an infection of the meninges, the membrane surrounding the brain. It is life-threatening and requires urgent treatment. One of the symptoms is a stiff neck – for this reason you should always seek medical advice if your child complains of neck pain. Other symptoms include:

- A distinctive, blotchy red rash that does not disappear when pressure is applied.
- Flu-like symptoms, such as appearing pale with a raised temperature.
- Headache, nausea and vomiting.
- Shying away from light – the eyes become over-sensitive to light as a result of the infection.

NOTE: if your child shows any of these symptoms, you need to seek urgent medical help. If you are in doubt, it is better to see a doctor straight away than to leave it too late. Meningitis can be very difficult to diagnose so there is no reason to feel foolish if it is a false alarm.

Treatment for neck strain or sprain

If the only symptom your child has is a sore neck, it is likely that it is a simple sprain.

- Paracetamol or ibuprofen liquid may help to ease the pain and reduce any inflammation, but seek medical advice first.
- A warm bath may help to ease the muscles of the neck.
- The doctor may advise that your child rests in bed with a warm hot-water bottle and some comfortable pillows.

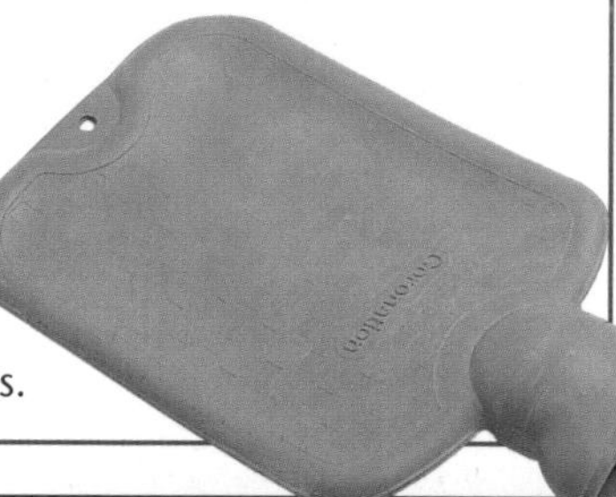

Emergency measures for a suspected neck fracture

If your child has had a fall or been involved in a car accident and displays the symptoms of a fractured neck, you must call an ambulance immediately as urgent medical treatment will be required. While you are waiting for the ambulance, there are a number of steps you can take to help your child.

1 Make sure that his airway is clear and that he is breathing normally.

2 If a fracture is suspected, do not move your child, unless he is in imminent, life-threatening danger. If you do have to move him, you will need someone else to help. Make sure that the back and neck are supported and roll your child like a log, keeping his neck and spine aligned, to a safe place.

3 If your child is moving, you may need to restrain him gently by placing a rolled-up blanket either side of him, or by placing a pillow either side of his head to stabilise it.

4 Continue to monitor your child's breathing and pulse until the ambulance arrives.

If you suspect a neck fracture, call an ambulance immediately and make sure your child is breathing normally.

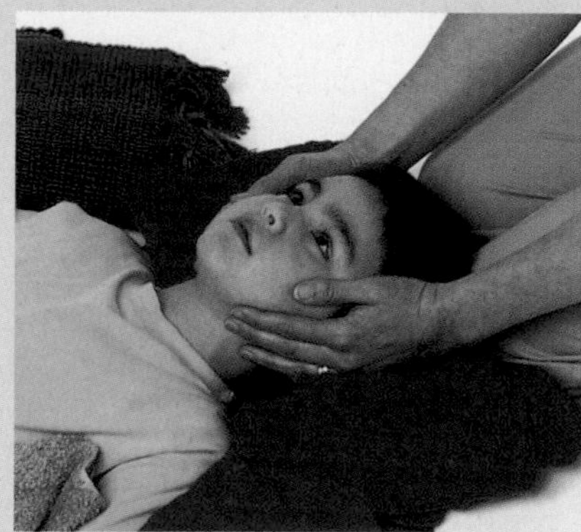

Hospital treatment

When the ambulance arrives, you will need to explain to the paramedics exactly how the injury happened. This will help them to assess the damage accurately.

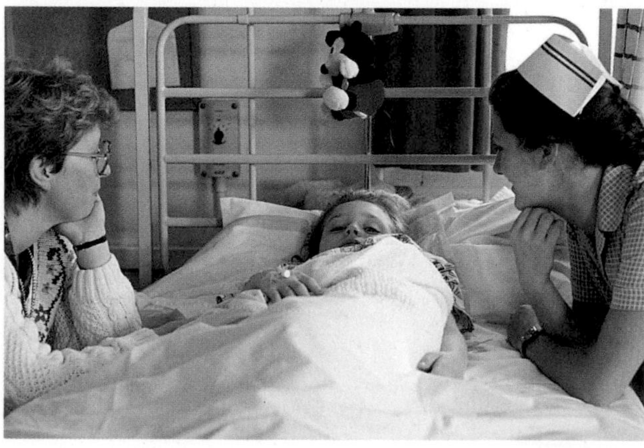

- If a broken neck is suspected, the paramedics will place a special collar around your child's neck. This stabilises the neck and prevents the head from moving.
- Your child will then be lifted on to a stretcher and transported to hospital in the ambulance.
- Once at the hospital, your child will be assessed for any nerve damage and an X-ray will be taken to confirm whether or not the neck is broken.
- Treatment will depend upon the extent of the injury. If the neck is broken, it will need to be re-aligned and fixed in place.

A neck injury can be very serious. Hospitalisation may be necessary to reduce the risk of further damage.

NOSE-BLEEDS

HOW NOSE-BLEEDS HAPPEN

Nose-bleeds are very common in young children, but they are rarely serious. The medical term for a nose-bleed is epistaxis, and the usual cause is damage to the blood vessels inside the nose.

- Tiny blood vessels in the nose can swell and burst, or become inflamed and damaged.
- These blood vessels are concentrated in an area of the nose called Little's area, towards the front of the septum (this is the area of gristle in the middle of the nose that separates the nostrils).
- The blood vessels moisten and warm the air that we breathe before it reaches the lungs, so they are very near the surface of the inner lining of the nose – and this makes them vulnerable to damage.

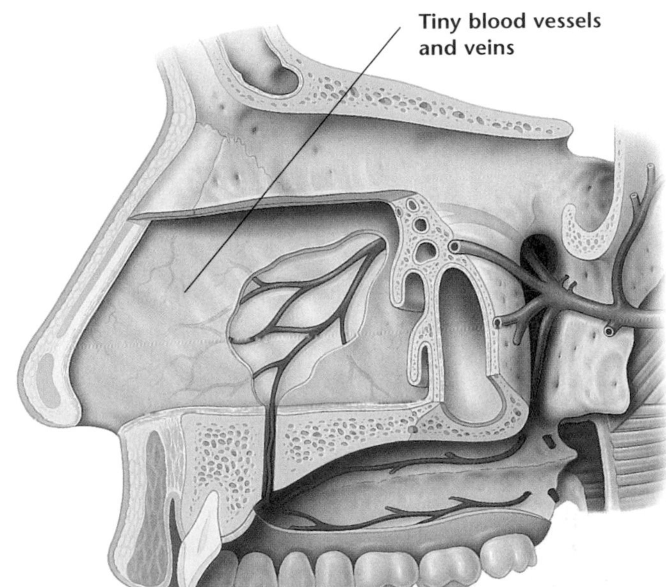

A nose-bleed is usually a result of damage to the tiny blood vessels found just inside the nostrils.

The causes

There are many types of nose-bleed, triggered by a variety of factors.

1 Most nose-bleeds are caused by the child picking her nose – a common childhood habit.

2 A foreign body may be stuck in the nose – children may put small items into their nostrils, where they can become stuck, leading to bleeding.

3 It's also possible for a nose-bleed to result from your child blowing her nose too hard, or sneezing violently if she has a cold.

4 Another type of nose-bleed is one resulting from an allergic reaction, such as hay fever or a reaction to a pet.

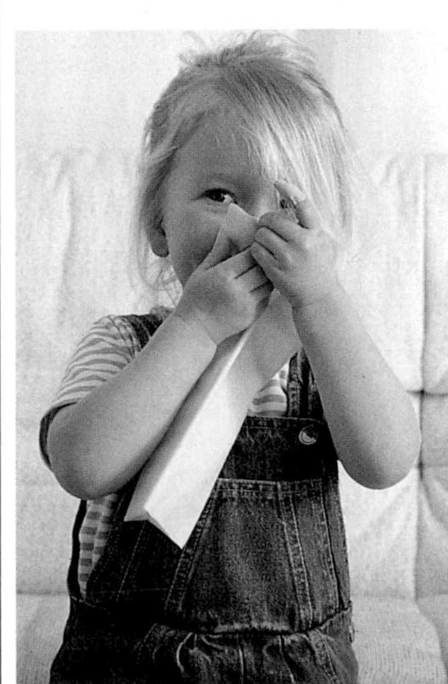

5 If nose-bleeds occur frequently, this could mean that the lining of your child's nose is particularly fragile or infected.

6 Nose-bleeds can indicate a serious health problem, such as a blood-clotting disorder or leukaemia, but this is very rare.

A nose-bleed may be caused by a physical injury, or may be due to something as simple as your child blowing her nose too hard.

A minor condition

Generally nose-bleeds are nothing to worry about – there is often less blood than you think.

- Nose-bleeds are frequent during the winter months, when colds, sinus infections and dry winter air can dry out the lining of the nose and make bleeding more likely.
- Even if the bleeding makes you anxious, don't panic – it may just be that your child has made it worse by rubbing or picking her nose.
- If your child suffers from a nose-bleed during the night, you may see dried blood on the pillowcase in the morning. Again, there is no reason to worry.

When to call the doctor

If pinching the nose fails to stop a nose-bleed and it seems particularly severe, or lasts for longer than half an hour, seek medical advice.

- You may be advised to take your child to your local accident and emergency department, where a doctor may stop the bleeding by packing your child's nose with gauze (never try to do this yourself).
- If your child's nose-bleed is due to a foreign object becoming stuck in her nose, don't attempt to remove it yourself, even if you can see it – you could end up pushing it further up her nose.
- Seek medical advice if your child gets a nose-bleed from a blow to the head or a fall.

How to treat a mild nose-bleed

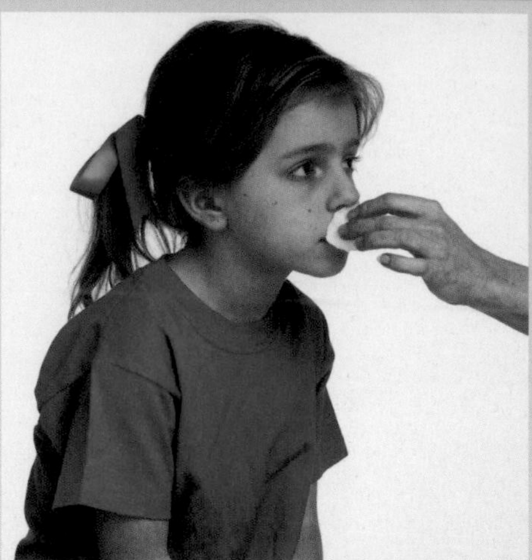

Once the bleeding has stopped, clean your child's nose with lukewarm water but don't insert the cotton wool into the nostril.

Don't panic if your child has a nose-bleed – the right treatment should stop it quickly.

1 Try to remain calm, even though your child's nose may appear to be bleeding heavily. If your child gets excited or upset, her agitation is likely to prolong and worsen the nose-bleed.

2 Don't tilt your child's head back as this could result in blood flowing down her throat, which may make her sick. Instead, get her to sit tilting her head forward – this will allow the blood to drain from her nose.

3 Gently pinch the soft part of your child's nose between your thumb and index finger for 10 minutes if possible, or get her to do it herself. Then gently release. If it is still bleeding, follow the steps for treating a severe nose-bleed.

4 Don't allow your child to blow her nose after you've stopped squeezing it, and don't be tempted to insert tissues or cotton wool into her nostril to clean it, as this could disturb any clots that have formed to stop the bleeding.

NOTE: your child is likely to have further light nose-bleeds over the following days, until the lining of her nose has fully healed.

How to treat a severe nose-bleed

If the treatment for a mild nose-bleed doesn't seem to be working, you will need to try a different approach.

1 Sit your child up at the table and place a bowl under her face for her to lean over.

2 If she has blood collecting in her mouth, encourage her to spit it out.

3 Pinch her nose very firmly just below the bridge, or get her to do it herself. Apply gentle pressure for 10 minutes. Don't be tempted to release the pressure to see if it has stopped the flow of blood – it is important that it remains constant.

4 Reassure your child and as she leans over the bowl remind her to breathe through her mouth, keeping it open so that any blood can drip into the bowl. If the bleeding persists for more than 30 minutes, seek medical help.

NOTE: a severe nose-bleed may result in your child vomiting blood that has been swallowed.

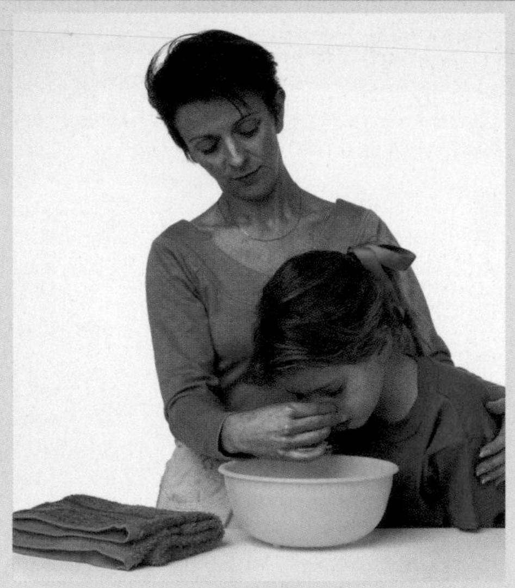

To treat a serious nose-bleed, your child should be seated with her head forward, while you gently pinch her nose for 10 minutes.

Medical treatment

If your child has severe nose-bleeds or they recur frequently, she may be referred to an ear, nose and throat specialist for further treatment.

- **Chemical cauterisation:** this may be recommended, particularly if your child's nose-bleeds seem to be occurring because the lining of her nose is very fragile. This involves using a chemical called silver nitrate, which is applied to the area of the nose that's been bleeding, using a cotton bud.
- **Electrical cauterisation:** this is used for more severe cases because the results of the chemical method are sometimes temporary. Your child will need to have a general anaesthetic.

Preventing nose-bleeds

There are several steps you can take to make the occurrence of nose-bleeds less likely.

- Dry air can dry out the nasal lining – if the air in your home is dry, or you have the central heating on, use a humidifier in your child's bedroom at night. Alternatively, place a bowl of water in her bedroom.
- Applying a small amount of petroleum jelly to the inside of your child's nose can relieve any dryness, but ensure that your nails are short.
- It's extremely difficult to convince a young child that she shouldn't pick her nose, so keep her fingernails trimmed so she's less likely to scratch the lining of her nose.

POISONING

POISONING IN BABIES AND CHILDREN

Children's boundless curiosity and their tendency to put objects in their mouths makes poisoning in the under-six age group very common.

- The majority of poisoning in children is minor, with no treatment required, because the substance is non-toxic or the amount swallowed is small. However, certain substances, such as iron and some anti-depressants, are very dangerous.
- Accidental poisoning usually happens at home. It may occur when you are visiting a house where no children live because the family may be less vigilant.
- Any disruption in the usual routine at home, such as a new baby or moving house, increases the risk of poisoning. This is because the child may be less supervised and harmful substances may be more accessible in the chaos.

Babies and toddlers are most at risk of poisoning because they often put things into their mouths. However, death from poisoning is rare in the UK (around 10 to 15 each year).

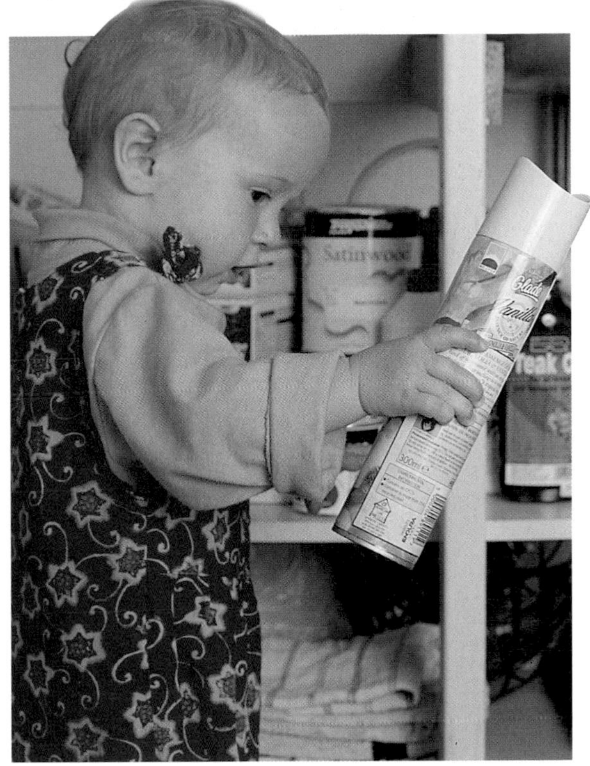

Common dangers

A poison is any substance that is harmful when swallowed or absorbed. Children are usually poisoned from consuming a dangerous substance.

Household products: assume that all household cleaning products are dangerous. Your child may eat them or spray them into her face. Paint thinner/remover, pesticides, petrol, paraffin and metal polishes should also be kept out of the reach of children.

Pills and medicines: anti-depressants, paracetamol and iron tablets are just some of the potentially lethal drugs adults may keep at home.

Cosmetics: even something as seemingly harmless as hair remover may be dangerous if it is taken by mouth.

Household and garden plants: dangerous species include arum lily, daffodil bulbs, deadly nightshade, foxglove and rhubarb leaves.

Tobacco and alcohol: just one cigarette can be lethal to a toddler if eaten. If a child drinks the dregs of an alcoholic drink left in a glass, she may be seriously affected.

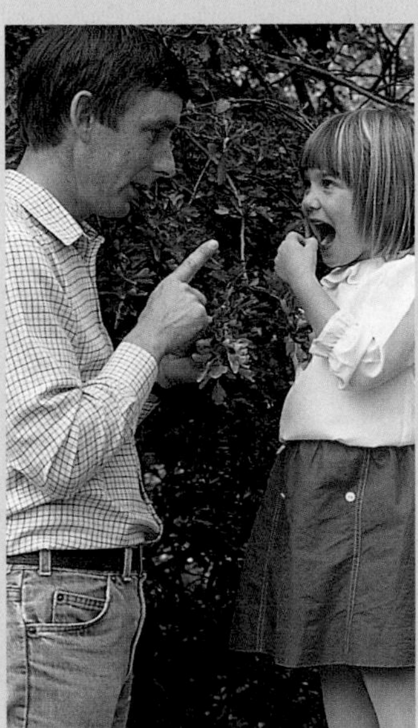

LEFT: Plants are often brightly coloured and irresistible to children. If you go on country walks, make sure your child knows about the dangers of poisonous plants.

Poison-proofing your home

- Keep all medicines in a locked cupboard. Never leave them on a bedside table or sideboard.
- Keep all alcohol, perfumes, cosmetics, detergents and bleaches out of reach.
- Buy medicines in child-resistant containers, but still keep them out of reach because the containers are not 100 per cent safe.
- Keep all products in their original containers. Don't decant them into milk jugs or drink bottles.
- Limit the amount of medication in the house; always throw away any that are out of date.
- Keep ashtrays and waste bins empty.
- Don't keep medicines in your handbag (a child raiding a handbag is a common cause of poisoning).
- Never call a medicine a sweet to entice your child to take it.
- Teach your child not to eat leaves, berries and mushrooms. Be aware of which plants are poisonous and remove them from your garden.

LEFT: Be extra vigilant with all cleaning products when your curious toddler is around. Keep them in a locked cupboard, well out of her reach.

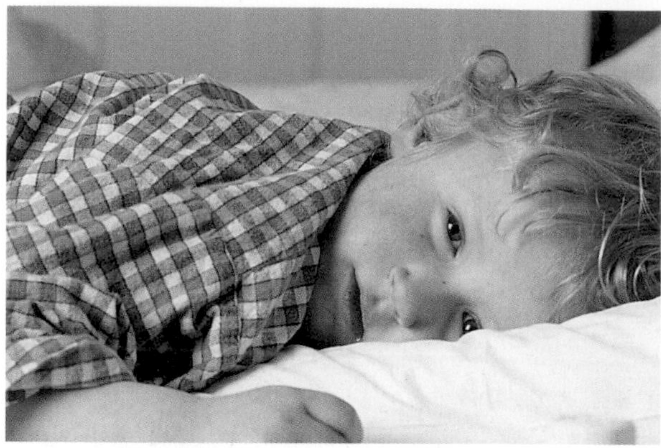

Signs of poisoning

A child who has been poisoned may suddenly develop unusual symptoms. These include:

- Staggering about as if he is drunk.

If your child seems drowsy or 'drunk', he may have swallowed a poison. Check for stains around his mouth and a strong odour on his breath.

- Burns around his lips and mouth.
- Stains of a substance around his mouth.
- A strong smell of a substance on his breath.
- Finding an opened or spilt bottle of pills.
- Being very sleepy before his usual nap time.

What to do

If you realise that your child has swallowed poison, stay calm. Remember the substance is probably harmless, especially if your child has only tasted it and spat it out.

- If your child is well and not distressed, ring your GP or local accident and emergency department. Tell them exactly what your child has taken and they may be able to telephone a local poisons information unit to establish the correct management.
- However, if your child seems unwell you need to call an ambulance immediately. If you know exactly what and how much of a substance your child has taken, write it down so that you can tell the doctor. Try to find some of the left-over substance to take to the hospital.
- Do not try to make your child sick. She may breathe in her vomit, which can cause more problems than the original poisoning. This is especially important if she has ingested any corrosive substances, such as bleach, which will do as much damage coming back up as it did going down.
- The doctor will want to know the time that the accident happened and the age and weight of your child.

Hospital treatments

A child who has ingested a poisonous substance may not require treatment, but if there is uncertainty about the quantity taken, overnight observation in hospital may be recommended.

1 Charcoal is sometimes given to a child as a drink. This absorbs the ingested poison in the stomach and therefore lessens the amount the child absorbs into the bloodstream. The problem is that charcoal tastes awful and most children refuse point blank to drink it.

2 Occasionally, a stomach wash-out may be performed. This is very rare and, as with medicine to make a child sick, has not been proven to help reduce the effects of the poison. This treatment may be performed for iron poisoning because the effects are very difficult to reverse once it has been absorbed into the blood.

3 Some drugs, such as iron and paracetamol, do have an antidote. The levels of the drug in the blood are measured four hours after swallowing it and then the antidote is given if the levels are high.

4 If a child has taken a corrosive substance, she may need an oesophagus examination to assess the internal damage.

If you suspect that your child has swallowed something poisonous, seek medical advice immediately. It will help speed up her treatment if you know exactly what she has consumed.

Serious side-effects

The effects of poisoning are often minor, but certain substances can be more damaging:

- Corrosive products, such as dishwashing powder, burn the gullet, which can cause permanent scarring and problems with swallowing.
- Some anti-depressants may cause heart rhythm problems, and paracetamol may cause liver failure.
- Some poisons affect the nervous system, causing a loss of balance, drowsiness, confusion, fitting, and sometimes lead to unconsciousness.

RASHES

RASHES IN BABIES AND CHILDREN

A rash on a baby or child rarely indicates a serious problem, but occasionally it is a warning sign.

- Rashes can be caused by allergic reactions or by infections. In most cases, allergic reactions are harmless, but when a rash is the result of an infection it can be a warning sign of a serious condition – especially if the infection responsible is meningitis.

- It is sensible to learn to distinguish harmless rashes from dangerous ones, taking into account other symptoms, although you should always consult your doctor immediately if you are in any doubt.

- If the rash is caused by infection, you may also need to consider whether isolation is necessary.

A child's rash caused by an infection may require an incubation period – consult your doctor to get a proper diagnosis.

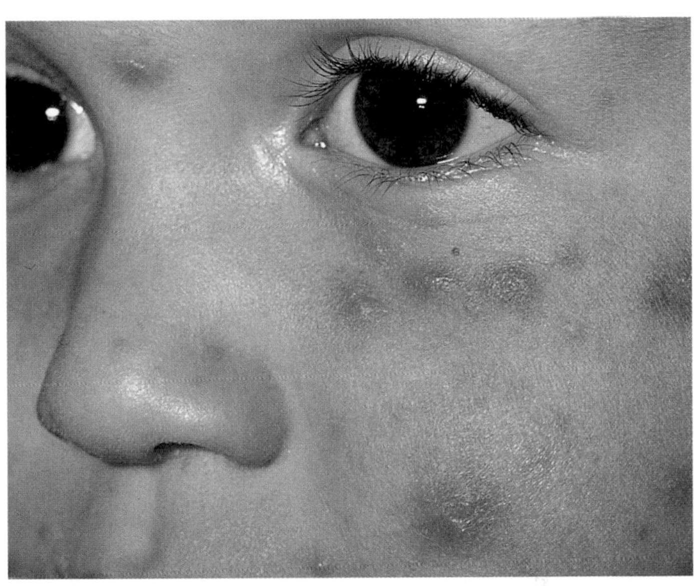

Recognising childhood rashes

It is generally impossible to take one look at a rash and know at once what it means. Rashes can erupt due to a variety of causes ranging from the raised temporary weals caused by stinging nettles to the purple spots associated with life-threatening meningitis. However, many of them have particular distinctive features that give clues to the problem.

Urticaria
This type of rash is usually caused by an allergy or a localised skin reaction to, for example, a nettle sting. It often develops very suddenly. The rash can be recognised by its distinctive irregularly shaped raised weals, which are surrounded by an inflamed red area. In a serious allergic reaction, urticaria may be accompanied by difficulty breathing and swelling of the face, particularly the lips and around the eyes.

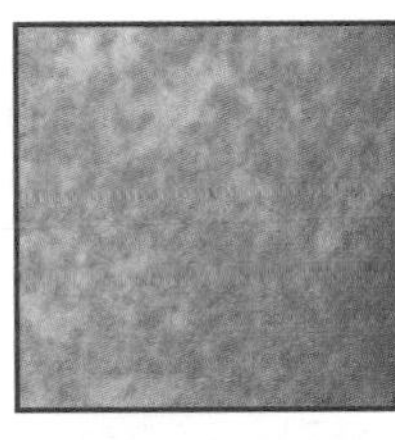

Measles
Measles is a viral infection that causes a lung infection and a non-itchy brown-pink rash about three days into the illness. There are also severe cold-like symptoms. Typically, the rash starts behind the ears and then affects the face and upper body. The rash consists of both raised and flat red patches on the skin that can be up to 2cm (¾in) in diameter. Small white spots, known as Koplik's spots, can also develop on the tongue.

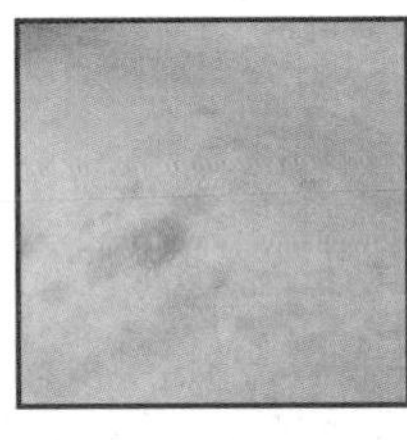

Roseola infantum
This illness causes a rapid temperature rise – somewhere between 39.5°C (103°F) to 41°C (106°F) – with swollen glands. As the temperature returns to normal, a pink rash with flat spots appears, first on the trunk and then spreads to the neck, arms and thighs. The flat spots turn white when the skin is pressed with a glass, which can also happen in early meningitis (see below).

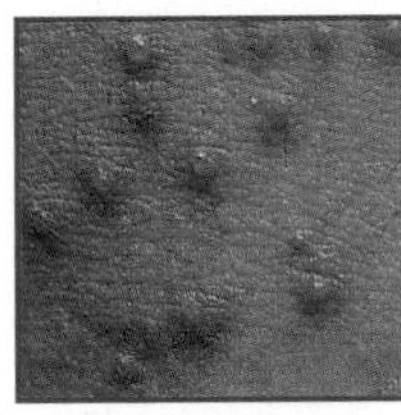

Chickenpox
This condition usually starts with a mild fever, headache and sore throat, with small raised red spots appearing on the head or upper body. The spots become fluid-filled and are extremely itchy and inflamed. Over a few days, the fluid in the spots becomes cloudy and they eventually crust over to form scabs.

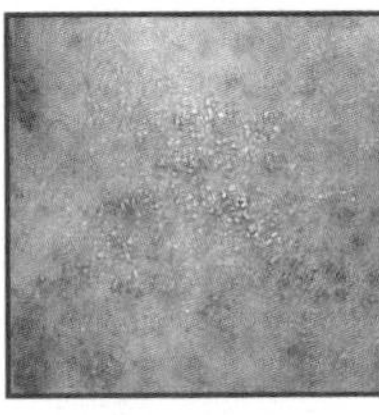

Rubella
Also known as German measles, the initial symptoms of this viral illness are a mild fever and swollen glands behind the ears, leading to a rash on the second or third day after infection. The rash consists of multiple tiny flat spots that eventually blend together to give a red 'blush' to the skin.

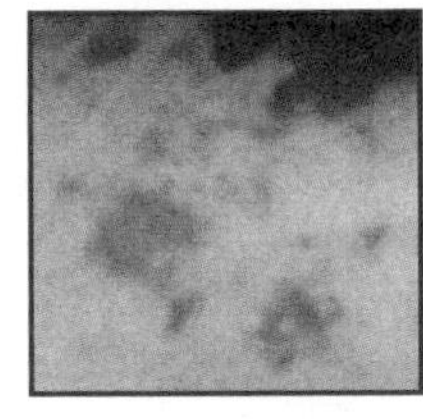

Meningitis and septicaemia
These are serious infections. Purple-coloured blotches may appear, which do not fade when pressed with a glass. In early meningitis, the rash can resemble that of measles, rubella or roseola and may turn white during the glass test. Other symptoms are a high temperature, vomiting and neck stiffness.

When to call the doctor

Seek urgent medical advice without delay in any of these situations:

1 If you suspect meningitis (see box below) or measles (see previous page).

2 If your child has a high fever – over 39.5°C (103°F) – or has a febrile convulsion.

3 If your child (especially a baby under nine months) has been unwell for over 48 hours with no sign of improvement.

4 If your child develops a rash and becomes rapidly unwell with a fever of 37.8°C (100°F) or more.

5 If your child repeatedly vomits and/or complains of a headache.

6 If you suspect an infectious disease (so that contact with any vulnerable patients in the surgery can be avoided).

7 If your baby is floppy or unresponsive.

Meningitis and septicaemia

Meningitis is an extremely serious infection to which children under five are particularly vulnerable. Septicaemia or blood-poisoning may occur alongside meningitis.

- Meningitis can be caused by either a viral or bacterial infection and at first the symptoms are similar. Viral meningitis is the most common type and is rarely serious. It usually follows an infection such as influenza, chickenpox, measles or mumps.

- Bacterial meningitis is rare and the most dangerous – it can be fatal. However, with early diagnosis and treatment, most children go on to make a full recovery.

- Symptoms include a high-pitched cry; refusing food; vomiting; fever; difficulty in waking; being floppy and lethargic; having bulging fontanelle; neck stiffness. These are common to many childhood illnesses, but in meningitis the child's condition deteriorates rapidly.

- A rash can develop at any time, although it does not always do so, and anywhere on the body. The skin is pale and blotchy with a pin-prick, purple-red rash that turns into bruise-like blotches.

- The rash caused by meningitis is unique but does not always appear when the disease strikes. If a rash appears anywhere on the body, press the side of a clear glass against it. If its colour does not fade, get urgent medical help so that antibiotics can be given without delay.

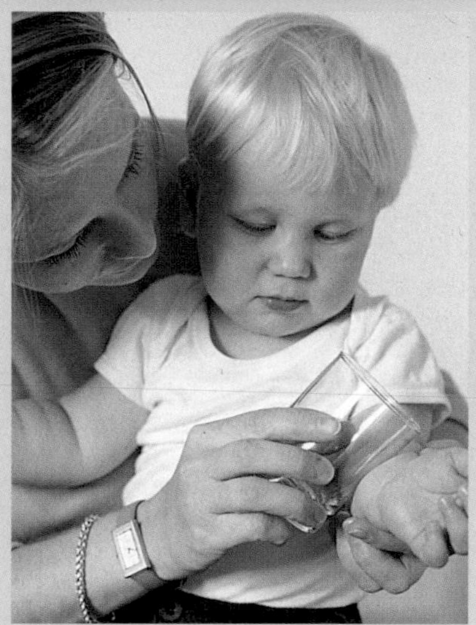

Hold a glass firmly against your child's skin – if the rash does not fade, you should suspect meningitis.

Allergic rashes

Allergic rashes occur when the skin comes into contact with an irritant or something to which a child is allergic.

- Any rash that appears on your child's skin as the result of contact with an irritant, such as a chemical in biological washing powder, baby wipes or soap, is known as contact dermatitis.

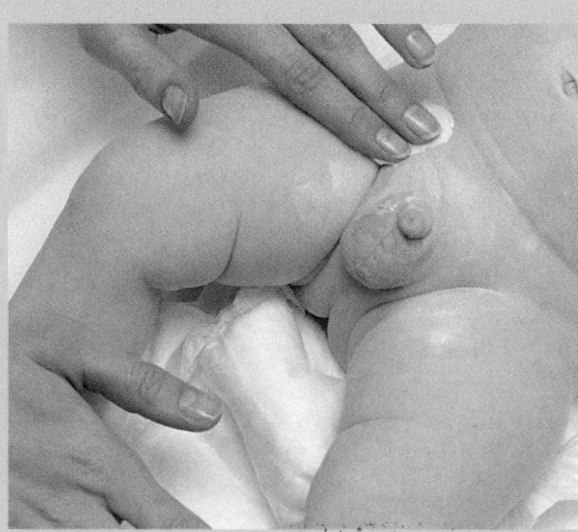

- The rash is usually red, lumpy and itchy and localised to the area of contact but otherwise the child should be well. Soothing creams are all that is usually required.

- Nappy rash, a form of contact dermatitis, is a common problem in babies under two. Clean your baby frequently and leave the nappy area open to the air as much as possible. Use barrier creams to reduce skin contact with irritants.

To prevent and treat nappy rash in your baby, apply a barrier cream over the area after every nappy change.

- Sometimes a nappy rash can become infected with thrush. The skin becomes bright red and there are white and red pimples. It can be treated with an anti-fungal cream.

- Hives is a common allergic skin complaint – nettle rash is a form of hives. It produces red weals that eventually become white with a red rim. These can itch and sting, but the child is otherwise well. Usually they disappear within 24 hours so long as the cause of the reaction has been removed. Treat with a soothing antihistamine cream.

RECOVERY POSITION

WHAT IS IT?

The recovery position is a comfortable, secure position that allows an unconscious or semi-conscious child to continue breathing freely until medical help arrives.

- The position keeps the head, neck and back comfortably aligned.
- It prevents the tongue from blocking the throat and, because the head is slightly lower than the rest of the body, any fluid is allowed to drain from the nose and mouth.
- Placing an unconscious child in the recovery position is the most effective way of preventing her from choking to death if she vomits.
- Knowing how to place a child safely and promptly in the recovery position can save her life.

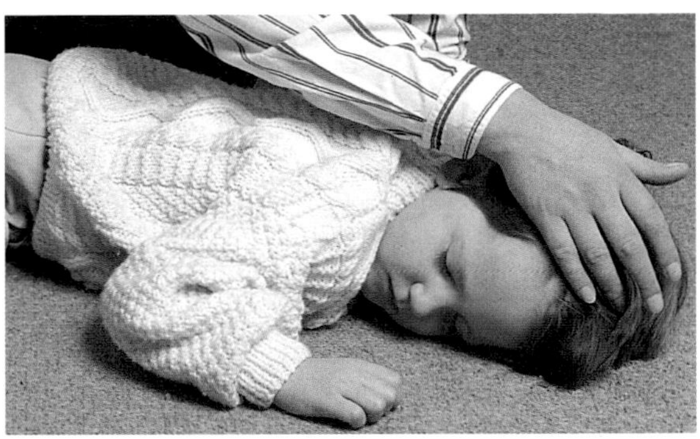

A child who is unconscious but breathing should be placed in the recovery position to await the arrival of qualified paramedics.

Initial precautions

The recovery position should be used as part of the emergency procedure designed to ensure that the child is kept in as stable a condition as possible. The emergency checklist known as DRABC should be carried out.

- **D (Danger):** check that neither you nor the child are in any danger from hazards such as traffic. Proceed when it is safe to do so.
- **R (Response):** ascertain whether or not the child is conscious and, if so, if she is aware of where she is. Quickly assess her for injuries and then cover her to maintain a stable body temperature.
- **A (Airway):** check the airway. Remove any foreign objects that may be blocking the airway.
- **B (Breathing):** check that the child is breathing properly. If breathing cannot be detected, perform mouth-to-mouth resuscitation.
- **C (Circulation):** check for signs of circulation, such as colour, movement and skin temperature. If there are no signs of circulation, give chest compressions.

When not to use the recovery position

In some situations, moving a casualty can be more dangerous than leaving her where she is.

1 It is not necessary to use the recovery position if the child is conscious.

2 Do not use the recovery position if the child has no pulse or is not breathing freely. Perform mouth-to-mouth resuscitation and CPR immediately.

3 If you suspect that the child may have a neck or spinal injury, do not try to move her. Do not place anything at all under her neck to prop her up. Await emergency help.

Modifications to the recovery positions

Sometimes, the recovery position may require a different procedure.

If your baby is unconscious but breathing, place her in your arms with her head tilted back.

- If the child is under the age of one, hold her in your arms so that the head is lower than the rest of the body and is tilted back to keep the airway clear. Try to keep the head, neck and back aligned at all times. If you suspect a neck or spinal injury, do not move the child unless her breathing is restricted or she needs to be quickly removed from a position of danger.
- If the child has limb injuries, it may not be possible for her to use her arms and legs as described in the step-by-step guide (overleaf). If possible, use rolled-up blankets to help support her and maintain the correct position.
- If the child has abdominal or chest injuries, it may still be necessary to place her in the recovery position. However, careful attention should be paid to be sure that no further damage occurs to the injured area.

A step-by-step guide to the recovery position

The technique described here for turning a casualty can be used on anyone over the age of one. The steps described assume that the child is found lying on her back. If she is already lying on her front or side, you will need to modify some of the steps. The main aim is to get the child into a position lying on her side from which she cannot accidentally roll in either direction.

1 Before starting the procedure, remove any fragile or bulky objects from the child's pockets.

2 Kneel beside the child and open the airway by tilting the head back and lifting the chin. Straighten the child's legs.

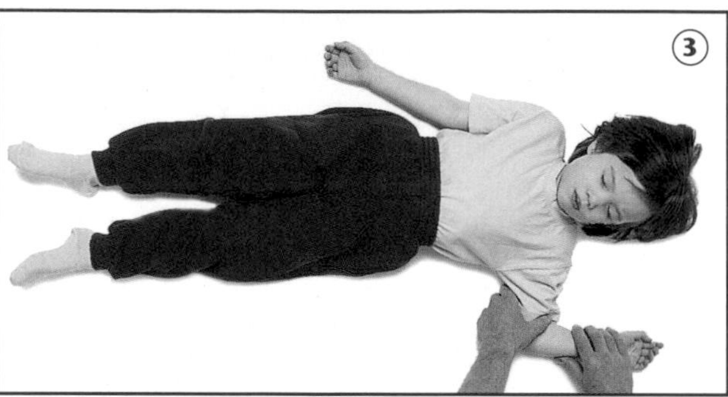

3 Place the arm nearest to you so that the upper part is at right angles to the body and the forearm is parallel to the head (as though the child had raised her arm to stop traffic).

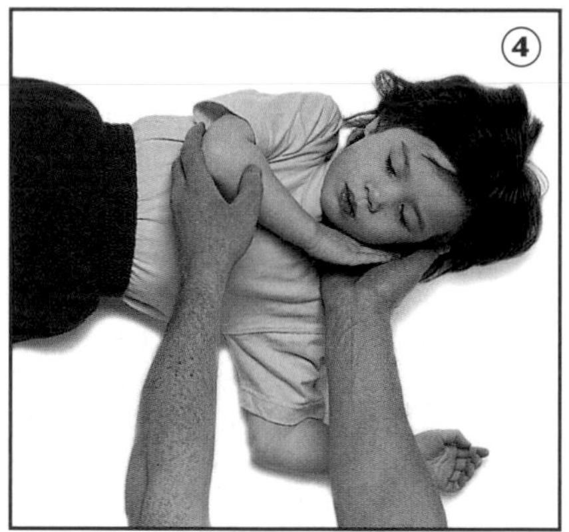

4 Bring the child's arm that is furthest from you across the chest. Then use the flat of your hand to hold the back of the child's hand against her cheek. This will help support her head.

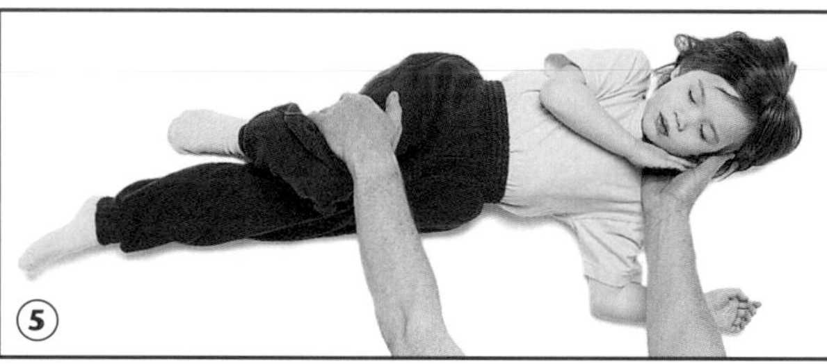

5 Using your free hand, hold the child's furthermost leg just above the knee and draw the leg up so that the knee is raised and the foot remains flat on the ground.

6 While still keeping the child's hand pressed against her cheek, pull the upper part of the raised leg towards you so that the child rolls on to her side. Use your knees to prevent the child from rolling too far. You can see from the picture that one of her hands is under her chin and one at her side.

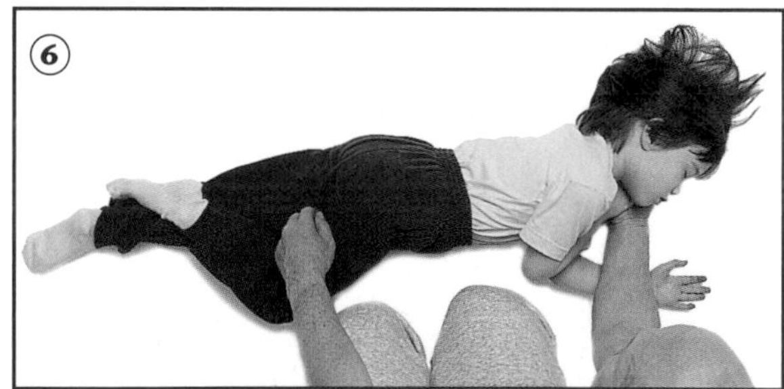

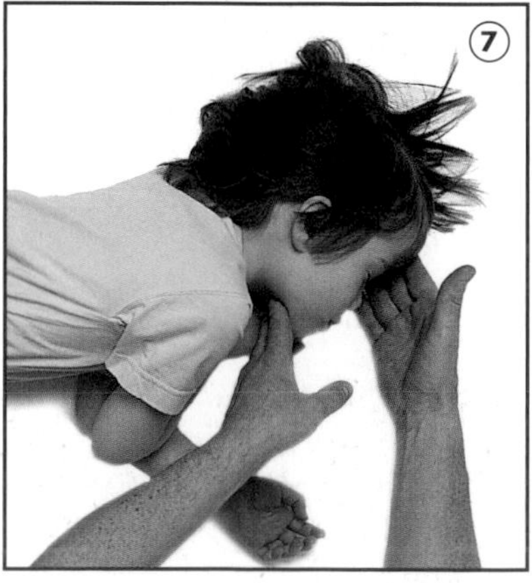

7 Ensure that the child's mouth is downward, and tilt the head back to keep the airway free. If necessary adjust the hand that is supporting the cheek so that the head cannot tilt forward again.

8 Adjust the upper leg (the one you pulled over) so that the knee and hip are bent at right angles to stop her rolling forward.

What to do next

- Call an ambulance, if this has not already been done.
- Check the child's breathing and signs of circulation regularly, if possible every three or four minutes, but at least every 10 minutes.
- If the child's pulse or breathing stop, turn her on to her back and commence CPR or mouth-to-mouth resuscitation.
- If the child starts to regain consciousness, try to keep her still and reassure her until medical help arrives.

RESUSCITATION

Should the unimaginable happen and your baby or child does become unconscious and stops breathing, it's vital that you stay calm and act quickly. It can take just a few minutes without oxygen for permanent brain damage to occur.

1 First, make sure that neither you nor your child is in any danger (from fumes, electricity or fire). Then open your child's airways and check that she is breathing and has signs of circulation. If she is not breathing but has signs of circulation, start mouth-to-mouth respiration immediately (see overleaf). If she has signs of circulation, start external chest compressions.

2 Get another adult to phone the emergency services. If you are alone, shout for help.

3 If your child has been involved in an accident, take steps to stop any severe bleeding by pressing down on to the wound and holding the injured part higher than the heart if possible.

4 Don't attempt to move your child if you are uncertain of her injuries, or if there may be damage to her neck or spine.

5 If your child starts to breathe on her own, place her in the recovery position. This is the safest position for her to be in, as it prevents her tongue from falling back into her throat and obstructing her airway. She also avoids the risk of choking if she vomits.

DRABC of resuscitation

Here is a quick way of remembering your priorities in an emergency:

D is for ***danger***. Check you and your child are safe.

R is for ***response***. Talk, shout and touch her gently to see if she wakes.

A is for ***airway***. Open your child's airway and, if possible, remove any obstruction.

B is for ***breathing***. Check breathing and be ready to start mouth-to-mouth respiration.

C is for ***circulation***. Check for signs of circulation and, if there are none, be ready to give chest compressions.

External chest compression

If your child is not breathing and there are no signs of circulation, you will need to start external chest compression.

Babies up to a year

- Lie your baby on her back on a flat surface, then slide one hand under her shoulders and grab the top of her arm. Locate the bottom of her breastbone with your other hand, then find the half-way point between this and the base of her neck.
- Using two fingers, press down just below this halfway point to a depth of about one third of the chest, then release.
- Make five compressions in rapid succession (about 100 per minute) then give one breath into her lungs as before. Do this for one minute then carry the baby to dial 999.
- Continue to make five compressions followed by a breath until her heart restarts or help arrives. Check her breathing and heartbeat every minute.
- When her heart starts beating, stop compressions but continue with mouth-to-mouth respiration until she breathes independently, or until help arrives.

One to seven year olds

- Locate the bottom of your child's breast bone, then find the halfway point between this and the base of her neck.
- Using the heel of your hand just below the halfway point, press to a depth of about one third of the chest, then release.
- Give five compressions at a rate of about 100 per minute, then breathe into her lungs once. Continue the sequence of five compressions to one ventilation for one minute. Then, if the child is small enough, carry her to the phone to ring 999. If you have to leave your child, restart the sequence when you return. If you think the breathing or heart may have restarted, stop and check.
- If her heart restarts, stop compressions, but continue with mouth-to-mouth respiration until she breathes independently, or until help arrives.

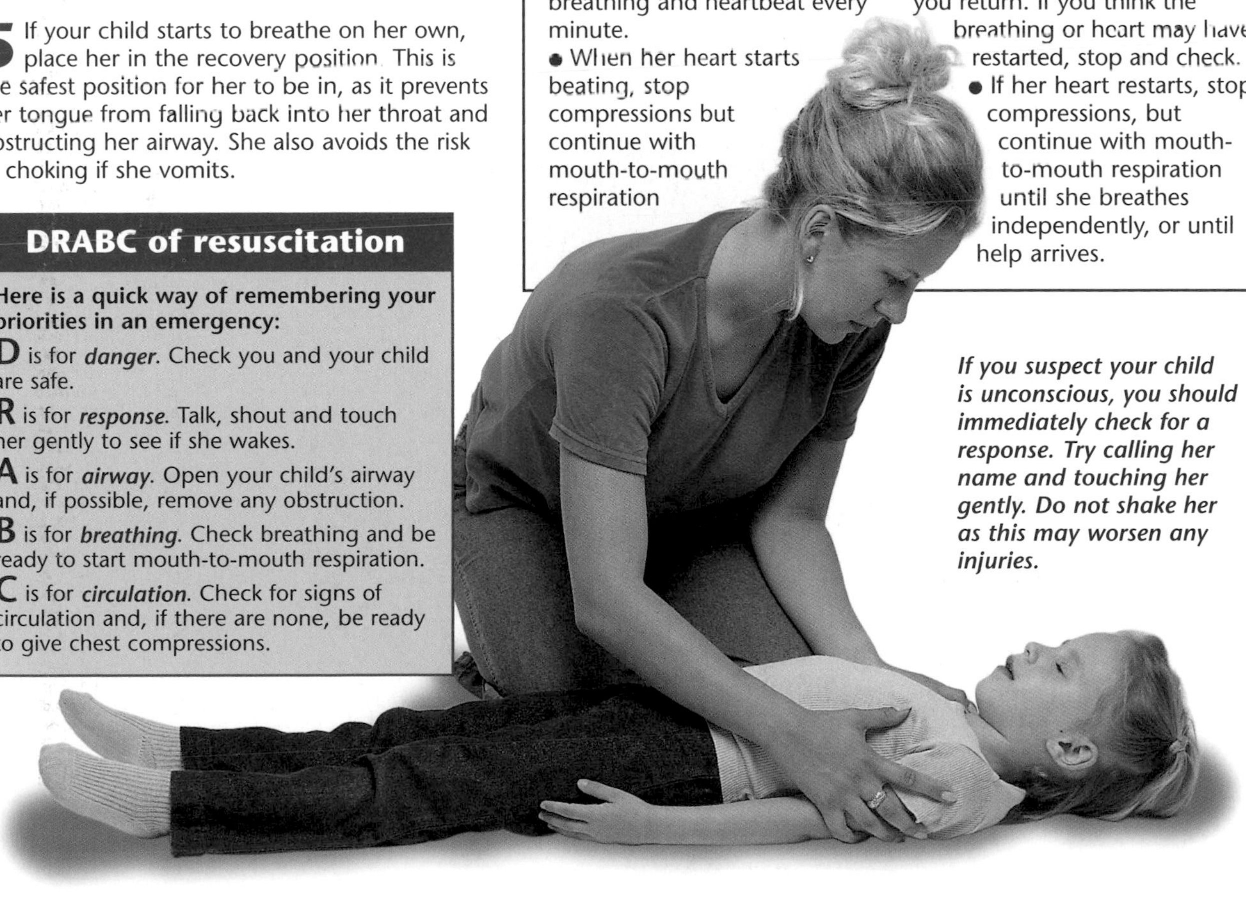

If you suspect your child is unconscious, you should immediately check for a response. Try calling her name and touching her gently. Do not shake her as this may worsen any injuries.

Mouth-to-mouth resuscitation step by step

Before you attempt to resuscitate your child, lay her on her back, with her arms by her sides, and kneel beside her. Ensure that someone has called the emergency services.

1 Open your child's airway by pressing gently on her forehead to tilt her head back. If there are signs of choking, check for any obstructions in the mouth. DO NOT put your fingers in her mouth. Check to see if she is breathing. Pinch the nostrils shut with one hand and support the chin with the other.

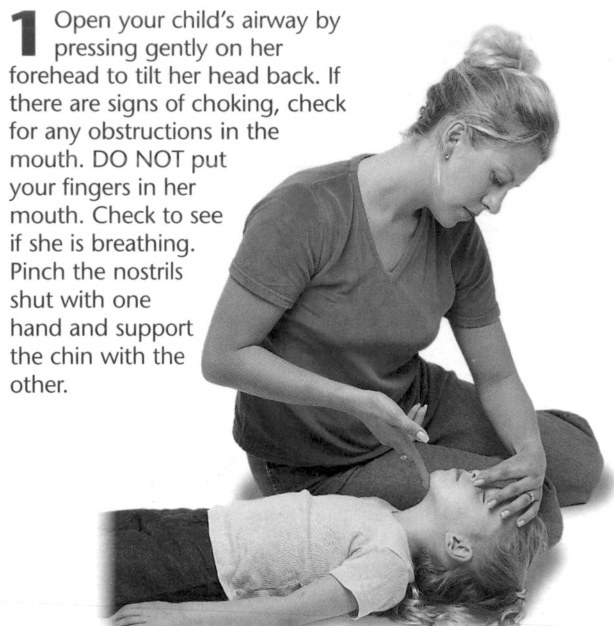

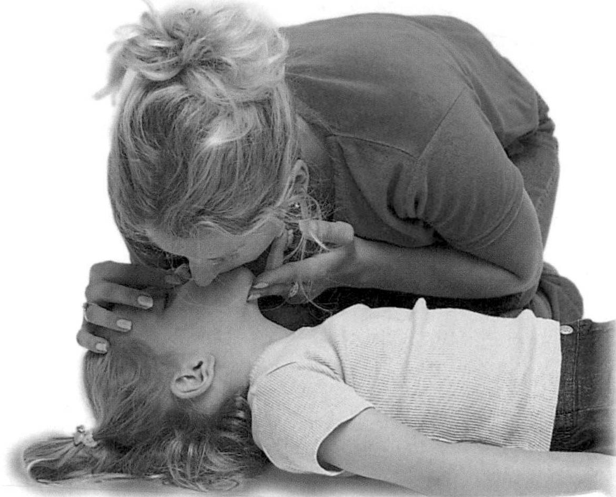

2 Seal your lips around your child's mouth and breathe gently but firmly into her lungs until you see her chest rise. Watch her chest fall before continuing. Give two effective breaths then check for signs of circulation.

3 To check for signs of circulation, look for colour, movement, coughing and skin temperature. Continue with mouth-to-mouth at a rate of 10 breaths per minute until the child starts breathing alone or the ambulance arrives.

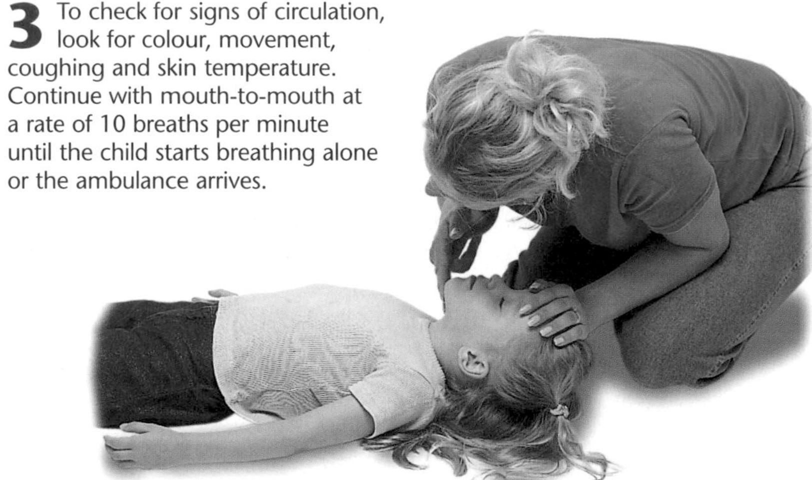

4 If your child is breathing independently, place her into the recovery position. This will ensure that her airway is kept open, allowing excess fluids, such as vomit, to run freely from her mouth and prevent her from choking.

Take a course

Excellent first-aid and lifesaving courses, run by first-aid companies, are available in most areas. Check the telephone directory for details. Make sure the teachers have been professionally trained.

Resuscitating a baby

The technique for resuscitating a baby is only slightly different from the technique used for an older child.

- You should still open the airway by tilting the head back, then put one finger under your baby's chin and tilt it up, taking great care not to press too hard, as her windpipe is soft and flexible and you may block or injure it.
- A baby's face is much smaller than a child's, so you should seal both her nose and mouth with your lips before you start artificial respiration.
- If your baby has no signs of circulation, you should start external chest compression immediately.

ROAD ACCIDENTS

WHAT TO DO AT THE SCENE OF AN ACCIDENT

When you first come across an accident, remember that the primary aim is to preserve life. This includes your life, the lives of any casualties and the lives of other road users.

- Call the emergency services when you have a good idea of how many casualties there are and if they are breathing.

- Make sure that it is safe for you to approach. Be aware of your limitations, but if necessary take charge of the accident scene until the emergency services arrive.

- If the accident is on a busy road, get someone else to help control the traffic. If possible, place a red warning triangle 100 metres or yards behind the accident.

- Check for the existence or possibility of fire. If an engine is running, switch it off if you can. Remove the ignition key and drop it on the car floor.

- Deal with any casualties that are not breathing or are bleeding severely.

- Do not move casualties any more than is necessary, unless they are in immediate danger.

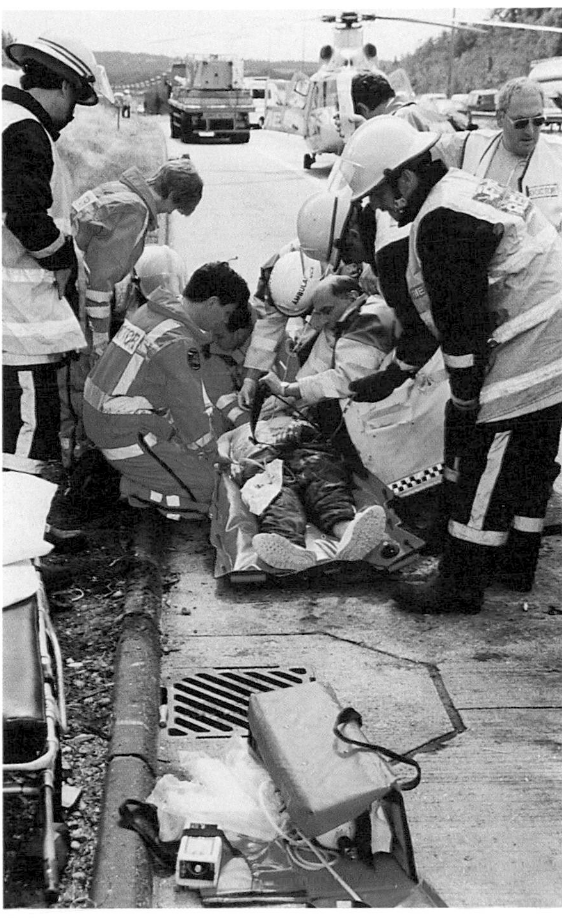

It may be necessary to take control of the accident scene until the paramedics arrive. Once they arrive, listen to their instructions and let them take over.

If you are involved in the accident

Be aware that your reactions and judgement may be impaired.

- If you have any children with you, try to get them clear of the accident as soon as possible. If they are injured, leave them where they are unless there is a good reason to move them.

- Get help, either by flagging down another vehicle or by using a telephone. If possible let someone else take charge.

- Try to remember what caused the accident as the police will need this information later. Do not leave the scene of the accident unless there is no other way of getting help.

Making an assessment and calling for help

It is useful for the emergency services to have some idea of the seriousness of the accident and what equipment is likely to be needed. You should try to make a rapid assessment of the accident scene.

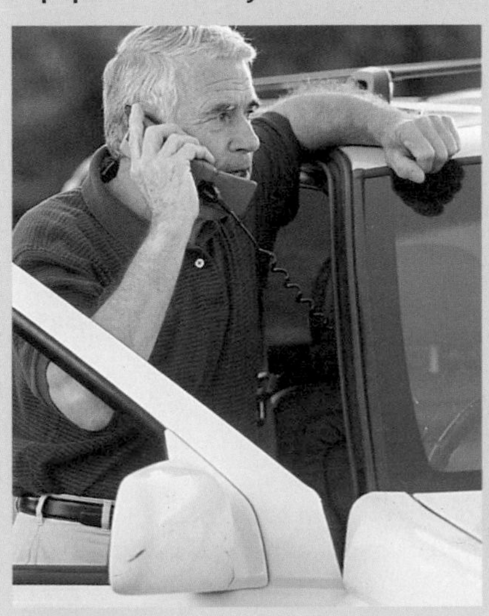

1. Keep calm and controlled and try to assess the situation as swiftly as possible.

2. Count the number of casualties and try to assess their condition. Check to see if casualties are unconscious and whether or not there is any serious bleeding.

3. Find a telephone and dial 999, or get someone else to do it. The European emergency number is 112.

Whether by land-line or mobile phone, it is important to report the accident to the emergency services as soon as possible

4. Ask for the police and give the location of the accident and, if possible, the number and condition of the casualties. Tell them if anyone is trapped in a vehicle. Give details of any possible hazards. Do not end the call until the control officer clears the line.

5. If you're using a land-line phone, don't worry if you are unsure of the location – the police will be able to locate the telephone you are using. If you are using a mobile phone, try to describe your surroundings, especially obvious landmarks. The police will contact the other emergency services.

Giving basic first aid

Casualties should be attended to according to the seriousness of their condition.

1 Use the treatment that is most likely to benefit the casualty, but follow the 'do no harm' rule. If possible the casualty should be kept still in the position that you find them.

2 First attend to any casualties that are unconscious and not breathing and then to any who are bleeding severely. Next attend to anyone who is unconscious. Then attend to anyone who is conscious with minor injuries. Deal with children first within these criteria.

3 Try to make sure that the casualty you are dealing with can breathe freely. Loosen any tight clothing around the neck and chest. If necessary, give artificial respiration.

4 Try to stop any severe bleeding, getting the casualty to help if possible so you can attend to others.

5 Talk to the casualties and keep them reassured that help is on the way. Try to keep bystanders away so that the privacy of the casualties is maintained as far as possible.

Removing a protective helmet

Only remove a motorcycle or bicycle helmet if it absolutely necessary to do so. In most circumstances a helmet is best left on because removing it may cause damage to the casualty's neck.

- You may have to remove a helmet in order to give artificial respiration. If there is anyone else around, get them to help you.

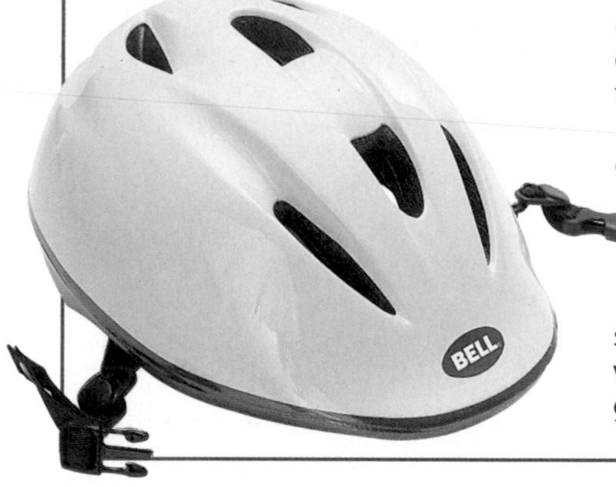

- Make sure that the neck is held carefully aligned with the spine while the helmet is being removed.
- If the helmet is an open-face type, such as a child's cycle helmet, first unfasten the buckle of the chinstrap, or cut through the strap itself. One person should support the casualty's neck and head with both hands, while the other grasps the rim of the helmet firmly, forcing the sides apart. It should then be possible to lift it gently away.
- If the helmet is a full-face type, first undo or cut the straps. Working from the base of the helmet, one person then eases their fingers under the rim, while the other supports the helmet with both hands. The first person can then support the neck, while holding the lower jaw. The other person tilts the helmet forward slightly so that it can pass over the base of the skull. Finally, the helmet is lifted off the casualty's head.

Dealing with bystanders

Bystanders may be frightened and feel helpless, especially if they have no first-aid training. If you need to ask a bystander to help or to stand back, do so in a firm but gentle way.

- An accident scene can be a distressing sight. Try to ensure that children not involved are removed from the scene as soon as possible. Get a responsible adult to help with this if possible.
- Some bystanders may have witnessed the accident, in which case the police may wish to interview them. Try to ensure that they stay in the vicinity.

Car safety

To minimise the possibility of injury in a car accident, you should always take safety precautions, particularly when travelling with children.

- Ensure that all passengers are wearing seat belts of the appropriate type. Small children should be strapped into properly fitted safety chairs or harnesses at all times. They should never be allowed to move around the car freely. Make sure that head restraints are properly adjusted.
- Make sure that child safety locks on the rear doors are engaged. Do not lock the doors so that they cannot be opened from the outside.
- Keep a first-aid kit and a small fire extinguisher in the car.

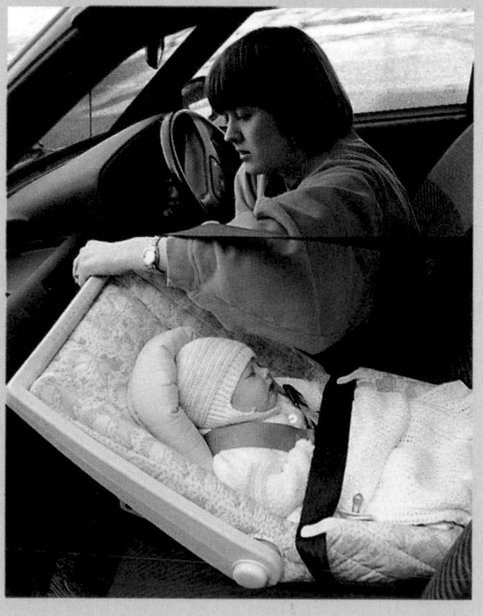

It's essential to ensure that all car passengers are securely strapped in, especially children and babies.

SCALDS

Preventing scalds

Of the many accidents that happen in the home, scalds are one of the most preventable. A few simple measures will help minimise the risk of potential disaster.

In the kitchen

- Avoid using a table-cloth. Little ones might be able to drag it and pull hot food and drink on top of themselves.
- Turn saucepan handles away from the edge of the cooker and, even better, cook on the back burners.
- You can buy guards that fix to the edge of the cooker to prevent pans from being pulled off.
- Don't try holding your baby and a hot cup of anything. Put the cup down before picking up your child.
- Avoid laying rugs in the kitchen, especially around the cooker area, because of the danger of slipping.
- Check where your child is before moving hot liquids around in the kitchen. Keep children out of your 'traffic path' when you are cooking.
- Kettles now have flexes no longer than 75cm (30in), but other appliances with cords, such as chip fryers and slow cookers, should be kept well away from the edge of kitchen surfaces.
- Make sure that anyone in charge of your child knows about safety in the kitchen, and in general, and that they always watch your child.
- Although microwaves are convenient for heating up baby's bottles, they will sometimes cause 'hot spots' in otherwise cold-feeling milk, which may burn the child's tongue or throat. Bottles should really be warmed up in hot water but, if microwaved, should be given a good shake and left to settle for a few minutes. All microwaved food should be well stirred before it is given to a child to distribute the heat evenly.
- Care should be taken with foods, such as doughnuts, that, while cool on the outside, could have piping-hot jam on the inside.

In the bathroom

- Never leave a child under five alone in the bath. Even an older child may turn on the taps as a game and cause a scald. The best taps are the 'push and turn' variety, which are more difficult for children to turn on.
- Unplug your phone or put the answerphone on when you are bathing your child so that you are not distracted.
- Run the cold water first.
- Ensure that your thermostat is at least as low as 15.6°C (60°F) – even this temperature can cause superficial burns in 10 seconds.

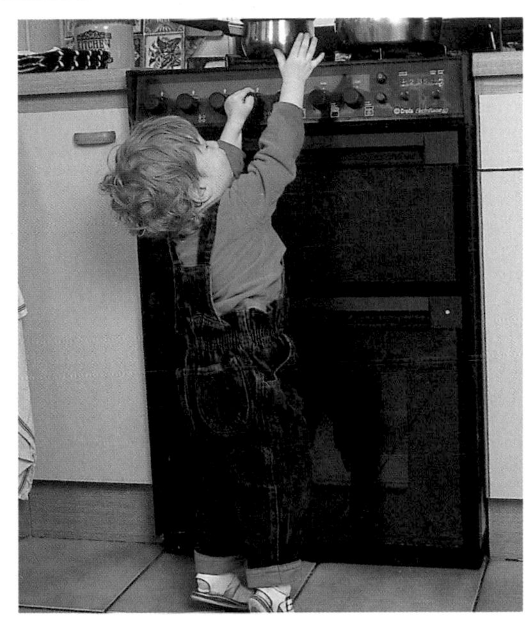

Out of reach

Of all children, toddlers are especially vulnerable to scalds. They are starting to explore their world, to climb and to reach for things, and this is when scalding accidents occur. A scald may be minor or serious but it is always painful any may lead to lifelong scarring, so be vigilant.

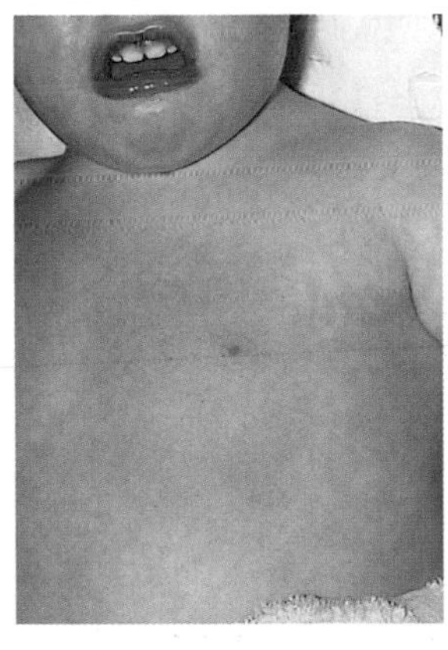

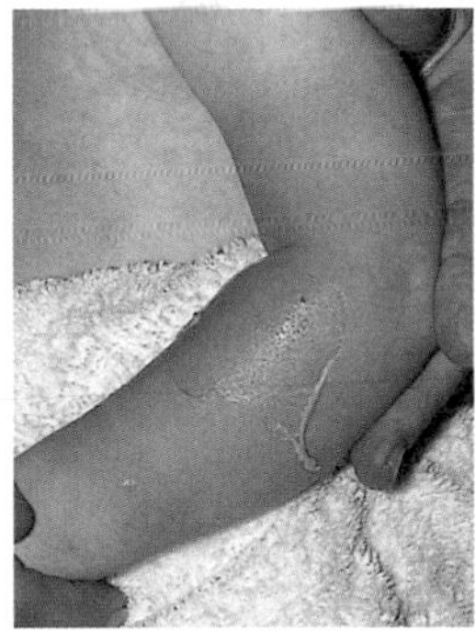

ABOVE: This young child is suffering from hot-water burns to the chest and arm. The area is cooled down and will be wrapped to prevent further pain, and to protect against infection.

ABOVE LEFT: This scalding accident has resulted in a superficial burn to the chest, which will heal without scarring.

When to call the doctor

Always take your child to your doctor or local accident and emergency department if:

- Your child has scalded his face, genitals or neck.
- Your child has scalded more than a palm-sized area.
- The skin is blistered, or has a 'dead' white bloodless appearance. This suggests more than just a superficial scald and there may be problems healing. Do not break any blisters. A doctor may decide to, but breaking a blister will make the wound very sore.
- After initially seeming a minor burn, the skin around the area becomes red and hot, or if your child develops a temperature. There may be infection brewing – covering the scalded area with a wet, clean towel will reduce the chances of this.

Treating scalds

Prompt action is extremely important if your child is scalded. It's vital to know what to do because the wrong action may result in further injury. The quicker you react, the less damage will occur and the less will be the pain and trauma for your child.

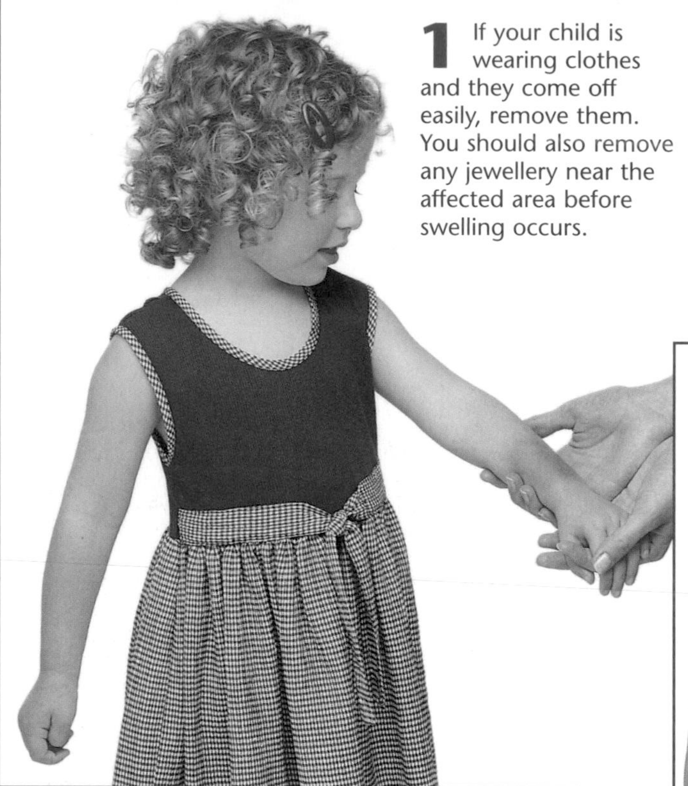

1 If your child is wearing clothes and they come off easily, remove them. You should also remove any jewellery near the affected area before swelling occurs.

Take care!

- **Never use ice, Vaseline or butter on a scald because they will continue to burn the skin.**
- **Do not try to remove your child's clothes if they are sticking to the scalded area because this will cause further damage to her skin.**
- **Make sure you have a complete first-aid kit and leave it in an accessible place.**

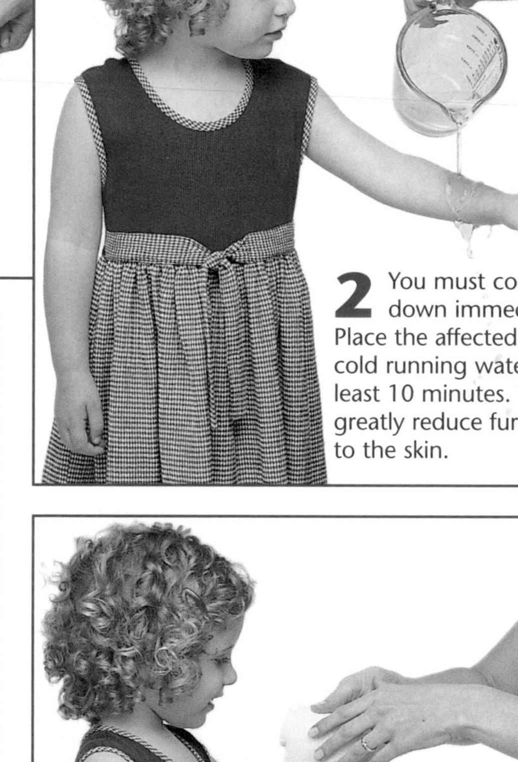

2 You must cool the scald down immediately. Place the affected area under cold running water for at least 10 minutes. This will greatly reduce further harm to the skin.

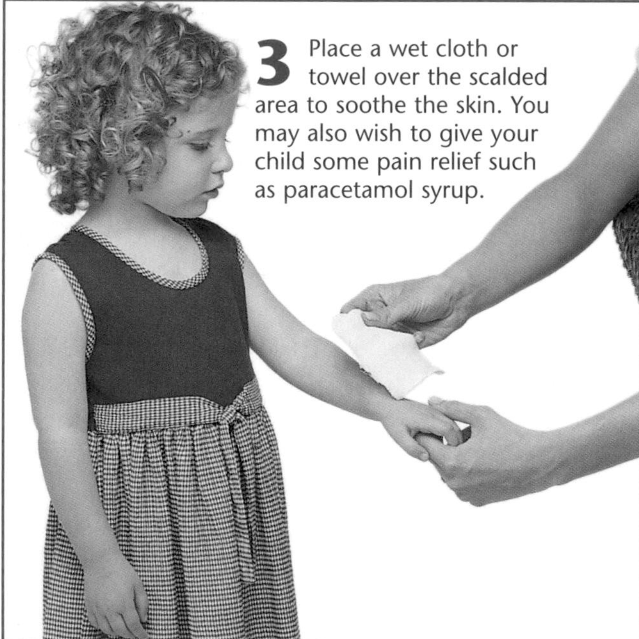

3 Place a wet cloth or towel over the scalded area to soothe the skin. You may also wish to give your child some pain relief such as paracetamol syrup.

4 Finally, loosely cover the scalded area with a clean piece of material or a sterile bandage. Do not pull this too tight because it may stick to the scald and damage the skin.

SHOCK

WHAT IS SHOCK?

Most people use the word shock to describe the emotional distress that can follow a traumatic event. When doctors use the term shock, however, they are referring to the potentially life-threatening state that can occur after a serious injury to the body.

- Shock can develop as a result of any situation in which the heart cannot pump blood effectively, or in which there is too little blood to pump.

- The result is that there is not enough blood circulating around the body, and even in mild conditions treatment is important to prevent damage to the body's organs. When first aid is given for shock, the whole body needs to be taken into account, not just the initial injury.

- A child is most likely to go into shock due to severe bleeding, or a severe burn or scald. These injuries require immediate medical treatment.

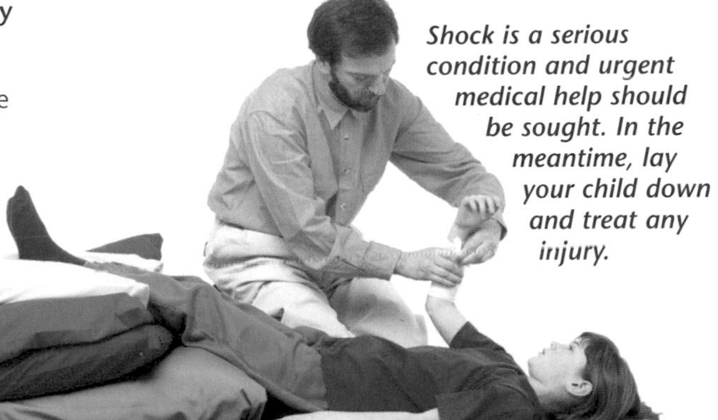

Shock is a serious condition and urgent medical help should be sought. In the meantime, lay your child down and treat any injury.

Causes of shock

Shock can be caused by any condition that impairs the circulation of blood. There are a range of conditions that may result in circulatory shock.

- **Serious bleeding:** this is the most common cause of shock in which blood loss reduces supply to the body's vital organs.

- **Electric shock:** this can affect the function of the heart, so that it becomes unable to pump any blood around the body efficiently.

- **Head injury:** may cause bleeding into the skull.

- **Severe burns:** these cause vital fluids to be lost through the skin, reducing blood volume.

- **Poisoning:** certain poisons affect the heart and/or lungs, preventing them from functioning normally.

- **Heatstroke:** this causes dehydration and can result in a serious drop in blood pressure.

- **Dehydration:** as water is lost from the body, blood volume is decreased.

- **Blood infection and meningitis:** infection affects the blood's ability to carry oxygen, and fluid is lost through the walls of the blood vessels.

Recognising the signs of shock

The symptoms of shock can be very varied, so if your child suffers an injury, no matter how mild, you should monitor him very closely for some time afterwards. Check for any signs of the following:

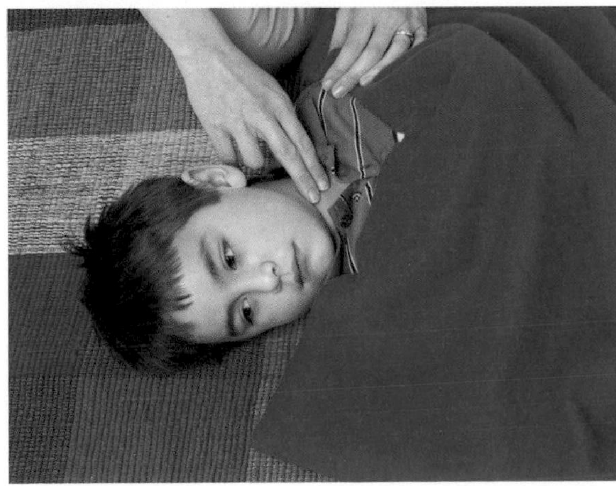

- An uncharacteristic change in behaviour; your child may become very quiet for example, or extremely distressed.

- Light-headedness or feeling faint.

- Pale, cold and clammy skin.

Early signs of shock include a rapid pulse and sweaty, clammy skin with a blue/grey tinge. Lay a blanket over your child and dial 999.

- A weak and irregular pulse.

- Irregular, rapid and shallow breathing.

There may also be the following symptoms:

- A vacant expression and enlarged pupils.

- Trembling and shivering.

- Nausea and vomiting.

- Loss of bladder or bowel control.

Emergency measures

It is essential to call an ambulance if your child has gone into shock because he will require urgent medical attention. While you are waiting for the ambulance, there are a number of things you can do to help alleviate your child's symptoms.

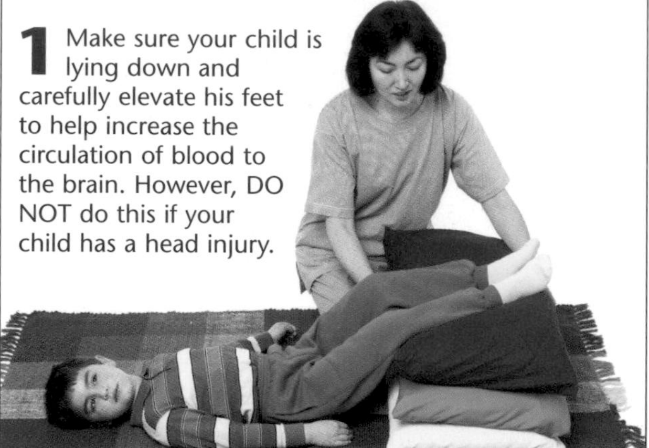

1 Make sure your child is lying down and carefully elevate his feet to help increase the circulation of blood to the brain. However, DO NOT do this if your child has a head injury.

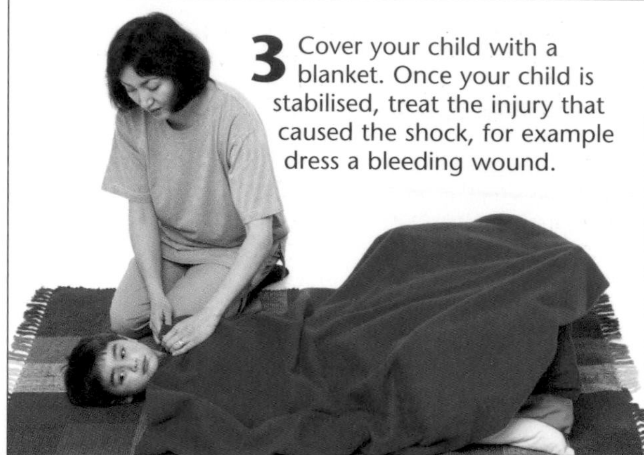

3 Cover your child with a blanket. Once your child is stabilised, treat the injury that caused the shock, for example dress a bleeding wound.

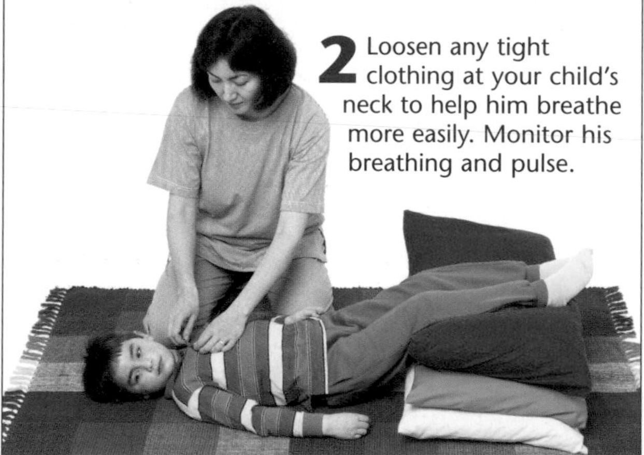

2 Loosen any tight clothing at your child's neck to help him breathe more easily. Monitor his breathing and pulse.

First-aid tips

- Do not move your child until the ambulance arrives, but gently loosen his clothing.
- If your child is thirsty, wet his lips with water. Do not give him any fluids if he has abdominal injuries.
- Speaking to your child in a reassuring voice may help to calm him down and reduce the effects of shock.
- Continue to check your child's breathing every 10 minutes until the ambulance arrives.
- Resuscitate your child if his breathing and pulse stop.

Hospital treatment

Once your child arrives at the hospital, the doctors will work quickly to restore the supply of blood and oxygen to his organs.

- This may mean giving your child oxygen via a face-mask, and administering intravenous fluids (putting him on a drip), or even performing a blood transfusion if blood loss is severe.
- Your child may also be given medication to help increase his blood pressure.
- Once the cause of the shock has been established, this will also be treated, for example surgery may be required to repair an internal wound, or antibiotics to combat infection.

ALLERGIC SHOCK

Allergic shock (anaphylactic shock) is a condition in which the body has a serious reaction to an outside factor, such as an insect bite or food.

- **Why it happens:** this is a life-threatening form of shock, caused by a severe allergic reaction (anaphylaxis). Some people are sensitive, so that certain substances such as penicillin, wasp stings or foods, such as nuts or shellfish, can cause their body to have a serious reaction. The allergic reaction leads to the person going into shock, and death can result within minutes if appropriate treatment is not given. The symptoms of this form of shock are far more pronounced than normal shock.
- **Symptoms:** the skin may become red and itchy and begin to burn; the face or tongue will swell; there will be difficulty breathing as the throat swells and the chest tightens and consciousness may be lost.
- **Treatment:** your child will require an injection of adrenaline to combat the allergic reaction. People who suffer from anaphylaxis are usually aware of their condition and so carry life-saving medication with them at all times, but a child will require help taking this. If your child suffers a severe reaction to anything for the first time, however, it is essential that you call an ambulance immediately. In the meantime, talk to him to keep him as calm as possible and give first aid to assist his breathing if necessary.

SPRAINS

WHY SPRAINS OCCUR

An active child is bound to have occasional minor accidents. Your child will be climbing, running and jumping with little thought about his own safety, so you may well have to deal with strains and sprains from time to time.

- Strained and sprained limbs usually occur due to sudden twists or an awkward landing. They come under the heading of 'soft tissue injuries', which are injuries to the ligaments, tendons and muscles that surround and support the bones.

- A strain is caused by sudden over-stretching of a muscle or a tendon, which is the fibrous band that anchors the muscle to a bone. A sharp pull or twist to the muscle may cause the muscle fibres to tear.

- A sprain happens when there is injury to a ligament, usually caused by sudden over-stretching. Ligaments are tough bands that hold bones together at joints. Sudden twisting of the joint makes the ligament stretch and possibly tear. The most common sites for a sprain are the ankles, knees and fingers.

A sprain or strain may result from a sudden or unexpected wrenching movement, and can partially tear or pull the ligament or joint.

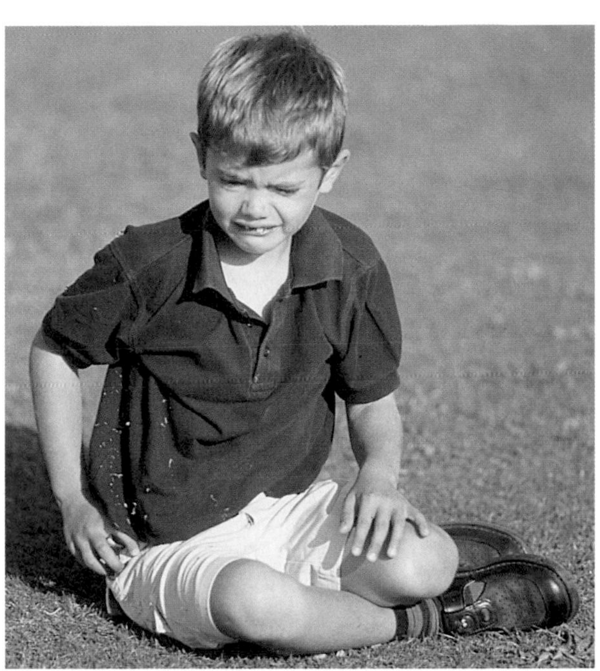

Recognising the signs

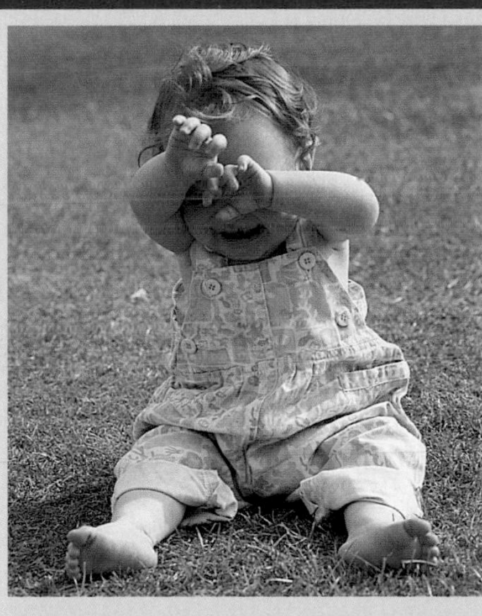

Most falls and bumps will result in nothing more than a few tears and are soon forgotten. If, however, your child has a strain or sprain, you may notice some obvious signs.

- **Pain or tenderness** in the area of the injury. A very young child will not be able to tell you where it hurts, so it is important to watch him carefully to see if he cries when a particular joint is used.

- **Swelling** of the affected area, either immediately or later.

A sprain in a baby can easily go unnoticed although she may point to the affected area. If your baby has had a fall and continues to cry and be distressed, seek medical advice.

- **Redness or bruising** in the area of the injury. This may not become apparent until several hours after the injury has occurred.

- **Reduced mobility** in the affected joint. Damage to ligaments does not prevent the joint working, as may be the case with a fracture, but the pain and swelling of a sprain may make it difficult to move. In the case of an ankle, leg or foot sprain or strain, the child will have difficulty putting full weight on it.

When to call the doctor

Most strains and sprains are minor and can be dealt with simply at home. However, a soft tissue injury can sometimes be more severe and there may even be a fracture – even medical staff find it hard to tell the difference between a sprain and a fracture. Seek medical advice if:

1. You think there may be a broken bone rather than a sprain; sometimes a bone will have made an audible snapping noise.
2. Pain is severe, and doesn't get better fairly quickly.
3. A joint looks misshapen or 'out of place' – this may be a sign of a dislocation.
4. Your child isn't moving the injured limb, or can't bear to put weight on it.
5. Symptoms don't improve, or they get worse, or if the child shows any signs of shock.
6. Bruising remains in the affected area for several days after the injury has occurred.

Giving first aid

Most sprains can be treated at home by giving basic first aid. An easy way to remember how to deal with a soft tissue injury is to think of the word RICE – which stands for Rest, Ice, Compression and Elevation. However, if in doubt seek medical advice.

- **Rest:** it is very important that the child rests the injured area so that it can begin to heal. Lay your child in a comfortable position and steady and support the injured area.

- **Ice:** if the injury has just happened, an ice-pack or a cold compress should be held against the injured area. This will help to reduce the pain, swelling and bruising. Never put ice directly on to your child's skin; make sure it is wrapped up in several layers of thin cloth. Apply the compress for approximately 10 minutes every two hours.

- **Compression:** applying a layer of padding, secured with a bandage, to the injured area will help to stop swelling and will also give added support and protection.

- **Elevation:** if you can raise the injured area this will reduce the blood flow and help to prevent further swelling and bruising. A sprained ankle should be lifted up and supported by a cushion while your child rests.

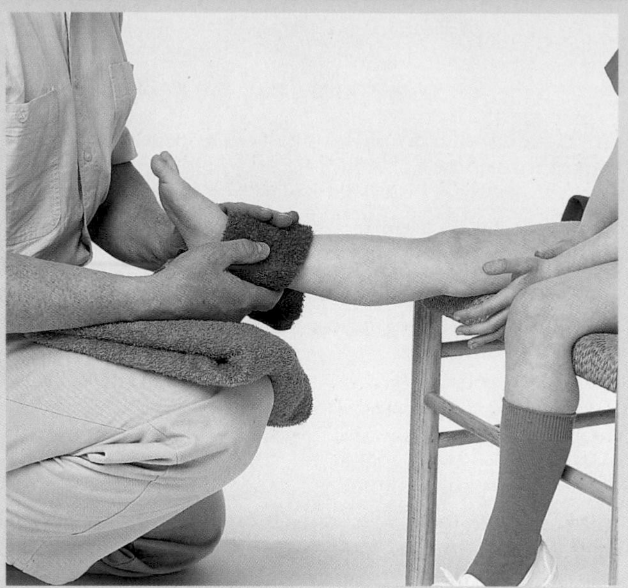

It is important to follow the RICE procedure to treat a sprain or strain initially. After supporting the limb, apply a cold compress to the area – soak a flannel in very cold water, wring it out and place it firmly over the injury.

Cold compresses

There are a number of ways to cool an injury.

1 Placing the affected area under cold running water for several minutes may help, especially if your child has an injured finger.

2 Soak a flannel or towel in cold water, wring it out and place it firmly over the injury and surrounding area. The cloth will need to be re-soaked every three to five minutes to keep it cold.

3 Make an icepack by putting ice cubes or crushed ice into a plastic bag then wrapping the bag in a cloth. This can be held against the injured area for 10 minutes, every two to three hours.

NOTE: a sealed bag of frozen vegetables can be used as an icepack in an emergency. Make sure you wrap the bag in several layers of cloth before applying to the injured area.

A pack of frozen vegetables wrapped in a cloth is an effective home-made compress. It is also possible to buy a ready-made compress.

Helping your child to recover

You can expect your child to recover fully from a strain or sprain, although this may take one to two weeks.

- Rest is the most important factor in healing a soft tissue injury. You and your child must be patient and allow the injured area plenty of time to recover properly.

- Pain relief may be necessary in the first day or two. Give liquid ibuprofen, but follow the instructions on the bottle carefully. Seek advice from a pharmacist if necessary.

- Gentle movement can begin when there is no more pain. Gradually increase your child's activity, but stop if the injury begins to hurt or swell again. When all his symptoms are gone your child can resume normal activities.

- You will notice that any bruising gradually changes colour from blue to purplish-black then yellow.

- Try to prevent a repeat of the injury by talking to your child about how it happened, or making any necessary changes to your safety arrangements around the house.

- Complications are unusual. Repeated sprains of the same area, which may happen in older children who play sport, may lead to weakness of that part of the body. Strapping the weak limb, especially during play, may be necessary to give extra support to the injured area.

SUFFOCATION

WHAT IS SUFFOCATION?

Suffocation occurs when the body cannot breathe in the amount of oxygen it needs. This may be because the airway is blocked, because the inhaled air is low in oxygen or because the air contains contaminants that affect the ability of the blood to absorb oxygen. Blockage of the airway is the most common cause of suffocation in children.

- Smothering can occur when the nose and mouth are covered.
- A child can be suffocated by strangulation, where the airway is squeezed by a tight band around the neck.
- The airway can also be blocked by choking, where a small object or morsel of food is inhaled into the windpipe.
- Children may also be at risk of being suffocated by lack of air if they climb or fall into confined spaces, such as car boots.
- Smoke or fumes, such as those caused by a house fire, may cause a child to be suffocated. Carbon monoxide, a poisonous gas given off by inadequately serviced gas heaters, is also a potential hazard.

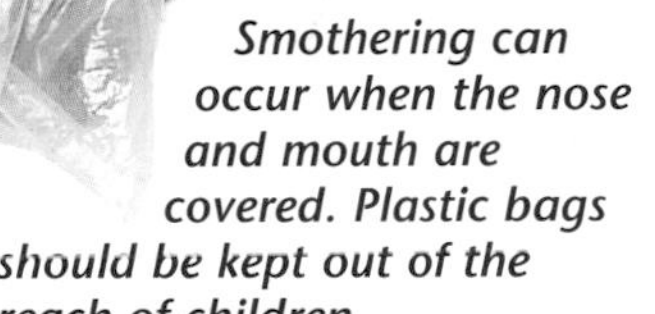

Smothering can occur when the nose and mouth are covered. Plastic bags should be kept out of the reach of children.

Preventing suffocation

Most causes of suffocation in children are preventable. If you are aware of the dangers, there are many things you can do to help keep your child safe.

- Remove hood cords and drawstrings from clothing to prevent playground accidents.
- Remove ribbons and strings from toys, and never attach toys or dummies to your child with string.
- Keep out of reach all cords for curtains and window blinds, especially those with loops.
- If you have a toy box, remove the lid, or make sure that it is not airtight, in case your child falls in.
- To avoid choking, keep small objects out of reach, check toys for detachable parts and supervise your child while he eats.
- Never allow your child to play with a deflated balloon or a plastic bag.

Safe sleeping

Sadly, every year some babies die by suffocation in the very place where they should be safest – their own beds. Following the official guidelines on sleep safety should help to reduce the risk of this terrible tragedy.

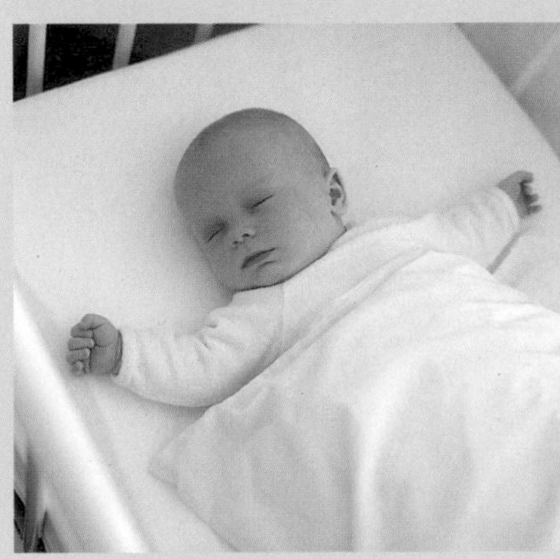

1 Lay your baby to sleep on his back, on a firm mattress.

2 Make sure your baby is in the 'feet to foot' position. This is where his feet touch the foot of the cot and prevents him wriggling under the covers.

Your baby's feet should be at the foot of the cot and the covers should reach no higher than his shoulders.

3 Make sure the mattress fits the cot, with no spaces around the edges where your baby may become wedged.

4 The cot bars should be less than 5cm (2in) apart to avoid your baby's head or body being trapped.

5 Do not place pillows, a duvet or sheepskin in the cot. These can cause overheating and increase the risk of suffocation.

6 Remove your baby's bib before laying him down.

First aid for smoke or fume inhalation

Smoke and fumes may contain toxic vapours or tiny particles, which can harm the delicate lining of the lungs. Carbon monoxide, which stops the blood from taking up oxygen, is particularly dangerous because it is colourless and has no smell. If your child has been exposed to smoke and fumes, take immediate action.

1 Quickly remove your child from the source of the smoke or fumes. Take great care – you cannot help your child if you are overcome by smoke yourself.

2 Once in the fresh air, your child will probably be able to clear his lungs with deep breaths and may need no further help. He should see a doctor to check that there has been no lung damage.

3 If your child is unconscious but breathing, place him in the recovery position. Call for an ambulance and stay by your child's side to monitor his condition.

4 If your child is not breathing, you should attempt mouth-to-mouth resuscitation and continue to administer this until the ambulance arrives.

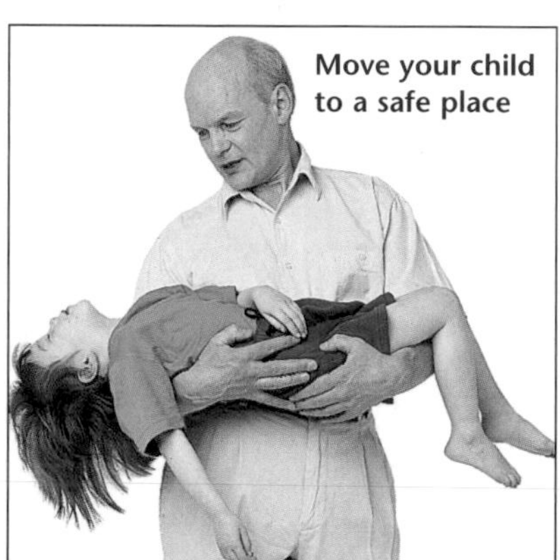

Move your child to a safe place

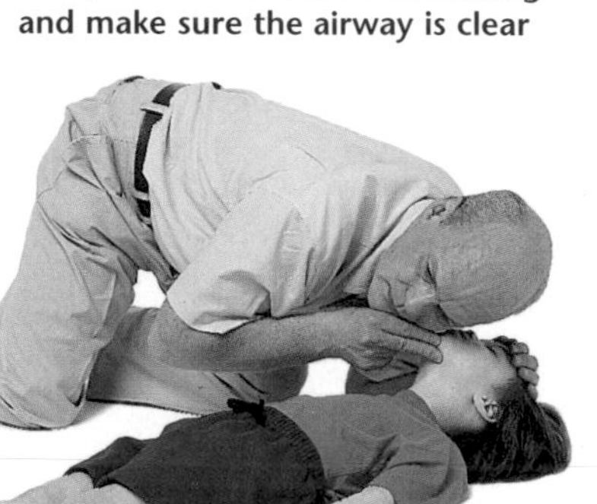

Look, listen and feel for breathing and make sure the airway is clear

Place your child in the recovery position and stay with him until the ambulance arrives

First aid for smothering or strangulation

Most cases of suffocation by smothering or strangulation occur in the home. Children have been smothered by soft bedding, plastic bags over the head and deflated balloons in the mouth. Strangulation may happen as a child slips while climbing out of a cot, or wriggles through bars that are too narrow for his head. Occasionally, clothing, and especially drawstrings around the neck, may catch on playground equipment.

1 Quickly remove any object that is smothering him. Remove or cut away any constricting band around the neck while supporting his body.

2 If you have found your child hanging, his spine may be damaged. Move him as little as possible to prevent further injury.

3 Send or shout for help immediately.

4 Check to see if your child is breathing. If not, attempt mouth-to-mouth resuscitation.

5 If your child is breathing but unconscious, place him in the recovery position.

6 Call for an ambulance. Even if your child seems to be unharmed, it is essential that he is examined by a doctor.

Make sure the airway is clear

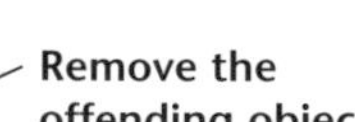

Remove the offending object

If you find your child being smothered or strangled, quickly remove the offending object while supporting his body. If he is not breathing, attempt resuscitation and call an ambulance.

INDEX

PICTURE ACKNOWLEDGEMENTS

Photographs: 9: Retna Pictures Ltd (Jenny Acheson) (b); 10: BPL (Jennie Woodcock) (tl); SRG (Sally Greenhill) (bl); 12: MBPL; 13: BPL (P.Cutler) (br); 14: BPL (A.Hampton) (cr); E.McNulty (tl); Family Life Picture Library (A.Williams) (bl); 15: MBPL (Frances Tout) (bl); WTPL (Anthea Sieveking) (tr); 16: Paul Dunn (cl); Rex Features Ltd (br); 17: BPL (Ian West) (tr); Retna Pictures Ltd (Jenny Acheson) (bl); 18: BPL (Jacqui Farrow) (bl); Angela Maynard Pictures (tr); 19: Retna Pictures Ltd (Jenny Acheson) (tr), (Sandra Lousada) (bl); 20: SRG (cl); SPL (Peter Arnold/Matt Meadows) (br); 21: SPL (Mark Clarke/Chris Priest) (tr); Bubbles (Jennie Woodcock) (b); 22: Getty Images UK/Stone (br); 23: BPL (Ian West) (bl); DK (cr); 25: SPL (Damien Lovegrove) (c); 26: BPL (Dr. Hercules Robinson) (bl), (Loisjoy Thurston) (tl); 27: BPL (Geoff Du Feu) (c); 28: BPL (Anthony Dawton) (bl), (Jacqui Farrow) (cr); 29: BPL (Rex Moreton) (br), (Ian West) (cr); 30: BPL (Ian West) (tr); 31: MBPL (Ian Hooten) (c); 32: BPL (Claire Paxton) (br), (Ian West) (tl); MBPL (Ian Hooten) (bl,cr); 33: St John Ambulance; 34: St John Ambulance; 37: SPL (Damien Lovegrove) (tr); 38: BPL (Loisjoy Thurston) (br); SPL (Holmes/James King) (tl); 39: SPL (Jim Selby) (bc); 40: BPL (David Robinson) (bl); SPL (CC Studio) (tr); 41: BPL (Ian West) (tr); MBPL (Paul Bricknell) (bl); 42: BPL (Ian West) (bl); SPL (Damien Lovegrove) (cr); 43: BPL (Ian West) (bl,cr); 44: BPL (tr); BPL (Moose Azim) (bl); 45: Medipics (Adam Scott) (bl); SPL (BSIP/Boucharlat) (t); 46: Medipics (Adam Scott) (cr); Janine Wiedel (b); 47: Medipics (Dr.Samira Sayed) (tr); WTPL (c,bl); 48: Medical Picture Collection (bc); Medipics (cr); SPL (Alexander Tsiaras) (tr); 49: SRG (bl); SPL (Will McIntyre) (tr); 50: WTPL (Anthea Sieveking) (blu); SRG (cr); 51: BPL (Loisjoy Thurston) (tr), (Jennie Woodcock) (cl); 52: BPL (Loisjoy Thurston) (tl); SPL (Dr.Linda Stannard) (br); 53: BPL (Moose Azim) (cr); SPL (Dr. P.Marazzi) (br,bc); 55: WTPL (Anthea Sieveking) (br); SPL (Dr.P.Marazzi) (tr); 56: SPL (Dr. P.Marazzi) (cl), (Hattie Young) (tr); 57: BPL (F.M.Magliocca /Prof. P.M.Motta) (bl); SRG (Sally Greenhill) (cr); 58: Medipics (cl); MBPL (br); 59: BPL (Frans Rombout) (tr); 60: BPL (Frans Rombout) (c); SRG (Sally Greenhill) (tr); 61: BPL (Loisjoy Thurston) (cl); 62: BPL (Loisjoy Thurston) (tr); 63: BPL (Ian West) (tr); 64: BPL (Toni Revan) (tr); SPL (Oscar Burriel) (b); 65: SRG (Sally Greenhill) (tr); MBPL (bl); 66: BPL (c); WTPL (A. Sieveking) (tr); MBPL (c); 67: BPL (Loisjoy Thurston) (bl); WTPL (Fiona Pragoff) (tr); 68: BPL (Loisjoy Thurston) (bl); SPL (Larry Mulvehill) (tr); 69: SPL; 70: SPL; 71: BPL (Ian West) (cr); SPL (Eye Of Science) (cl); 72: BPL (Rex Moreton) (bl), (Lucy Tizard) (br); 73: SPL (Biophoto Associates) (bl); 74: SPL (Richard Hutchings) (br), (Gary Parker) (tl); 75: BPL (Martin Jackson) (tr), (Loisjoy Thurston) (bc); 76: MBPL (Nick Cole) (tr); SPL (Hattie Young) (bc); 77: BPL (F.Rombout) (tr); TWPL (bc); 78: SRG (Sally Greenhill) (bc); 79: Medical Illustration Services (Zena Holloway) (tr); SPL (Kaye Mayers) (bl); 80: BPL (Loisjoy Thurston) (tr); 81: SPL (CNRI) (bl), (Doug Plummer) (tr); 82: SPL (Leca/BSIP) (bl), (Alexandra Tsiaras) (cr); 83: BPL (Loisjoy Thurston) (bl,tr), (Ian West) (br); 84: BPL (Loisjoy Thurston) (cr), (Ian West) (bl); 85: DK; 86: BPL (Jacqui Farrow) (bl); DK (t); 87: BPL (br); 88: Family Life Picture Library (Angela Hampton) (br); SPL (cl); WTPL (c); 89: Medipics Photo Library (Kevin Harrison) (tr); SPL (Chris Priest) (bl); 90: SPL (Simon Fraser) (tl); 93: BPL (Jennie Woodcock) (cr); SPL (Dr.P.Marazzi) (bl,cl); 94: BPL (Ian West) (br); Getty Images UK/Stone (Chris Everard) (bl); SPL (Bsip Edwige) (tl); 95: BPL (Frans Rombout) (tr); SPL (CNRI) (cl); 96: BPL (Loisjoy Thurston) (tr); MBPL (Ruth Jenkinson) (br), (Eddie Lawrence) (bl); 97: BPL (Jennie Woodcock) (bl); 98: BPL (Dr.Hercules Robinson) (tl), (Frans Rombout) (br); 99: BPL (Frans Rombout) (bl,tr); 100: SPL (Jerrican/Gable) (tr), (Salisbury District Hospital /Department Of Clinical Radiology) (bl); 101: BPL (Pauline Cutler) (bl); SPL (CDC) (cr); WTPL (bl); 102: BPL (Loisjoy Thurston) (cr); SPL (Dr. P Marazzi) (bl); 103: BPL (Loisjoy Thurston) (br); SPL (Eddie Gray) (cl), (Damien Lovegrove) (tr); 104: SPL (Mark Clarke) (bl); 105: A. Maynard (tr); SPL (Dr. Jeremy Burgess) (br), (Mark Clarke) (bl); 107: WTPL (A.Sieveking) (cr); MBPL (bl); 108: SPL (Simon Fraser) (cr), (Mehau Kulyk) (c); 109: BPL (Jennie Woodcock) (b); SPL (Dr H.C. Robinson) (t); 110: SPL (James Stevenson) (tl), (Hattie Young) (cr); 111: SPL (Saturn Stills) (cr); 112: SPL (Aron Haupt) (c); 113: BPL (Loisjoy Thurston) (bl); SPL (Dr P Marazzi) (t); 114: BPL (Loisjoy Thurston) (t), (Jennie Woodcock) (b); 115: BPL (Ian West) (tr); MBPL (bc); 116: Image State-Pictor (br); MBPL (cl); SPL (James Stevenson) (tr); 117: BPL (Ian Lever) (bl); WTPL (cr); 118: BPL (Loisjoy Thurston) (bl); SPL (Custom Medical Stock /Scheikhorn) (cr); 119: SPL (Colin Cuthbert) (b), (Geoff Tompkinson) (t); 120: SPL (Michael Abbey) (tl), (Simon Fraser) (cr), (National Cancer Institute) (tl); 121: MBPL (M.Wyndham) (tr); PRHPL (Dr.Gopal) (bc); SPL (Dr. P.Marazzi) (c); 122: BPL (C.Rout) (tr), (L.Thurston) (bl); 123: BPL (William Crees) (bl); Angela Maynard Pictures (Angela Maynard) (cr); 124: Retna Pictures Ltd (Philip Reeson) (tr) 125 Meningitis Trust (br); Public Health Laboratory Service (tr); 126: BPL (Jacqui Farrow) (C); SPL (James Prince) (bl); 127 WTPL (br); SPL (bc), (Lowell Georgia) (bl), (Saturn Stills) (tr); 128: SPL (Mark Clarke) (cl), (Saturn Stills) (tr); 129: BPL (bl); 130: Getty Images UK/Stone (tr); MBPL (cl); 131 BPL (Jacqui Farrow) (bl); Robert Harding Picture Library Ltd (International Stock /Richard Pharaoh) (cr); 132: SPL (Colin Cuthbert) (tl), (John Greim) (bc); 133: BPL (Jennie Woodcock) (bl); MBPL (tr); 134 BPL (Loisjoy Thurston) (tr); SRG (cl); 135: BPL (Jacqui Farrow) (tr); 136: BPL (bl); SPL (Dr.Kari Lounatmaa) (tr); 137: SPL (bl), (Stevie Grand) (tr); 138: SPL (Will & Deni McIntyre) (cl), (Hank Morgan) (clu), (Ron Sutherland) (br); 139: BPL (Ian West) (cr); Retna Pictures Ltd (Sandra Lousada) (br); SPL (c); 140: BPL (David Robinson) (tr); SPL (E. Gueno) (bl); 141: MBPL (Paul Mitchell) (bl); WTPL (Anthea Sieveking) (tr); 142: BPL (Dr.Hercules Robinson) (bl), (Loisjoy Thurston) (cr); 143: SPL (Michael Abbey) (tr), (Mark Clarke) (bl); 144: WTPL (Medical Photographic Library) (tr), (Anthea Sieveking) (bl); 145: BPL (Amanda Knapp) (tr), (Dr.P Marazzi) (bc); WTPL (cl); 146: SPL (St Bart's Hospital) (tl), (Sue Ford) (bc); 147: WTPL (Anthea Sieveking) (tr); WTPL (bl); 148: BPL (Jennie Woodcock) (cr); SPL (Charron/Jerrican) (tl); 149 Impact Photos Ltd (cr); 150: SPL (St Bartholomew's Hospital) (cr), (Saturn Stills) (bl); 151: SPL (Mark Clarke) (bl); WTPL (tr); 152 Retna Pictures Ltd (John Powell) (br), (Philip Reeson) (tl); 153: BPL (Dr.Hercules Robinson) (tr); SRG (bc); 154: MBPL (Ian Hooten) (bl); SPL (Saturn Stills) (tr); 155: BPL (Angela Hampton) (tr), (Jennie Woodcock) (bl); 156: BPL (Nick Hanna) (br), (David Robinson) (cl); 157: SPL (Scott Camazine) (tr); WTPL (bc); 158: Retna Pictures Ltd (Sandra Lousada) (tr); SPL (bl); 159: BPL (Jennie Woodcock) (cr); SRG (Sally Greenhill) (bl); 160: SPL (Ron Sutherland) (br), (Sheila Terry) (tl); 161: SRG (Sally Greenhill) (b); WTPL (Anthea Sieveking) (t); 162: MBPL (Ian Hooton) (t); WTPL (b); 163: Retna Pictures Ltd (Juliette Antoine) (bl); SPL (D. Phillips) (tr); 164: BPL (Richard Yard) (bl); SPL (Mark Clarke) (c); 165 DK (tr); MBPL (Ian Hooten) (bl); 166: BPL (Frans Rombout) (bl), (Loisjoy Thurston) (cr); 167: BPL (Ian West) (cr); SPL (bl); 168: BPL (Ian West) (tl); Getty Images UK/Stone (cr); 171: BPL (Loisjoy Thurston) (bl); SPL (Chris Priest) (tr); 172: BPL (Frans Rombout) (bl); SPL (Chris Priest) (tr); 173: SPL (Jeremy Burgess) (cl); 174: SPL (Dr.P Marazzi) (tl); WTPL (Anthea Sieveking) (br); 175: Ardea London Ltd (tr); WTPL (cl); 176: Ardea London Ltd (bl); SPL (Saturn Stills) (tr); 178: BPL (John Powell) (tr); Retna Pictures Ltd (Ken Bank) (bc); 179: DK (bl); Robert Harding Picture Library Ltd (tr); 180: SPL (Dr. P.Marazzi) (tc); 181: BPL (Loisjoy Thurston) (bl), (Ian West) (tr); SPL (Mark Clarke) (br); 182: DK (c,cr); 183: SPL (Dr. Hercules Robinson) (tr); WTPL (Anthea Sieveking) (bl); 184: DK; 185: DK (cr); SPL (Dr.P.Marazzi) (bl); 186: DK; 187: BPL (Jacqui Farrow) (cr); DK (bl); 188: BPL (John Howard) (cr); DK (bl,br); 189: DK; 190: DK(t); WTPL (bl); 191: WTPL; 193: BPL (Ian West) (bc); MBPL (Paul Mitchell) (tr); 194: WTPL (Anthea Sieveking) (br); 195 BPL (Jennie Woodcock) (bl); WTPL (br); 196: DK (cl); SPL (Dr.P Marazzi) (br); 197: WTPL (Anthea Sieveking) (c,tr); 198: DK (cl,bl); 199: DK (c); WTPL (Anthea Sieveking) (bl); 200: DK; 201: BPL (Geoff du Feu) (bl), (Loisjoy Thurston) (cr); 202: DK (Andy Crawford/Steve Gorton) (cr,cu,cl); SPL (Erik Hilderbrandt) (br); 203: SRG (Sally Greenhill) (bl); SPL (Mark Clark) (cr); 204: BPL (Jennie Woodcock) (bl); SPL (David Parker) (tr); 207: Retna Pictures Ltd (Sandra Lousada) (bl); Robert Harding Picture Library Ltd (tr); 208: WTPL (bl); SPL (bc), (Jim Selby) (tr); 209: BPL (Jacqui Farrow) (cr), (Ian West) (cl); Retna Pictures Ltd (Ewing Reeson) (br); 210: Retna Pictures Ltd (Philip Reeson) (bl); WTPL (cr); 211: BPL (Loisjoy Thurston) (bc); MBPL (Paul Mitchell) (cr); 212: BPL (Frans Rombout) (br); DK (tr,cl); 213: BPL (Jennie Woodcock) (bl); DK (tr); 214: BPL (Jacqui Farrow) (cr); Retna Pictures Ltd (bl); 215: SPL (Simon Fraser) (cr), (Thomas/Jerrican) (bl); 216: BPL (Jennie Woodcock) (bl); DK (cr); 217: WTPL (Anthea Sieveking) (bl); 218: DK (tl,cr); 219: BPL (Ian West) (bl); Angela Maynard Pictures (tr); 220: BPL (David Robinson) (cr), (Loisjoy Thurston) (tl); 221: BPL (Loisjoy Thurston) (cr); Meningitis Trust (bru); SPL (c), (Dr. P.Marazzi) (cru), (John Radcliffe Hospital) (cl); WTPL (bc); 222: MBPL (Ian Hooten) (cr); 223: BPL (Jacqui Farrow) (tr); DK (bc); 224: DK; 227: Image State-Pictor (bl); WTPL (tr); 228: WTPL (Anthea Sieveking) (br); 231: DK; 232: DK; 233: BPL (Jennie Woodcock) (bl); Retna Pictures Ltd (Philip Reeson) (tr); 234: DK (tr); 235: BPL (Frans Rombout) (bl); DK (c); 236: DK.

Cover, title page and all other photographs by Belinda Banks.

Illustrations: 39: Jane Fallows (cr); 55: Roger Coultard (bl); 78: M.McClement (c); 90: WTPL (Amanda Williams) (bc); 98: Matthew McClement (cl); 149: Andrew McLoughlin (bc); 217: Michael Courtney (cr).

KEY (positions): b = bottom; bc = bottom centre; bl = bottom left; br = bottom right; cl = centre left; c = centre; cr = centre right; t= top; tc = top centre; tl = top left; tr = top right; u = upper.

KEY (library abbreviations): BPL = Bubbles Picture Library; DK = Dorling Kindersley Photo Library; MBPL = Mother & Baby Picture Library; SPL = Science Photo Library; SRG = Sally & Richard Greenhill; WTPL = The Wellcome Trust Photo Library.